Quick Reference Index to Health and Self-Care (SC) Teaching

Clinical Manual of Maternity Nursing

Jean D. Neeson, R.N.C., M.S.N., N.P.

Director, Women's Health Nurse Practitioner Program,
and Associate Clinical Professor,
Department of Family Health Care Nursing
School of Nursing
University of California, San Francisco

Associate Clinical Professor
Department of Community and Family Medicine
School of Medicine
University of California, San Diego

J.B. Lippincott Company *Philadelphia*

London Mexico City New York St. Louis São Paulo Sydney

Acquisitions Editor: Paul R. Hill
Developmental Editor: Eleanor Faven
Indexer: Angela Holt
Art Director: Tracy Baldwin
Design Coordinator: Anne O'Donnell
Designer: Katharine Nichols
Production Coordinator: Charlene Catlett Squibb
Compositor: Circle Graphics
Printer/Binder: R. R. Donnelley

Library of Congress Cataloging-in-Publication Data

Neeson, Jean D.
Clinical manual of maternity nursing.

Includes indexes.
1. Obstetrical nursing. 2. Perinatology.
I. Title. [DNLM: 1. Obstetrical Nursing.
2. Perinatology—nurses' instruction. WY 157.3 N382c]
RG951.N43 1987 610.73'678 86-21360
ISBN 0-397-54496-0

The authors and publisher have exerted every effort to ensure that drug selection and dosage set forth in this text are in accord with current recommendations and practice at the time of publication. However, in view of ongoing research, changes in government regulations, and the constant flow of information relating to drug therapy and drug reactions, the reader is urged to check the package insert for each drug for any change in indications and dosage and for added warnings and precautions. This is particularly important when the recommended agent is a new or infrequently employed drug.

Preface

Clinical Manual of Maternity Nursing is a concise guide to the clinical practice of maternity nursing, designed to be used by both the practicing nurse and the student. The manual complements *Comprehensive Maternity Nursing: Nursing Process and the Childbearing Family* but can be used with any maternity nursing text. Its handy size makes it a pocketable reference book for the busy nurse, providing both quick aid for problem solving and the background information needed in caring for the childbearing family.

The first chapter discusses terminology and the statistics of mortality, morbidity, risks, and genetics. Emphasizing a strong family approach, the chapter considers trends in family-centered nursing and discusses customs and practices of various ethnic groups.

Chapters 2 through 11 thoroughly cover such important topics as female anatomy and hormonal control, reproduction, sexuality, family planning, adaptations of pregnancy, fetal development, labor and delivery, and the postpartum period. Assessment and care of the normal and high-risk neonate are stressed. These chapters are designed to provide basic background information that is of value both for quick reference and for client teaching. The essential clinical data are topical, timely, and practice oriented, and special attention is given to self-care.

Chapters are heavily weighted toward the dual function of nursing assessment and intervention. Nursing process predominates, and probable nursing diagnoses, nursing objectives, and evaluation are discussed in detail.

Chapter 12 discusses some 45 procedures and medical tests useful as clinical reference and for patient teaching.

The goal of this clinical manual is to supply a wide range of information in a manner that is definitive, succinct, easy to read, and rapidly accessible. To facilitate quick access, the Table of Contents provides two levels of headings, a list of possible nursing diagnoses follows the Table of Contents, and in addition to the main index at the back of the book, there is also a quick reference index at the front. The Appendixes provide information on normal lab values and on drug effects and contraindications for mother, fetus, and newborn in a handy tabular format. The book's content is enhanced by the use of 32 illustrations from Childbirth Graphics, Ltd., Rochester New York.

Jean D. Neeson

Contents

Appendix

Possible Nursing Diagnoses Related To

1
Contemporary Maternity Nursing

MATERNAL AND INFANT MORTALITY

Health care is often evaluated by examining statistics on mortality and morbidity in a given population. In maternity care statistics on birth rate, maternal and infant mortality, and birth weight are the major indicators of health.

- *Birth rate* is reported as the number of live births per 1000 in a given population.
- *Birth weight* is an important indicator of health. Low birth weight is associated with higher infant mortality. A birth weight of less than 2500 g is considered to be low birth weight. The average birth weight for infants born in the United States in 1980 was 3360 g (7 lb 7oz).
- *Infant mortality rate* is expressed as the number of deaths under 1 year of age per 1000 live births. Nearly two-thirds of infant deaths in the United States are related to low birth weight. Other contributing factors are congenital anomalies and sudden infant death syndrome (SIDS). About 10% of infant deaths occur on the first day after birth and 70% during the first 28 days after birth.

PSYCHOSOCIAL ASPECTS OF CHILDBEARING

Nursing Objectives in Psychosocial Care

- To assess psychosocial factors that affect a person's readiness for parenthood
- To identify risk factors associated with early or delayed child-bearing and to implement supportive nursing care as needed
- To assess a patient's cultural perspective in relation to child-

bearing and how that perspective will affect nursing care during pregnancy, labor, birth, and the postpartum period
- To recognize areas in which cultural variations are likely to occur in birth practices
- To incorporate patient and family practices into the plan of nursing care wherever possible

---

Psychosocial Readiness for Childbearing

Psychosocial readiness for childbearing is defined as the ability to cope with the demands and complete the tasks of pregnancy, childbirth, and parenthood. Psychosocial readiness for childbearing has been achieved when the prospective parent has the following characteristics:

- The capacity to establish and maintain intimate relationships
- The ability to give and to care for another human being
- The ability to learn and to adjust patterns of daily life
- The ability to communicate effectively with others
- An established sexual identity

Early Childbearing: Adolescent Childbearing

- Approximately 1.2 million teenagers in the United States become pregnant each year, representing 20% of births.
- Of today's 14-year-olds, one in four will become pregnant while still a teenager; one in seven will choose abortion.
- The rate of first births among women aged 15 to 19 fell from about 54 per 1000 in 1979 to about 40 per 1000 in 1980.
- Although fewer adolescents are bearing children, more are becoming pregnant and are having abortions.
- The proportion of adolescent births out of wedlock increased from 43% in 1970 to 62% in 1980.
- The birth rate among unmarried adolescents aged 15 to 17 years increased from 17 per 1000 in 1970 to 21 per 1000 in 1980.
- Nearly one-third of adolescents aged 15 to 17 are sexually active, and 70% of females have intercourse before the age of 20.
- The mean age at first intercourse is 16.2 years for girls, 15.7 years for boys.
- Teenage pregnancy has become a major health concern.

Perinatal Risk Factors for Adolescent Pregnancies

- Perinatal risk is greater for adolescents, aged 14 years and younger.
- Middle adolescents, 15 to 17 years, and young adults 18 years and older, have more positive perinatal outcomes when other risk factors are controlled for.
- There is little evidence to suggest that youth or physiologic immaturity alone are related to poor maternal and neonatal outcomes. Factors such as inadequate prenatal care, nutritional deficiencies, noncompliance with health regimens, and adverse social conditions are more critical.
- Factors placing teenagers at additional risk include: lower socioeconomic status; poor nutritional habits; lower prepregnancy weight; delays in seeking and receiving prenatal care; and infection and sexually transmitted diseases.
- Specific perinatal risks include iron deficiency anemia; preterm and small-for-gestational age births; preeclampsia, eclampsia, and chronic hypertension; chorioamnionitis; postpartum endometritis; and neonatal septicemia.
- Psychosocial risks include single motherhood; stress of childrearing; marital instability; uninvolved partner or other lack of support; limitations on educational attainments; early entry into the work force; less-skilled, lower-paying jobs; and family stress and a divorce rate two to four times greater than that found in more mature couples. The teenage father may encounter negative reactions from persons who regard him as the "guilty" party. Even though he feels tremendous responsibility for the pregnancy, he is without resources.

Delayed Childbearing

Since 1980 an increasing number of women over age 30 have become pregnant for the first time. Between 1970 and 1980 the rate of first births to women aged 30 to 34 years climbed from 7.3% per 1000 women to 12.8% per 1000 women. Among white women the proportion who were still childless at age 30 increased from 14% in 1970 to 17% in 1980.

Causes of Delayed Childbearing

- In the over 40 age group, contraceptive failure, usually caused by ineffective contraception and irregular menstrual cycles (the woman may be multiparous)

- In the 30-to-35-year-old age group, conscious delay of pregnancy
- A woman's motivation for pregnancy after age 30 may stem from the feeling that time is running out; the hope that pregnancy will keep her youthful; a secure relationship with her partner; and improved financial status.

Perinatal Risk Factors for Delayed Childbearing

- Second-trimester abortions
- Chromosomal abnormalities
- Twinning
- Low-birth-weight infants, especially in the primigravida
- Labor abnormalities
- Increased fetal and neonatal deaths associated with chronic maternal hypertension; placenta previa; uterine inertia; and a greater number of breech births.
- Increased risk during pregnancy among women over age 30 results from underlying medical problems that increase with age rather than from maternal age alone.
- Postnatal physical and psychosocial manifestations among women over age 30 may include:
  - Slower physical recovery from childbirth
  - Increased fatigue
  - Greater expectations for their maternal role than younger mothers
  - Decreased self-confidence approximately 8 months after birth
  - Loss of occupational satisfaction
  - Greater emotional investment in motherhood

TRENDS IN FAMILY-CENTERED MATERNITY CARE

Research on long-term psychological benefits of family-centered maternity care has been inconclusive. However, research has shown that families are pleased with short-term gains of family-centered care.

Benefits of Family-Centered Care to the Hospital and Care Providers*

- Positive first-family contact with hospital, which increases likelihood of return for future care
- Increased continuity of care, better staff utilization, and improved working relationships among staff

* Adapted from Jennings A: Family Centered Maternity Care: An Alternative Obstetrical Approach. Chicago, American Hospital Association, 1978

- Lower staff turnover
- Valuable ongoing staff education program
- No increase in costs over traditional care
- No evidence of increased complications due to changes in care

Benefits of Family-Centered Care to the Family

Birth Options and Alternatives

Families have the right to make choices about pregnancy and birth care. Options for care should be carefully weighed by the family and the nurse to help achieve the goal of a healthy mother and baby. Family involvement includes the father's participation in prenatal classes and delivery. Other family members are also encouraged to participate actively in such activities.

Participation by Fathers in Vaginal and Cesarean Births
The father is actively involved in the cesarean birth. He supports the mother and remains with her throughout the operation. He may also be the first person to present the infant to the mother. As integral members of the birthing team, many fathers experience personal satisfaction and increased self-esteem.

Support People for Labor and Birth
Support for the laboring woman may be carried out by persons other than family members.

Participation by Siblings
A family's decision to include a child at the birth is often based on cultural attitudes, the parents' desires, and support by health care providers. Children are prepared for this experience in special birth classes.

Options in Childbirth Setting

In-Hospital Alternative Birth Centers (ABCs) ABCs have homelike furnishings with equipment stored out of sight. The woman usually labors, delivers, and recovers in the same room. Women who use ABCs are low risk patients. Early discharge (within 24 hours) is provided.

Freestanding Birth Centers Freestanding birth centers are located outside the hospital. These homelike facilities are designed for families who anticipate a normal labor and delivery and who want to participate actively in their own prenatal care. This low-cost comprehensive care is delivered by nurse midwives, physicians, and nurses. A back-up hospital facility is available if complications arise. Early discharge is routine, and nursing follow up at home may be provided.

Single-Room Maternity System The single-room maternity system was devised to replace the traditional maternity unit/alternative birth center and is now common in hospitals that serve both low-risk and high-risk patients. The system consists of a central service area that contains all the equipment, both routine and emergency, and services necessary for the woman's entire hospital stay. Single birthing rooms surround the service area. A primary care nurse is assigned to the family from the woman's admission to discharge. The system's many advantages arise from its ability to provide comprehensive medical care to obstetric patients in a single setting.

Home Births With the increasing use of obstetric technology, the number of home births appears to be increasing. Families choosing home birth are usually those who desire to have more control over the birthing process, who wish to deliver in familiar surroundings, and who want their family and friends close by during and after birth. Women choosing this option must be low-risk patients. Birth attendants may include a physician or nurse midwife who must inform the family about the benefits and risks of home birth, offer comprehensive prenatal care and delivery services, and provide for back-up hospital care in the event of problems.

PRACTICES RELATED TO PREGNANCY AND BIRTH IN VARIOUS ETHNIC GROUPS IN THE U.S.

Most cultures view pregnancy and birth not as an illness *per se* but as a period of increased vulnerability and risk. Many birth practices appear to be aimed at decreasing this risk by protecting the mother and unborn baby from supposed harmful influences. Cultural beliefs about the relative risks of pregnancy and the intrapartal and postpartum periods also differ from the dominant American view that the birth is the period of highest risk and the postpartum period is of much less concern.

Black Americans

- Black women view pregnancy as a normal healthy state.
- Children born to single mothers are cherished and are not stigmatized.

- Children born to adolescents are often raised by the grandmother as her own.
- The extended family, particularly the adolescent's mother is a source of significant support.
- Many women prefer the maternal grandmother to be their labor support person rather than the baby's father.
- During pregnancy women may avoid "acid" or "strong" foods to prevent having a hard-to-manage infant.

Mexican Americans

- Mexican women may view pregnancy as a natural event requiring no medical care under usual circumstances.
- The woman and fetus are considered vulnerable to outside bad influences.
- During pregnancy women may wear a *cinta* (a belt with keys attached) or a *muñeco* (a knotted cord around the abdomen) to prevent birth complications.
- Women may avoid drinking milk and may stay physically active to help prevent a large baby and a difficult delivery.
- Female family members are often present during labor and birth. Among more traditional couples fathers rarely participate.
- Breastfeeding practices differ, and women may believe that colostrum is unclean and refuse to breastfeed until the second day after birth.
- Women may observe a 40-day resting period after birth called *la cuarentina* during which dietary and activity restrictions, including prohibition of sexual intercourse, are followed.
- Mothers may bind the infant's umbilicus to prevent "bad air" from entering. Mothers may resist allowing the umbilicus to air dry.

Filipino Americans

- During pregnancy and the postpartum period the mother may observe traditional activity and diet patterns.
- Hot, spicy, or salty foods may be avoided during pregnancy, and satisfying food cravings may be seen as important in preventing premature birth.
- Pregnant and postpartum women are encouraged to decrease their activity, a practice that may be misinterpreted as laziness or noncompliance by hospital staff.
- Politeness, ease in social interaction, and deference to family authority, particularly the mother's mother, may create misunderstandings between the staff and family.
- The mother may smile and agree that she understands certain health care instructions but may not adhere to the recom-

mendations and instead follow tradition as encouraged by her mother.
- Women are socialized toward motherhood at an early age, and the extended family may have an important role in child care.

Asian Americans

Japanese Americans

- Japanese Americans value highly deference and politeness, emotional reserve, conformity, and allegiance to family.
- Traditional families may show strong male dominance, and the extended family may be important in daily life. Birth of a male child may confer high status on the mother.
- Western medicine tends to be well accepted, and pregnancy is viewed as a state of health that requires little change in normal activities.
- The mother is expected to satisfy infant needs immediately and to maintain very close contact with the infant.

Chinese Americans

- The customs related to childbearing in this group may vary according to the length of time the parents' families have lived in the United States and their educational level.
- Beliefs in the value of maintaining physical and spiritual balance during pregnancy and the postpartum period may be present.
- Herbal teas may be used as tonics during pregnancy, and certain foods may be avoided.
- An example of the importance of balance in maintaining health is the custom of "doing the mother," a period of 40 days after birth during which the woman is advised to stay in the house, to rest, and to avoid unnecessary activity. During this time the woman may avoid contact with water, reflecting the belief that she has an excess of cold in the body and will be vulnerable to arthritis and other body aches later in life if she becomes chilled during the postpartum period.

Southeast Asian Americans (Vietnamese, Cambodian, Laotian, Hmong)

- Women of reproductive age who have lost many relatives to war (deaths, refugee camps) may desire to have a large family; consequently, birth control information may be refused.
- Various religious, such as Catholicism, Buddhism, Confucian-

ism, and spiritualist beliefs may influence a woman's childbirth practices.

- Women are stoic and may consider crying out or complaining during labor and delivery to be shameful, especially in the presence of a man. This may result in unexpected, imminent births.
- Politeness and deference to authority is a strong cultural tradition evidenced by avoidance of eye contact and social and physical contact and affirmative answers to questions regardless of the woman's true feelings.
- Squatting may be the preferred position for birth.
- Women are taught to conserve body heat during childbirth and the postpartum period and will need extra warmed blankets and drinking water without ice.
- Bathing after childbirth may be considered risky due to the chance of becoming chilled.
- Women may consume only "hot" traditional foods from home during the early postpartum period.
- The woman's activities may be restricted for 40 to 60 days after birth, during which time other female relatives assume household and infant care responsibilities.

Arab Americans

- Arab Americans may adhere to either Christianity or Islam but have common cultural practices.
- Childbearing is a major role for women, whose domain is primarily the home and family.
- Infertility in a married woman is grounds for divorce in some Arab countries.
- Male children are highly valued; the sex of the infant may appear to be more important to the parents than the infant's health.
- The husband is involved in all aspects of his wife's care, and often the woman will defer to him in decisions about her care.
- Arab women are expected to be modest and deferential, and it is considered normal for these women to moan and cry during labor. Few request anesthesia.
- Advance preparation for the birth and the infant is avoided for fear of attracting the "evil eye." Compliments about the infant are avoided for the same reason.
- A traditional mistrust of written agreements may present difficulties when informed consent for medical procedures must be obtained. Trust is more readily placed in verbal agreements, especially with others of similar background.
- Visiting by the extended family during the postpartum period is considered an obligation.
- Children are included in all aspects of family life, and women may have a strong desire to have older children greet the newborn in the hospital.

GENETICS

There is an ongoing need to identify women with increased risk of having a child with a serious genetic disorder so that they can be offered genetic counseling and appropriate genetic testing. Nurses are needed to actively identify and refer high-risk patients and their families to appropriate professionals and to meet the special psychosocial needs of those women who must deal with genetic disorders and congenital anomalies. Nurses, as primary providers of health services, are in a unique position to meet these challenges.

- *Genetics* is the science of heredity.
- Genes are the coded sequences of information by which cellular organisms regulate their embryologic development, metabolic functioning, growth, and reproduction.
- Approximately 1 in 50 newborns (2%) has a major congenital abnormality.
  - Environmental factors such as infection and nutritional deficiences may be underlying causes in 60% of these abnormalities.
  - About 40% are thought to be hereditary.
- In over 60% of first-trimester spontaneous abortions, the conceptus has a chromosomal abnormality.

Nursing Objectives in Genetics

- To screen patients and families for genetic susceptibility to congenital abnormalities
- To identify patients who need referral for genetic counseling
- To support patients who have given birth to a child with a genetic abnormality
- To provide long-term sensitive care to families with genetic disease

---

Possible Nursing Diagnoses Related to Genetics

- At-risk pregnancy related to maternal/paternal genetic predisposition; recurrent abortions; deformed infant; fetal or neonatal risk; or retarded infant.
- Anticipatory grieving related to potential abnormality or loss of the fetus/newborn.

Implementation of nursing objectives for genetic counseling involves an effort to ensure that all patients, regardless of socioeconomic status, have access to genetic services. Additional efforts must be made to educate all health professionals about the psychological needs of patients with genetic disease to protect these patients from insensitive care.

Burden of Genetic Diseases to Family and Community

- Financial cost to family
- Decrease in planned family size
- Loss of geographic mobility
- Loss of career opportunities and job flexibility
- Decreased opportunities for siblings
- Loss of family integrity
- Social isolation
- Lifestyle alterations
- Disruption of husband–wife relationship
- Threatened family self-concept
- Coping with intolerant public attitudes
- Psychological damage
- Physical health problems
- Loss of dreams and aspirations
- Reduction in contributions to the community by affected families
- Cost of institutionalization to society
- Cost to society of other family members' needs stemming from the affected individual
- Cost of long-term care
- Need for housing changes

Etiology of Genetic Disorders

Genetic disorders are classified into three main etiologic categories:

- *Chromosome disorders* demonstrate a change in the number or structure of an individual's chromosome complement.
- *Single gene disorders* are caused by a mutation at the gene level.
- *Multifactorial disorders* are abnormalities that are due to an interaction of environmental and genetic factors.

Chromosome Disorders

Changes in chromosome number or structure are a significant cause of fetal wastage in pregnancy. In newborns such changes lead to congenital abnormalities and severe mental retardation.

- *Monosomy* is the absence of a single chromosome and is almost always lethal to the embryo.
- *Trisomy* is the presence of an extra chromosome and is also usually incompatible with life. Trisomies involving the smaller chromosomes are found in living newborns with congenital defects and mental retardation.

Numerical chromosomal disorders are summarized in Table 1-1.

Causes of Chromosomal Abnormalities

The internal and environmental events that lead to the formation of chromosome abnormalities are not clearly understood. Radiation, drugs, viruses, toxins, and chemicals are known to induce chromosome damage. However, it is extremely difficult to determine the cause in individual cases. Women exposed to these environmental hazards during their first trimester should be referred for genetic counseling to explore the possibility of increased risks to their fetus.

The most significant factor predisposing a fetus to chromosomal abnormalities (most commonly Down syndrome) is increasing maternal age. As Table 1-2 shows, the risk of having a child with Down syndrome rises substantially with the mother's age. Common medical practice dictates that all women who will be 35 years or older at the time of delivery be counseled and offered prenatal testing to determine the karyotype of their fetus.

Single-Gene Inheritance in Familes

- Single-gene traits refer to those genetic diseases that are caused by a gene mutation at a single locus (site) on a chromosome.
- There are four basic patterns of single gene inheritance:

  Autosomal dominant
  Autosomal recessive
  X–linked dominant
  X–linked recessive

Multifactorial Inheritance

Many isolated birth defects and common genital malformations are now believed to be the result of multifactorial inheritance. This category of genetic disorders is defined as those traits and disorders that arise as a result of the interaction of many genetic factors or the interaction of genetic and environmental factors.

Assessment

Pedigree

The patterns of inheritance may be pictorially represented on a diagram called a pedigree. The pedigree, developed during assess-

(*text continues on pg. 18*)

Table 1-1 Summary of Numerical Chromosomal Abnormalities

Type	Synonym	Incidence	Diagnostic Features at Birth	Prognosis	Detection
Autosomal Monosomy					
		Rare, usually incompatible with fetal survival.			
Sex Chromosome Monosomy					
XO	Turner syndrome*	1/10,000 live female births; most common chromosomal abnormality in spontaneous abortions (18%)	Edema of hands and feet; increased incidence of coarctation of the aorta; somatic abnormalities may be few, and condition often is not recognized at birth.	Normal intelligence; sterile	Buccal smear for X chromatin bodies may be negative. Endocrine levels are abnormal. Syndrome is usually revealed in adolescence by presence of short stature, ovarian streaks, and

Table 1-1 Summary of Numerical Chromosomal Abnormalities (*continued*)

Type	Synonym	Incidence	Diagnostic Features at Birth	Prognosis	Detection
Sex Chromosome Monosomy					
					amenorrhea. Estrogen at puberty may aid development of secondary sex characteristics.
Autosomal Trisomy					
		Usually incompatible with fetal survival			"Older" mother is at higher risk for offspring with these syndromes.
Trisomy 13	Patau syndrome	1/20,000 live births	Microphthalmia (very small eyeballs); cleft lip; postaxial polydactyly (extra digits);	Severe mental retardation; 50% die within first year of life	Karyotype analysis confirms diagnosis.

			microcephaly; malformed ears; congenital heart defects; urogenital defects; polycystic kidneys		
Trisomy 18	Edwards syndrome	1/8000 live births	Micrognathia (small jaw); clenched fist with 2nd and 5th fingers overlapping the 3rd and 4th; rocker-bottom feet; low-set, malformed ears; congenital heart defects.	Severe mental retardation in all cases; death usual in first few months.	Karyotype analysis confirms diagnosis.
Trisomy 21	Down syndrome	1/800 live births; most common chromosomal disorder	Typical round face with flat profile; protruding tongue; epicanthal folds	Mild to severe retardation; increased incidence of leukemia	Karyotype analysis confirms diagnosis; "older" mother is at higher risk for offspring with this syndrome.
Sex Chromosome Trisomy					
XXX	Triple X syndrome	1/1000 female births	None	Usually normal intelligence but slightly increased incidence	"Older" mother is at higher risk for offspring

Table 1-1 Summary of Numerical Chromosomal Abnormalities (*continued*)

Type	Synonym	Incidence	Diagnostic Features at Birth	Prognosis	Detection
Sex Chromosome Trisomy					
				of mental retardation; fertile, with normal offspring	with this syndrome. Buccal smears may reveal triple-X karyotype.
XXY	Klinefelter syndrome	1/1000 live male births	None	Usually normal intelligence; mild mental retardation does occur; sterile	Feminine characteristics appear in puberty, including gynecomastia. Typically, sufferer is tall and gangly with small testes and underdeveloped facial and body hair. Breast reduction

				may be advised for psychological and cosmetic reasons.
XYY	1/1000 live births	None	Rarely, may be associated with some intellectual impairment; fertile.	Syndrome may remain undetected until revealed on karyotyping. In persons with XYY syndrome, sperm count may be reduced, plasma testosterone levels may be high.

*Turner syndrome can also be the result of other chromosomal abnormalities, but these are extremely rare.

Table 1-2 Risk of Down Syndrome by Maternal Age

	Frequency of Down Syndrome	
Maternal Age	*Fetuses*	*Live Births*
–19		1/1550
20–24		1/1550
25–29		1/1050
30–34		1/700
35	1/350	1/350
36	1/260	1/300
37	1/200	1/225
38	1/160	1/175
39	1/125	1/150
40	1/70	1/100
41	1/35	1/85
42	1/30	1/65
43	1/20	1/50
44	1/13	1/40
45–	1/25	1/25

(Thompson JS, Thompson MW: Genetics in Medicine, Philadelphia, WB Saunders, 1980)

ment and history taking, provides a quick reference source for other members of the genetic team and helps determine which members of the family need further examination and testing. Common symbols used in pedigree charting are shown in Figure 1-1.

Newborn Genetic Screening

Newborn genetic screening aims to identify those presymptomatic newborns affected with a genetic metabolic disease so that preventive treatment can be initiated before permanent damage is done.

Classic newborn screening involves obtaining a specimen of cord blood, newborn nursery blood, newborn follow-up blood, or newborn follow-up urine.

Microbiologic assays screen for:

- Phenylketonuria (PKU)
- Maple syrup urine disease
- Galactosemia
- Homocystinuria
- Tyrosinemia

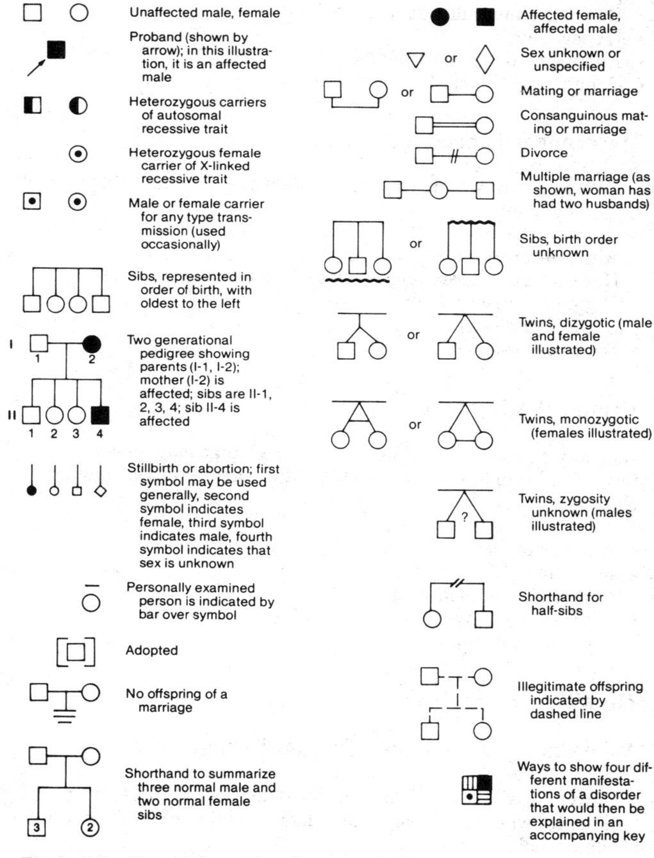

Figure 1-1 Commonly used pedigree symbols.

These screening tests are not diagnostic. An abnormal test must be confirmed by further testing. Other screening tests may also include those for genetic disorders such as:

- Congenital hypothyroidism
- Hemoglobinopathies
- Alpha-antitrypsin deficiency
- Cystic fibrosis

- Duchenne muscular dystrophy
- Hyperlipidemia
- Adenosine deaminase deficiency
- Congenital adrenal hyperplasia

Maternal Serum Screening

Most common disorders that can be identified with maternal serum screening are:

- Alpha-fetoprotein
- Heterozygous screening for detection of mutant genes
- Tay–Sachs disease
- Sickle cell disease
- Beta thalassemia

Prenatal Diagnosis

As many as 200 different genetic diseases that may develop in the fetus can be diagnosed accurately by a variety of techniques including:

- Amniocentesis
- Fetoscopy
- Chorionic villi sampling
- Ultrasonography
- Chromosome analysis

Genetic Counseling

Who Should Be Offered Prenatal Diagnosis?

- Gravidas who will be 35 years or older at time of delivery
- Clients who previously have had a child with chromosome abnormality
- Couples in whom either parent is a known balanced translocation chromosome carrier
- Couples in whom both partners are carriers for a diagnosable metabolic or structural autosomal recessive disorder
- Couples in whom either partner or a previous child is affected with a diagnosable metabolic or structural dominant disorder
- Gravidas who are known or presumed carriers for a serious X–linked recessive disorder
- Couples who have a previous personal or family history (i.e., first-degree or second-degree relative) of a neural tube defect
- Clients who exhibit extreme anxiety or concern

Components of Genetic Counseling*

- Initial interview
- Family history, pedigree preparation and analysis, other histories
- Assessment of client—physical examination, etc
- Establishment of an accurate diagnosis
- Confirmatory or supplementary tests or procedures:

Chromosome analysis	Developmental testing
Biochemical testing	Dermatoglyphics
X-ray films	Electromyography
Biopsy	Prenatal diagnosis
Lineage analysis	Immunologic testing

- Literature search and review
- Consultation with other experts
- Compiling of information and determination of recurrence risk
- Communication of the results and risks to client and family
- Discussion of options
- Review and questions
- Referrals—for example, amniocentesis, specialists
- Follow up
- Evaluation

Nursing Intervention†

- Provide referral for genetic counseling.
- Plan, implement, administer, or evaluate screening programs.
- Provide health teaching.
- Monitor and evaluate clients.
- Work with families under stress caused by problems related to a genetic disorder.
- Coordinate care and services.
- Manage home care and therapy.
- Follow up on positive newborn screening tests.
- Interview clients, assess needs, take family histories, and draw pedigrees.
- Reinforce genetic counseling information.
- Support families during counseling and decision making.
- Recognize the possibility of a genetic component in a disorder and take appropriate referral action.

* Order may vary depending on the reason for initial referral.

† Adapted from Cohen FL: Clinical Genetics in Nursing Practice. Philadelphia, JB Lippincott, 1984

2
Reproduction, Sexuality, and Fertility/Infertility

SEXUAL DIFFERENTIATION

Genetically, sex is determined at conception. For the first 6 weeks of gestation the conceptus remains sexually undifferentiated; that is, its gender is neither male nor female, and there is no anatomic difference. The gonads are bipotential, which means they can differentiate into either testes or ovaries. Two paired, primitive duct systems form in both male and female embryos at this time, the müllerian ducts and the wolffian ducts. Reproductive structures in one sex correspond to similar structures in the other sex because they both arise from the same embryologic tissue. The embryologically equivalent structures are called homologous.

Development of Male Reproductive Organs

- Primitive gonads develop into testes by the eighth week if the H–Y antigen (controlled by the Y chromosome) is present.
- Fetal androgen production must be present for further development of the male structures from the wolffian ducts.
- The male embryo produces müllerian duct-inhibiting substance and androgens that cause shrinking of the müllerian, or female duct system.
- The male hormones (androgens) testosterone and dihydrotestosterone cause masculinization and stimulate development of the wolffian ducts and the male internal and external reproductive organs.
- The genital tubercle develops into the penis.

Development of Female Reproductive Organs

- Differentiation of the primitive gonads into ovaries does not depend on hormones.
- Ovaries develop about the 12th week of embryonic life, and the müllerian duct system forms the uterus, fallopian tubes, and inner third of the vagina.

- The wolffian duct system (male) shrinks into tiny remnants, since testosterone is not present.
- Between the 7th and 14th week of development, the female external genitalia begin to differentiate.
- A small amount of testosterone in the female embryo assists in the development of the clitoris, vulva, and vagina.
- The genital tubercle develops into the glans in the clitoris.

By the 12th to 14th week of gestation, the biologic sex of the fetus is fairly well established, as shown in Table 2-1.

THE FEMALE REPRODUCTIVE SYSTEM: STRUCTURE AND FUNCTION

Female Reproductive Structures

External	Internal
Vulva (pudenda)	Vagina
Mons pubis	Uterus
Clitoris	Fallopian tubes
Labia majora	Ovaries
Labia minora	Supporting structures of the female pelvis
Vestibule	Bony pelvis
Urethral meatus	Perineum
Vaginal orifice and Skene's glands	Accessory organs
Bartholin's glands	Breasts
Perineum	

External Female Genitalia

The term *vulva,* also known as the pudenda, refers to all externally visible structures from the pubis to the perineum, as shown in Fig. 2-1.

The *mons pubis,* also known as the mons veneris, is the fatty cushion that lies over the pubic bone and is the most visible external organ. It is covered with coarse, curly hair and acts to protect the pubic bones beneath it.

The clitoris is a small, cylindrical, erectile body just below the mons pubis. It contains an abundance of blood vessels and nerve endings. It is highly sensitive to touch and fills with blood and becomes erect with sexual stimulation. It is homologous to the male penis.

The labia majora are two folds of adipose tissue that converge at the mons pubis and extend to the junction of the posterior commissure. Their outer surfaces are covered with curly hair while their inner surfaces are smooth and hairless. In nulliparous

Table 2-1 Sexual Development in the Fetus

	Characteristic	Male	Female
Fertilization	Chromosomal complement	XY	XX
6th Week	Gonadal development	Testes	Ovaries
6th Week	Androgen level	High	Low
8th Week	Internal ducts		
	Wolffian	Form vas deferens and associated glands	Degenerate
	Müllerian	Degenerate	Form vagina, uterus, and fallopian tubes
12th to 14th Week	External anatomy		
	Genital tubercle	Forms penis	Forms clitoris
	Swellings and folds	Form scrotum and lower shaft of penis	Form major and minor labia

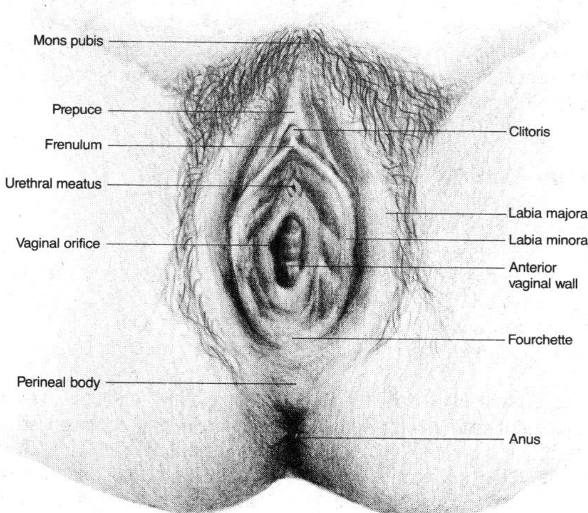

Figure 2-1 External female genitalia. (Childbirth Graphics)

women and in children, the labia are approximated and conceal the underlying structures. In multiparous women, the labia become less full and remain separated. After menopause they shrink and may disappear.

The labia minora are two thin, hairless folds that lie between the labia majora and are richly supplied with blood vessels and sensitive nerve endings. Both the labia majora and the labia minora contain numerous genital corpuscles that contribute to overall sexual stimulation. Anteriorly they converge to form the frenulum of the clitoris and the clitoral prepuce. At their posterior junction they form the posterior fourchette.

The *vestibule* is an almond-shaped area bordered by the labia minora, extending from the clitoris to the posterior fourchette. Six orifices are in this area:

- The urethral meatus is the external opening of the urinary tract.
- Skene's glands open on either side of the urethra. They secrete mucus and frequently are infected when gonorrhea is present.
- The vaginal opening is located at the inferior portion of the vestibule and varies in size and shape among women.
- Bartholin's glands are located in the lower vestibule and arise on either side of the lateral margins of the vaginal orifice. When the ducts become blocked, a cyst or abscess may form and become infected.

The *perineum,* sometimes referred to as the obstetric perineum, is the small area of muscle and fasciae that lies between the vulva and the anus. Support of this area is primarily provided by the urogenital and anal triangles, which may become traumatized during childbirth.

Internal Female Reproductive Organs

The *vagina* serves three purposes:

- It is the excretory duct of the uterus through which its secretions and menstrual blood flow.
- It is the female organ of copulation.
- it is the canal through which an infant is born.

To accommodate these functions the vagina is structured as a musculomembranous tube lined with transverse, corrugated, and distensible mucosa (Fig. 2-2). At its terminal end the circumference is attached to the uterine cervix; its posterior wall is attached high on the posterior cervix, causing a pouchlike area to be formed beneath it, the posterior fornix. Similar but smaller spaces surrounding the lateral and anterior vaginal attachments are called the lateral and anterior fornices. These areas are important because their thin-walled tissues allow access for vaginal palpation of the uterus and adnexa.

Mucosa of the vaginal wall is lined with stratified squamous epithelium. When stimulated by estrogen this layer of cells maintains the normal acidic vaginal ecology. Maintenance of this ecol-

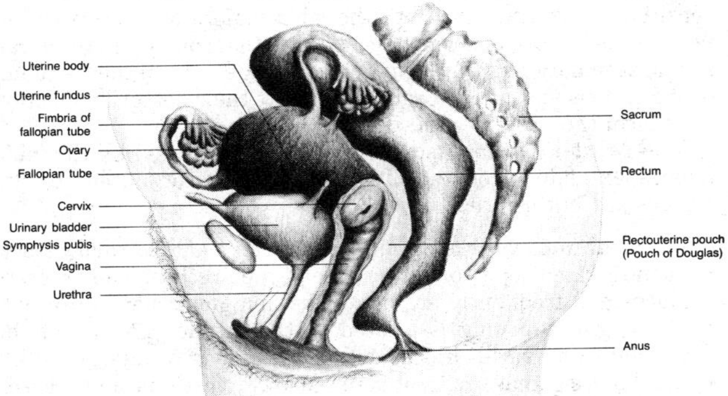

Figure 2-2 Internal female reproductive organs. (Childbirth Graphics)

ogy depends on a delicate physiologic balance of hormonal and bacterial action.

The nonpregnant *uterus* is located in the lower pelvis and lies between the urinary bladder anteriorly and the rectum posteriorly. Shaped like an inverted, flattened pear, its anatomic subdivisions include two major but unequal parts. The triangular upper portion of the uterus is called the body or corpus, and the lower portion is called the cervix (Fig. 2-3). The dome-shaped upper segment of the uterine body that is located between the insertion points of the fallopian tubes is called the fundus. The isthmus is the area that lies between the uterine body and the cervix, above the internal os of the cervix. During pregnancy the isthmus takes on special significance and becomes larger, softer, and more compressible. One of the signs of early pregnancy, known as Hegar's sign, is the softening of the isthmus between the uterine body and the cervix.

The *cervix* is the portion of the uterus that lies below the isthmus. The portion that protrudes into the upper vagina normally appears pink but may appear purplish during pregnancy. Prior to childbirth the cervical os appears small and round; after childbirth the os becomes a transverse slit.

The *fallopian tubes* extend from the superior portion of the uterus to the region of the ovaries. After the ovum is released from the ovary, it is drawn into the fallopian tube. Sperm entering the tube from the uterus are moved along to meet the ova.

The *ovaries* lie on either side of the uterus in the true pelvis and are attached to the posterior broad ligament of the uterus. Func-

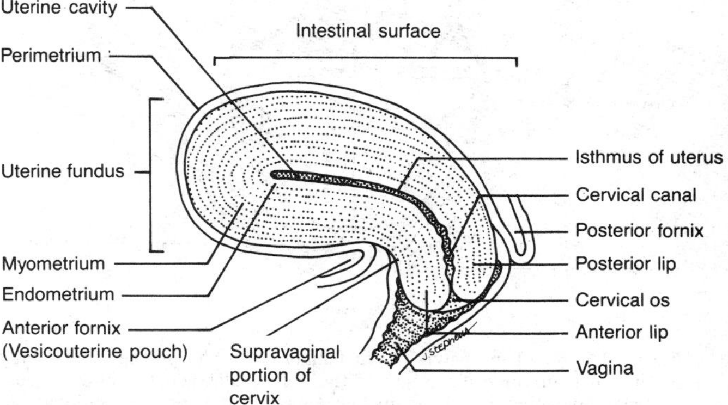

Figure 2-3 Cross section of the normal uterus. (Childbirth Graphics)

tions of the ovaries include production and secretion of estrogen and progesterone.

Supporting Structures of the Female Pelvis

These structures include the bony pelvis, perineum, and pelvic floor muscles. The female pelvis is especially adapted to childbearing, and its dimensions must be adequate to permit delivery of the infant's head. The pelvis is divided into two parts by the linea terminalis (Fig. 2-4). That portion lying above this line is the false pelvis (pelvic brim); the portion lying below the line is the true pelvis which contains the pelvic inlet, midplane, and outlet. The ischial spines in the midpelvis represent the shortest diameter of the pelvis through which the infant must pass. See Figure 2-5.

Perineum and the Pelvic Floor Muscles

The perineum is the region lying between the pubic arch anteriorly and by the sacrum and coccyx posteriorly. The underlying muscles of the pelvic floor support the pelvic contents. The urogenital diaphragm, composed of the pubococcygeal muscle, is constructed

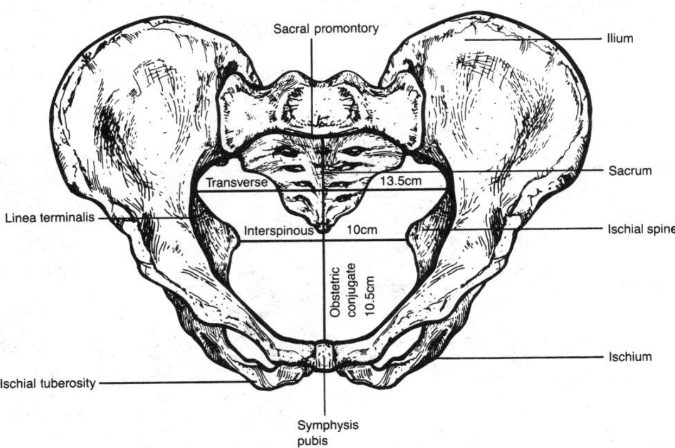

Figure 2-4 The bony pelvis. Adult female pelvis showing the anteroposterior and transverse diameters of the pelvic inlet and the interspinous (transverse) diameter of the midpelvis. Normally the obstetric conjugate is greater than 10-cm. (Childbirth Graphics)

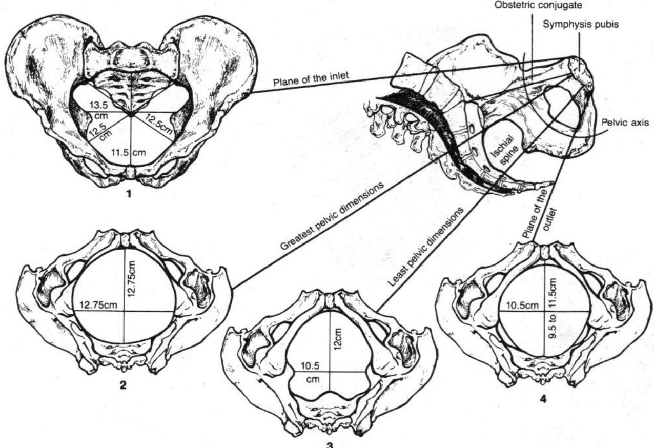

Figure 2-5 Planes and diameters of the bony pelvis. The cavity of the true pelvis resembles an obliquely truncated curved cylinder with its height greatest posteriorly. Note the curvature of the pelvic axis. (Childbirth Graphics)

to adapt and expand for childbirth. These muscles are stretched to their limit during childbirth and may never regain their previous strength or integrity.

Accessory Organs: The Breasts

The breasts are modified sweat glands that are highly specialized mammary glands located in the superficial fasciae of the pectoral region. The nipple is surrounded by the pigmented areola and contains Montgomery's glands, which secrete a protective lubricant during breastfeeding.

During pregnancy marked changes occur in the size, shape, and sensitivity of the breasts in preparation for milk production. Each breast consists of about 20 irregular lobes of secreting and adipose tissue. Each lobe has one lactiferous duct that converges at the areola of the nipple. Alveoli are milk-secreting glands contained in each lobe and that terminate in the ducts. The alveoli and adjacent ducts are surrounded by myoepithelial cells that contract to squeeze milk into the reservoir called the ampulla (lactiferous sinus) as shown in Figure 2-6. See Chapter 4 for more information on the physiology of breastfeeding.

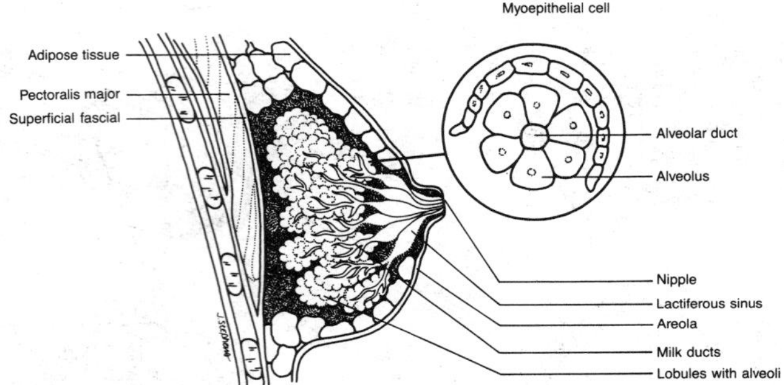

Figure 2-6 Breast structure and action of the myoepithelial cell during breastfeeding. Under the influence of prolactin, the alveoli secrete milk. When the baby begins to suck, oxytocin is released and causes the myoepithelial cells to contract and squeeze milk into the ducts during the "let-down" reflex. The milk flows into the lactiferous sinus, where it collects for immediate use by the infant. (Childbirth Graphics)

HORMONAL CONTROL OF THE FEMALE REPRODUCTIVE CYCLE

Sex hormones, produced by the endocrine glands, are chemical compounds that produce profound physiologic effects in target organs of the female reproductive system. The female hormonal system consists of three separate hierarchies of hormones and activities:

Level 1: The hypothalamus secretes gonadotropin-releasing hormone (GnRH) to the pituitary in response to signals received from higher centers in the central nervous system (CNS) or from the external environment. Rather than controlling the menstrual cycle, the hypothalamus responds to positive or negative feedback from the ovarian hormones.

Level 2: The anterior pituitary hormones, follicle-stimulating hormone (FSH) and luteinizing hormone (LH), are secreted to stimulate the ovary in response to stimulus from the GnRH of the hypothalamus.

Level 3: The ovarian hormones estrogen and progesterone are secreted in response to stimulation from FSH in the follicular phase and from LH in the luteal phase of the menstrual cycle.

The primary hormones of the female reproductive system include estrogen, progesterone, and the gonadotropins, FSH and LH (Table 2-2). The influence of the female hormones on the body and the menstrual cycle are shown in Table 2-3.

(*text continues on pg. 36*)

Table 2-2 Female Hormones

Hormone	Description
Estrogen	Hormone produced by ovarian follicles, corpus luteum, adrenal cortex, and placenta during pregnancy. It is associated with "femaleness." The three principle types are: 1. Estrogen E_1 (estrone)—the estrogen of menopause, oxidized from estradiol. (It is the second most active type, with a relative potency of 10.) 2. Estradiol E_2—the estrogen of reproductive-age women and the most potent type (relative potency 100) 3. Estriol E_3—the estrogen of pregnancy, formed from estradiol and estrone in liver, uterus, placenta, and estrogen precursors from the fetal adrenal gland. (It is the least potent estrogen with a relative potency of 1.)
Progesterone	Hormone secreted by the corpus luteum of the ovary, adrenal glands, and placenta during pregnancy. It is the hormone of the luteal phase of the menstrual cycle and of pregnancy.
Gonadotropins (FSH and LH)	Hormones that, when stimulated by GnRH from the hypothalamus, are released from the anterior pituitary gland to stimulate follicular growth and development, growth of graafian follicle, and production of progesterone
GnRH	Hormone that acts on the pituitary gland to release LH and FSH in response to feedback from the ovarian follicle destined to ovulate
Prolactin	Hormone produced by the pituitary gland, which, in association with estrogen and progesterone, stimulates breast development and formation of milk during pregnancy. (Stress of any kind can also stimulate prolactin release in the nonpregnant woman.)

Table 2-3 Influence of Female Hormones on the Body and Menstrual Cycle

Organ/System	Action of Estrogen	Action of Progesterone	Action of Gonadotropins
Uterus	• Increases excitability of myometrium • Causes proliferation of endometrium • Increases amount of cervical mucus and produces ferning and spinnbarkeit • Causes uterine growth in pregnancy	• Promotes secretory changes in endometrium • Decreases amount of cervical mucus and renders it impermeable to sperm • Causes loss of ferning • Promotes coiling of uterine arteries • Promotes disposition of glycogen in endometrium • Causes menstruation to occur when conception has not taken place • Reaches peak of activity 1 week after ovulation	• None
Fallopian Tubes	• Influences activity of tubal musculature	• Decreases tubal contractility in later luteal phase • May be important to transport of fertilized ovum into uterus	• None

Vagina	• Causes proliferation and cornification of vaginal epithelium • Maintains optimum acidic *p*H of 3.5 to 4.2 in vagina	• Causes change from cornified superficial cells to intermediate and basal cell predominance	• None
Mammary Glands	• Promotes development and growth of ductal system, gland buds, and nipples • Partially responsible for lobular and alveolar growth and deposition of fatty tissues • Promotes increased production of prolactin in pregnancy	• Promotes development of lobules and alveoli during pregnancy in preparation for lactation • Causes retention of subcutaneous fluid and swelling of breasts before menstruation	• None
Ovaries	• Interact with gonadotropins to stimulate growth of ovarian follicle and release of ovum • Produce estrogen • May be responsible for LH surge at menstrual midcycle	• Possibly involved in ovulation	*FSH* • Initiates and stimulates development of ovarian follicles • Promotes estrogen production and secretion by ovarian follicles

Table 2-3 Influence of Female Hormones on the Body and Menstrual Cycle (*continued*)

Organ/System	Action of Estrogen	Action of Progesterone	Action of Gonadotropins
Ovaries			*LH* • Causes final growth of graafian follicle • Causes steroidogenesis in conjunction with FSH • Stimulates ovary • Aids in formation of corpus luteum from ruptured follicle • Promotes production of progesterone by the corpus luteum
Skin	• Diminishes sebaceous activity of skin • Increases water content of skin	• May increase sebaceous activity of skin	• None

Cardiovascular System	• Increases blood flow • Increases amount of angiotensin, Factor V, and prothrombin in blood	• None	• None
Secondary Sexual Characteristics	• Responsible for female contours of fat deposition and axillary and public hair	• Partially responsible for breast development	• None
Thermogenic Activity		• Increases the basal body temperature about 0.4° to 0.6°C after ovulation, identifying luteal function • Influences deposition of glycogen in endometrium to furnish nutrients for implantation and support of fertilized ovum	• None • None
Metabolism	• Causes sodium and water resorption from kidney tubules • Affects calcium metabolism and bone growth	• None	• None

Menstrual Cycle

- *Menstruation* is defined as the bleeding and physiologic shedding of the uterine endometrium that occur at approximately monthly intervals from menarche to menopause.
- *Menarche* is the term used to describe the first menstruation of the pubescent female. It is a major event in the progression from childhood to maturity.
- *Puberty* is the period during which an individual becomes capable of reproduction.

Tanner Stages of Progression from Childhood to Maturity

Tanner Stage I (Prepuberty)

- Neither breasts nor pubic hair has developed.
- Vaginal mucosa is thin, red, and dry.

Tanner Stage II (Average Age 10 to 11 Years)

- Breast buds appear as diameter of areola increases.
- Labia majora become more vascular and wrinkled; fine, downy pubic hair develops.
- Vaginal mucosa becomes thicker, pink, and moist.
- Uterine fundus enlarges.
- Hips begin to widen with distribution of body fat.
- Height spurt begins.

Tanner Stage III (Average Age 11 to 12 Years)

- Breasts continue to enlarge.
- Pubic hair on labia majora becomes darker, coarser.
- Labia minora enlarge.
- Vaginal length increases, the mucosa thickens, and a white discharge may appear.
- The uterus continues to enlarge, and fallopian tubes increase in diameter.
- Sebaceous glands of the face become active (acne may appear), and axillary sweat glands begin to function.
- Rapid skeletal growth begins and achieves peak height velocity.

Tanner Stage IV (Average Age 12 to 13 Years)

- Breasts enlarge and areolae form mounds separate from the rest of the breast tissue.
- Pubic hair covers the mons pubis and perineum.
- Vagina and uterus enlarge.
- Menarche occurs.
- Linear growth decelerates.

Tanner Stage V (Average Age 13.5 to 15 Years)

- Breasts and genitals reach adult proportions.
- Pubic hair grows on thighs.
- Linear growth ceases.

Normal Menstrual Cycle

The menstrual cycle can be considered as two inter-related cycles. One cycle takes place in the ovary and depends on the other, which occurs simultaneously in the uterus. This unique mechanism cyclically affects the endometrium, making it ready for the development of the fertilized egg at the precise time of the month when the egg is present. The ovarian and menstrual cycles are summarized in Table 2-4.

FUNCTIONS OF THE NURSE THAT PROMOTE SEXUAL HEALTH

Every nurse should ask herself whether or not she feels comfortable dealing with sexual health concerns in patient care. The nurse who desires to explore the sexual concerns of clients must acquire specialized knowledge and skills. The nurse who is uncomfortable with the subject of sexuality should refer clients to sexual health resource professionals.

Even though the nurse may not wish to become an expert on human sexuality, familiarity with the principles of human behavior as they relate to sexuality is important. Nursing functions that promote sexual health, listed in order of increasing requirements for skill and knowledge, are outlined here:*

1. Facilitation of a milieu conducive to sexual health
2. Provision of anticipatory guidance
3. Validation of normalcy
4. Education
5. Counsel for clients who must adapt to changes in their usual forms of sexual expression
6. Provision of intensive therapy for clients with complex problems
7. Consultation with other helpers

* Woods NF: Human Sexuality in Health and Illness. St. Louis, CV Mosby, 1984

(*text continues on pg. 40*)

Table 2-4 Ovarian and Menstrual Cycle

Follicular/Proliferative Phase (Estrogen Dominant)	Ovulation (Gonadotropin Surge)	Luteal/Secretory Phase and Menses (Progesterone Dominant)
Early Follicular Phase (Ovarian)—2 to 6 Days • Rise in FSH levels, beginning day 24, due to estrogen decrease in previous luteal phase • Early growth of ovarian follicles *Advanced Follicular Phase (Ovarian)—7 to 16 Days* • Stimulation of graafian follicle by FSH • Continued follicular growth with increased production of estradiol, reaching a peak before ovulation • Stimulation of FSH and estradiol of rapid rise in LH production after day 10 (positive feedback)	• LH surge at midcycle, —requiring estradiol concentration over 200 pg/ml —exposure to estrogen for a minimum of 50 hours • Rupture of follicle, usually within 24 hours of LH peak • Ovulation (occurs only if mature follicle [adequate estrogen] is present) • Modest rise in FSH (may be necessary for normal corpus luteum development) • High gonadotropin levels lasting only 24 hours • Precipitous drop in estrogen, probably due to luteinization of follicle	*Luteal/Secretory Phase* • Initial sharp drop of estrogen (time from midcycle LH surge to menses is consistently about 14 days in 90% of women) • Plasma level of progesterone of 3 mg/ml produced, reliable evidence of ovulation at peak (8 to 9 days post-ovulation) • Formation of corpus luteum (CL) from follicle remnants after ovulation; synthesis by CL of androgens, estrogens, and progesterone • Stimulation by progesterone growth of endometrium, with coiling, enlargement, and spiraling of arteries in preparation for implantation of fertilized ovum

- Decline in FSH just prior to ovulation in response to increased estrogen from developing follicle (negative feedback)
- Secretion of estradiol, primarily by follicle that will ovulate
- Increase of preovulatory progesterone production to 2 to 3 ng/ml
- Atresia of all but dominant ovarian follicle caused by androgen production late in phase

Proliferative Phase (Uterine)

- Estrogen stimulation, producing
  —Proliferation of endometrium and myometrium
  —Increased vascularity, vasodilation, and rhythmic contraction of uterine blood vessels
  —Increased uterine motility in nonpregnant uterus in preparation for effect of progesterone after ovulation

- Shift from estrogen to progesterone dominance

- With fertilization the CL is maintained and progesterone production reaches a plateau at 9 to 13 days after ovulation, implantation occurs 6 to 8 days after ovulation
- Secretion of human chorionic gonadotropin by the implanting blastocyst (maintains steroidogenesis of CL until the 6th to 10th week of gestation, when the placenta takes over)
- Without fertilization, maintenance of CL is maintained by LH for 14 (±2) days
  —Inhibition of LH secretion by high progesterone levels
  —Decrease in estrogen production after degeneration-stimulating FSH secretion
- Degeneration, scarring, and eventual disappearance of the CL taking place over a 3-month period
- Rise in FSH levels beginning day 24 to stimulate early follicular development for the new cycle

Menstrual Phase

Menstruation, with sloughing off of the endometrium

Nursing Objectives in Sexual Health

- To obtain a brief sexual history of the couple's desires, sexual pattern, and concerns
- To obtain objective information about the status of the current pregnancy and relevant past reproductive history
- To make a nursing diagnosis by assessing areas where information, specific suggestions, and support would be helpful
- On the basis of the information given, to offer specific suggestions and to evaluate their effectiveness

Possible Nursing Diagnoses Related to Sexual Health During the Prenatal Period

- Alteration in comfort related to nausea and vomiting, heartburn, and potential infection
- Potential alteration of increased or decreased libido related to verbalization of the problem, alteration in sexual activity and perceived role
- Altered body structure or function related to change of interest in self and others
- Lack of knowledge or misinformation related to alteration in achieving sexual satisfaction, inability to achieve desired satisfaction

Counseling the Pregnant Couple about Sexuality

Many pregnant couples seem to lack knowledge about sex during pregnancy and immediately after birth and are hesitant about broaching the subject. The nurse must remember that each couple is unique and that a multitude of factors affect the sexual relationship during pregnancy. Consequently, sexual feelings and desires, the frequency of intercourse, and the degree of sexual enjoyment vary widely among couples.

Problems in Sexual Activity

First Trimester

- Nausea and vomiting after the sixth or seventh weeks of pregnancy may interfere with sexual feelings.

- Breast tenderness, which is common in early pregnancy, can make breast stimulation during arousal especially painful.
- Excessive tiredness caused by hormonal changes can curtail sexual interest.
- Fear of miscarriage creates anxiety and can cause couples to avoid all sexual expression, even cuddling. When a previous pregnancy has been lost or bleeding has occurred in the current pregnancy, sexual activity may be viewed as a threat to the fetus. This may, in fact, be true. But when the danger has passed, the couple should be reassured that they can safely resume sexual activity.

Second Trimester

- At about the fourth month of pregnancy, tissues around the inside the vagina "ripen" and become engorged from increased vascularity and blood volume to the area. The tissues remain this way throughout pregnancy and may cause the woman to be in a constant state of early arousal.
- Due to congestion of the pelvic organs caused by pressure from the growing fetus, some women feel a constant need for sexual outlet. Some women may feel guilty about this increased sexual drive; however, both partners should be reassured that the feeling is normal.
- The resolution phase takes longer and is less complete, adding to the feelings of congestion.
- As the pregnancy progresses the abdomen continues to enlarge, and the "missionary position" (man–on–top) becomes uncomfortable for the pregnant woman. At this point couples may wish to try other positions that prevent abdominal pressure or deep penetration.
- Vaginitis, pressure on the abdomen, or penile thrusting against the cervix may cause painful intercourse (dyspareunia).
- Fetal movement may decrease the couple's desire for sex.

Third Trimester

- The pregnant woman may experience heartburn and indigestion and, possibly, hemorrhoids, any of which may inhibit sexual interest.
- Following orgasm the uterus may have a sustained contraction that lasts for a minute or more. Some women perceive this as pleasurable; others fear that it will endanger their fetus. However, no reported evidence exists for the latter.
- As pregnancy progresses the woman may feel awkward or beautiful and may direct her sexual interest accordingly.
- Fatigue and its associated problems may return in the third trimester due to lack of sleep and the physical strain of carrying the fetus.

Nursing Interventions

Self-Care Teaching: Sexual Activity During Pregnancy

First Trimester

- Breast tenderness and other changes are temporary.
- Decrease breast fondling.
- Wear a bra during sex if the breasts are tender.
- Use a coital position during intercourse to prevent undue pressure on the breasts.
- Avoid sex when tired.
- If orgasm or sexual intercourse has been prohibited, use other means to express love, such as hugging, massage, together activities.
- Never have sex on an empty stomach.

Second Trimester

- Increased lubrication may cause hygienic concern. Wash genitals with warm water and avoid deodorant soaps and douches.
- A back rub after orgasm may ease discomfort.
- Try creative sexual positions during intercourse.
- Heightened or decreased interest in sex is normal.
- Masturbation and orgasm are acceptable in an uncomplicated pregnancy.

Third Trimester

- Sex may be more comfortable in the upright position.
- Alternatives to intercourse may become necessary.
- Remind your partner of the increased need for cuddling and holding.
- Sustained tonic contraction has not been shown to hurt the fetus.

Self-Care Teaching: Sexual Activity During the Postpartum Period

- For both vaginal and cesarean deliveries, sexual intercourse may be resumed at approximately 3 to 4 weeks postpartum.
- Do not resume sexual intercourse until vaginal bleeding has stopped to prevent introduction of infection at the placental site.
- Check for healing of the episiotomy and perineum by inserting a finger or tampon into the vagina.

- Sexual arousal may cause milk to leak from the breasts. Nursing the baby before sexual activity or wearing a bra with absorbent pads during intercourse may help.
- If additional lubrication is necessary, advise the woman to use contraceptive cream or a natural vegetable oil (safflower or soy, for example). K-Y jelly dries too quickly.
- Prolong foreplay to encourage lubrication.
- Communicate openly with your partner.
- Use alternative forms of sexual expression (mutual masturbation, massage, oral sex).
- Do not take baths for 2 to 3 weeks to avoid spreading bacteria from other parts of the body to the vaginal opening.
- Begin Kegel exercises immediately after birth. Do them whenever you urinate and frequently during the day to strengthen pubococcygeal muscles and to tighten the vaginal opening.
- Take Sitz baths 3 times daily to help heal the episiotomy.
- Examine the perineum with a good light and mirror within a few days of delivery, then again 3 weeks later to reassure yourself that it is healing. If something does not look right, contact a physician immediately. Problems can be resolved more easily when treated early.
- Your body and its response to intercourse do return to "normal." Some women feel they will never have sex again.
- Wear a bra 24 hours a day as soon as possible after delivery to help decrease engorgement.
- Encourage your partner to avoid putting pressure on sensitive breasts, especially during the night when the baby is sleeping for longer periods without feeding and breasts are full.
- Set priorities realistically. For example, arrange your schedule so that you nap when the baby does.
- Nap at least 30 minutes every day or at least lie down.
- If you're depressed, get help from friends and family. If the depression lasts longer than 3 days, professional help may be necessary.
- Once the baby is weaned, your sex drive will return to normal.
- Place the baby in another room or behind a screen during intercourse.
- Use music to soothe the baby during intercourse.

FERTILITY/INFERTILITY

Nurses play a crucial role in helping couples who are concerned about their fertility. Persons with infertility problems need emotional support, guidance, advocacy, education, and appropriate referrals for adequate care. Nurses contribute to each of these critical areas by providing skilled nursing care and by working with the infertile couple and the family unit.

Nursing Objectives in Fertility Concerns

- To help clients understand factors that may contribute to their fertility problems
- To create an atmosphere in which couples may discuss emotional responses to their fertility problem and use available sources of emotional and informational support
- To explain clearly treatment procedures and alternatives and the prognosis for successful treatment
- To encourage clients to maintain normal activities of daily living with a minimum of disruption in family relationships

Possible Nursing Diagnoses Related to Fertility Concerns

- Ineffective individual coping related to stress of infertility
- Ineffective family coping related to actual or perceived loss of childbearing function
- Disturbance in self-concept related to inability to conceive
- Sexual dysfunction related to stress of infertility

Fertility

Fertility patterns are dependent on many factors. The nurse must understand the physiologic processes underlying male and female reproductive potential and conception to deliver effective care to those who want to control their fertility by either avoiding pregnancy or achieving it.

- Maximum fertility in both men and women is achieved at age 24.
- Twenty-five percent (25%) of young fertile couples will conceive during the first month of unprotected intercourse.
- About 80% of young fertile couples will conceive by the end of 1 year of unprotected intercourse.
- Between 10% and 15% of couples remain childless after 1 year of trying to become pregnant.
- Among women aged 35 to 39, because of an increased incidence of reproductive tract disorders and irregular ovulation, only 52% will become pregnant.

Normal Process of Conception

Sperm Production

- Mature, healthy spermatozoa must be produced and deposited into the vagina for conception to occur.
- Sperm production depends on follicle-stimulating hormone (FSH) and luteinizing hormone (LH). These gonadotropic hormones are released from the pituitary gland and stimulate the production of testosterone by the testes.

Transport

- Sperm deposited into the vagina must be transported through the cervical mucus into the fallopian tubes.

Capacitation

- Capacitation is the process during which the surface characteristics of the sperm are changed to release enzymes that enable them to penetrate the ovum.

Ovulation

- Normally one ovarian follicle, known as the graafian follicle, is destined to ovulate. When the ovum it contains is released into the fallopian tube, it is ready to be fertilized.

Fertilization

- The ovum is fertilized early in its journey through the fallopian tube.
- When one sperm has penetrated the ovum, the zona pellucida blocks the entry of other sperm.

Implantation

- When the fertilized ovum attaches to the uterine wall and penetrates the maternal circulatory system, implantation has occurred.

Infertility

- *Infertility* is the inability to conceive and carry a pregnancy to viability after at least 1 year of regular sexual intercourse without contraception.
- *Primary infertility* is an inability to conceive and carry a pregnancy to viability with no previous history of pregnancy carried to live birth.
- *Situational infertility* applies to men and women without partners and to homosexual men or women whose lifestyle precludes the occurrence of contraception.
- *Sterility* denotes a total and irreversible inability to conceive.

Causes of Infertility

Biologic Causes: Female (40%)
- Vaginal: abnormalities, infections, sexual dysfunction, highly acidic vaginal *p*H
- Cervical: hostile environment (insufficient estrogen or infection), incompetent cervix
- Uterine: abnormalities, hostile environment that does not allow implantation and survival of blastocyst
- Tubal: adhesions, scar tissue due to pelvic inflammatory disease (PID); endometriosis
- Ovarian: anovulation, irregular or infrequent ovulation, secretory dysfunction, inadequate luteal phase

Biologic Causes: Male (40%)
- Anatomic abnormalities/congenital factors
- Inadequate sperm production/maturation: maternal diethylstilbestrol (DES) ingestion, varicocele, testicular inflammation, heat exposure, sexually transmitted disease, radiation exposure, stress, certain drugs
- Inadequate motility of sperm: same as above
- Blockage of sperm in male reproductive tract: same as above
- Inability to deposit sperm: problems with ejaculation

Interactive Causes (20%)
- Situational causes (lack of a partner; homosexuality)
- Unexplained causes (10% to 15%)

Assessment

Detailed Medical, Social, and Family History

- Duration of infertility
- Primary or secondary infertility
- Frequency of sexual intercourse

Female History
- Regularity, duration, and frequency of menstruation
- Premenstrual signs and symptoms
- History of vaginal discharge, cervicitis, pelvic infections, surgery, and accidents
- General physical condition
- Illnesses, allergies, and drug intake
- Significant family history
- Prior use of contraceptives, including type, duration, and complications
- Information on maternal use of DES

Male History

- History of mumps, orchitis, diabetes mellitus, herniorrhaphy
- History of exposure to x-rays or toxic substances
- Exercise patterns, exposure to heat
- History of maternal use of DES

Complete Physical Examination

- Complete examination for both partners.
- Pelvic examination of the woman particularly important

Diagnostic Procedures Used for Fertility Workup

Male Factors: Evidence of Normal Ejaculation and Sperm Production

Semen Analysis: Microscopic examination of semen sample. Done early in the workup since it is a simple test that provides valuable information and may obviate more invasive procedures. Done after 48 to 72 hours of abstinence from orgasm (less time may result in a false low sperm count).

Favorable clinical findings

- Normal amount of ejaculate (3 to 5 ml: range 1 to 7 ml)
- No agglutination of sperm. (Agglutination suggests infection or autoimmunity)
- Normal seminal fluid; semen liquifies
- Sperm count showing greater than 20 million cells with at least 50% motility 2 hours after ejaculation and more than 60% normal appearing

Female Factors: Evidence of Normal Pelvic Anatomy and Tubal Functioning

Hysterosalpingogram: Dye is injected through the cervix into the uterus with fluoroscopic visualization of spread of dye through the fallopian tubes.

Favorable clinical findings

- Patency of fallopian tubes demonstrated by dispersal of dye from the cervix and uterine cavities up into the peritoneal cavity
- Absence of abnormalities in uterine cavities and fallopian tubes

Laparoscopy: Direct visualization of pelvic structures using telescope and light source inserted through a small abdominal incision

Favorable clinical findings

- Normal pelvic structures and absence of signs of infection, adhesions, endometriosis, or lesions

Female/Interactive Factors: Evidence of Normal Hormonal Cycle and Receptivity to Sperm

Basal Body Temperature (BBT) Measurement: Oral temperature taken daily before arising throughout several menstrual cycles. Provides overall assessment of cyclic hormonal changes (Fig. 2-7).

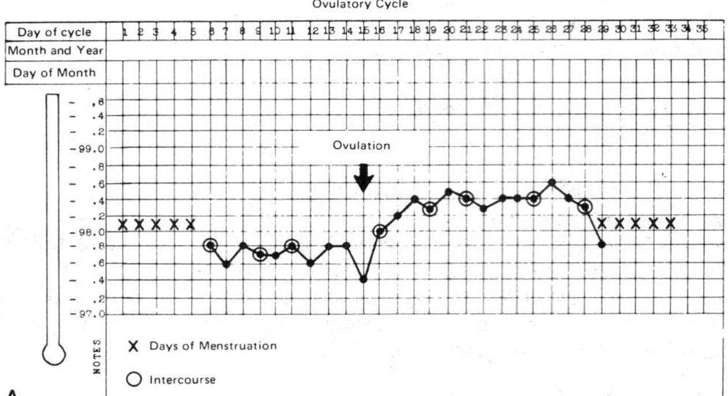

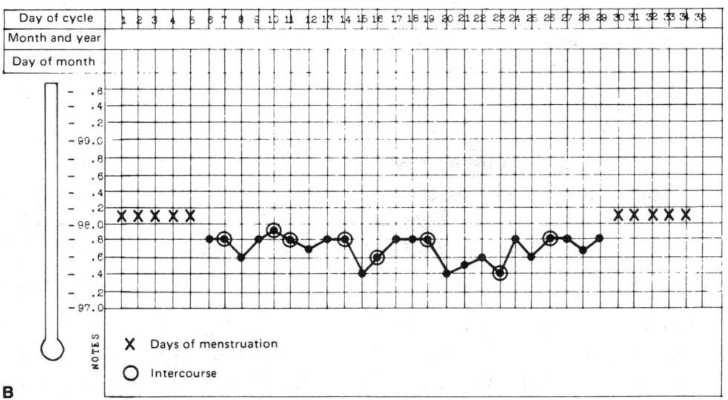

Figure 2-7 Basal body temperature records suggesting (A) ovulatory and (B) anovulatory cycles. As a rule, intercourse on day 16 (A) would be expected to be fruitful; but, as is shown here, this is not always the case. An indirect method of determing ovulation, the basal body temperature chart shows a biphasic pattern, with temperatures below 98°F for the first half of the menstrual cycle, and above 98°F for the second half of the cycle in ovulatory women. (Danforth DN [ed]: Obstetrics and Gynecology, 4th ed. Philadelphia, JB Lippincott, 1982)

Favorable clinical findings

- Biphasic pattern with persistent temperature elevation for 12 to 14 days prior to menstruation

Postcoital Test: Vaginal examination within 8 hours after intercourse during the time of presumed ovulation to determine whether normal ovulatory changes occur in cervical mucus and whether sperm survive in vaginal environment.

Favorable clinical findings

- Cervical mucus suggestive of ovulation. Microscopic ferning pattern is present. (See Chap. 12 and Fig. 12-1). Mucus is watery, slippery, abundant. Spinnbarkeit is present.
- Presence of normal live and motile sperm in cervical mucus

Serum Progesterone Measurement: A blood sample is used to determine whether serum progesterone peaks during midportion of the second half of the menstrual period (days 22 to 24).

Favorable clinical findings

- Serum progesterone at 3 to 4 ng/ml in early luteal phase, 10 ng/ml at midluteal phase

Endometrial Biopsy: Endometrial tissue is collected during vaginal examination in the second half of the menstrual cycle (days 22 to 24) to determine presence and adequacy of secretory tissue. Secretory tissue is present if ovulation occurs and peaks at midphase of second half of menstrual cycle (luteal phase).

Favorable clinical findings

- Biopsies at different points in menstrual cycle showing development of endometrium consistent with phase of cycle

Immunoassay Tests: Immunologic tests with semen and male/female serum

Favorable clinical findings

- Absence of antibody reaction

Treatment for Infertility

Once the cause of infertility has been diagnosed, treatment that involves the male partner, the female partner, or both may be instituted.

Female Infertility: Treatment of Vaginal, Cervical and Uterine Problems

- Vaginal treatment includes eradication of vaginitis when appropriate, sexual therapy for problems such as vaginismus, and surgical correction of structural or anatomic abnormalities when possible.
- Cervical treatment includes detecting and treating cervicitis, improving the *p*H of the cervical mucus and enhancing its ferning and spinnbarkeit, artificial insemination to bypass the cervix and vaginal secretions, and cerclage for an incompetent cervix.
- Uterine treatment includes surgical removal of uterine myomas (fibroids), and reversal of Asherman syndrome.
- Tubal treatment includes treatment for endometriosis, microsurgery for tubal blockage, and *in vitro* fertilization.
- Ovarian treatment usually requires the induction of ovulation with medications. The major drugs used are shown in Table 2-5.

Male Infertility

The goal of treatment in male infertility is to:

- Achieve an adequate sperm count, motility, and morphology
- Have sperm penetrate the egg to achieve fertilization
- Remove environmental hazards that cause decreased sperm production (oligospermia)
- Surgically correct a varicocele
- Artificially inseminate the woman when the male has retrograde ejaculation
- Use a split ejaculate for artificial insemination when sperm count continues to remain low

Interactive Causes of Infertility

A variety of treatments are attempted for interactive causes of infertility and include:

- Condom therapy for 6 months if infertility is due to the woman's manufacture of antibodies to her partner's sperm
- Sexual counseling or education for couples with sexual problems
- Various treatments when a specific cause of infertility cannot be found in hope that one might be successful
- Emotional support for the couple who chooses to stop the fertility workup and to consider other options. Help in selecting an appropriate option, including adoption, deciding to be childfree, artificial insemination, *in vitro* fertilization, embryo transplantation, and surrogate mothering

Table 2-5 Medications Used to Induce Ovulation

Medication	Method of Use	Disadvantages and Side-Effects
Clomiphene citrate	Increases secretion of FSH and LH, which stimulate follicle growth. Administered orally, 50 mg/day to 250 mg/day, from day 5 to day 9 of menstrual cycle. Ovulation should occur 5 to 10 days after the last dose.	Antiestrogenic—may cause poor cervical mucus. Other complications are vasomotor flushes, abdominal distention, bloating, pain, soreness, breast discomfort, nausea and vomiting, visual symptoms (spots, flashes), headaches, dryness or loss of hair, ovarian enlargement.
Human menopausal gonadotropin and Human chorionic gonadotropin (HCG)	Stimulates follicle growth. Administered IM daily for 7 to 10 days during first half of menstrual cycle. After the ovaries have been stimulated, HCG is administered IM to induce ovulation.	Ovarian hyperstimulation. Multiple pregnancies. Expensive. Sometimes requires repeated ultrasounds to rule out ovarian enlargement.
Bromocriptine	Inhibits pituitary secretion of prolactin, thus preventing suppression of pulsatile secretion of FSH and LH. Administered orally, 25 mg/day, until pregnancy occurs (some practitioners do not administer it during luteal phase because of possible teratogenic effects).	Nausea, diarrhea, dizziness, headache, fatigue

Nursing Intervention for Psychological Responses to Infertility

Nurses should be sensitive to the effects of infertility on the couple desiring children. They can help to lessen the emotional impact of the problem by understanding some of the anxieties these couples face, such as:

- Feeling of being "out of control," which adds to the couple's difficulties in resolving their feelings about their infertility
- Cultural beliefs that childbirth is expected and childlessness is pitied
- Feeling that the infertile person is inadequate or is being punished for previous wrongdoing
- Profound effects on self-image, sexuality, and sexual relationships
- Stress from the many procedures necessary for the workup; the need to engage in sexual intercourse "on schedule"; the repeated cycle of raised hopes followed by disappointment

The infertile couple may display the following sequence of response:

1. Disbelief and denial
2. Anger
3. Optimism
4. Desperation
5. Depression
6. Acceptance

NOTES

3
Family Planning

The currently available methods of contraception, their methods of action, effectiveness, and contraindications are discussed in this chapter. Also included is information on permanent contraception and elective abortion.

Overall Objectives in Family Planning

- To avoid unwanted pregnancies
- To regulate intervals between pregnancies
- To decide the number of children in the family
- To control the time at which births occur in relation to the parents' ages
- To facilitate wanted births for women with fertility problems
- To avoid pregnancy in women with serious disease who would be placed at additional risk by pregnancy
- To provide women who are carriers of genetic disease with the option of avoiding pregnancy

---

The overall goal of family planning is to improve the health of the mother, baby, and family. Child spacing, limitation of family size, and timing of the first birth are recognized preventive health measures.

In addition to the overall objectives of family planning, there are nursing objectives for this specialty.

Nursing Objectives in Family Planning

- To be sensitive to the woman's/couple's need for birth control
- To remain objective in discussing birth control methods, including sterilization and abortion

- To orient the woman to all birth control methods
- To present comprehensive information on the woman's chosen birth control method
- To enable the woman to make an informed decision
- To encourage the woman to seek help when questions or problems arise
- To be available for consultation when the woman seeks advice or for help when problems occur

---

Possible Nursing Diagnoses in Family Planning

- Alterations in effective family planning related to lack of knowledge about reproductive functions, inability to use a specific birth control method, belief that pregnancy will not occur (especially teenagers), correct use of contraceptive method with pregnancy occurring, dislike of chosen contraceptive method
- Noncompliance related to lack of knowledge

METHODS OF CONTRACEPTION

Although there is no perfect method of contraception, all sexually active, fertile couples must use some form of birth control or expect to become pregnant within 6 months to 1 year.

Current Methods Available for Contraception

Hormonal methods
IUDs (Progestasert only)
Mechanical barriers: diaphragm, condom, cervical sponge, cervical cap
Chemical barriers: foam, creams, jellies
Natural family planning
Surgical sterilization: male and female
Abortion for unwanted pregnancy

Contraceptive Risk

The hazards of contraception are meaningful only when compared with the alternative risk of uncontrolled fertility. All common methods of contraception present fewer risks than pregnancy and childbirth. An exception is the use of the pill by women over 35 years of age who smoke.

Assessment

Patient History

- Menstrual history
  - Regular or irregular patterns
  - Amount of blood loss
  - Discomfort during or between periods
- Reproductive history
  - Past pregnancies, abortions, and complications of pregnancy and delivery
  - Past use of contraception, including method, length, satisfaction, side effects, and reasons for discontinuation
  - History of gynecological surgery
- Sexual history
  - Record of sexually transmitted diseases, vaginal or pelvic infections, coital history, and attitude toward sex
  - Frequency of sexual intercourse, number of partners
  - Personal hygiene
  - Woman's comfort in touching her own body and discussing her sexuality
- Health history
  - Illnesses, disorders, allergies
- Family history
- Social history
  - Daily activities, coping patterns, family life
  - Aspirations for the future
  - Reliability and judgment
- Nutritional history
- Review of systems

Physical Examination

- Identify conditions that would contraindicate particular contraceptives
- Baseline data for later re-evaluation: blood pressure, weight and height; eye examination and examination of head and neck; breast examination; abdominal examination; pelvic examination; examination of extremities
- Speculum examination
- Bimanual examination

Laboratory data

Baseline laboratory studies should include urinalysis, complete blood cell count (CBC), Pap smear, gonorrhea culture, VDRL test, pregnancy test, and a wet mount where vaginal infection is suspected. Blood clotting studies may also be ordered when appropriate.

Oral Contraception

The combination oral contraceptive pill contains both estrogen and progesterone in various amounts depending on the manufacturer. The pill's mode of action is its effect on the hypothalamus, which effectively suppresses ovarian function to prevent ovulation. Estrogen suppresses ovulation, ovum transport, and maintenance of the corpus luteum. Progestin influences ovulation, cervical mucus, capacitation, ovum transport, and implantation.

Noncontraceptive Health Benefits of Oral Contraceptives

See Table 3-1.

Factors in Pill Selection

Age

- Women under 30 years of age who have no contraindications are good candidates for pill use.
- Women over 35 years of age who smoke should not use oral contraceptives, regardless of health status.

Pill Type

- Pills containing 35 μg or less of estrogen should be used initially.
- Adjustment of pill type can be made if minor side-effects become a problem.

Motivation

- For healthy women who desire the most effective contraceptive method, the pill is a good choice.
- Women with relative or possible contraindications who insist on pill use should be referred to a physician.
- Women must remember to take a pill daily.
- Ambivalence about pill use may be caused by cultural or religious beliefs.
- Women who prefer spontaneous sexual activity would probably be more interested in the pill than in other methods of contraception.

Resources

- Resources should be readily available for follow-up appointments and care if problems should arise.
- The expense of this method may preclude its use by women with inadequate finances.

Table 3-1 Noncontraceptive Health Benefits of Oral Contraceptives

Benefit	Cause
• Decreased iron deficiency anemia: 50% less than in nonusers of oral contraceptives • Decreased menstrual flow: Decreased menorrhagia Decreased intramenstrual bleeding	• Decreased endometrial proliferation during each menstrual cycle, resulting in increased iron stores
• Less pelvic inflammatory disease	• Decreased menstrual bleeding to act as culture medium • Less dilation of cervical canal during menstruation • Hostile cervical mucus, which deters pathogens from entering uterus • Weaker uterine contractions, which decrease spread of infection
• Reduced incidence of benign breast disease Incidence decreases with longevity of use Incidence decreases when progestin dose increases and estrogen dose stays the same	• Protection provided by progestin component; mechanism unknown
• Decreased incidence of benign ovarian cysts	• Suppression of cyclical ovarian activity
• Protection from ectopic pregnancy	• Decreased incidence of pelvic inflammatory disease, which would lead to blockage of fallopian tubes • Prevention of ovulation
• Decreased incidence of rheumatoid arthritis	• Cause unknown
• Decreased risk of endometrial cancer	• Regular endometrial sloughing, caused by progestin contained in combined oral conceptive pills

Table 3-1 Noncontraceptive Health Benefits of Oral Contraceptives (*continued*)

Benefit	Cause
In addition, oral contraceptive use: • Decreases menstrual cramps • Decreases length of menstrual period • Regulates menstrual periods • Eliminates mittelschmerz • Diminishes fear of pregnancy • Can be helpful in the treatment of acne, ovarian cysts, endometriosis • May increase sexual enjoyment • Decreases premenstrual tension	

Side-Effects of Oral Contraception Due to Hormonal Imblance

See Table 3-2

Contraindications to Oral Contraceptive Use

Absolute Contraindications

- Thrombophlebitis, thromboembolic disorders, cerebral vascular disease, coronary occlusion; a history of these conditions; or conditions predisposing to these problems
- Markedly impaired liver function
- Known or suspected carcinoma of the breast
- Known or suspected estrogen-dependent neoplasia, especially carcinoma of the endometrium
- Undiagnosed abnormal genital bleeding
- Known or suspected pregnancy
- Obstructive jaundice in pregnancy (although not all patients with this history will develop jaundice on the pill)
- Congenital hyperlipidemia (because estrogen increases the risk of cardiovascular death in these patients)
- Obesity in women who smoke and are over 35 years old

Relative Contraindications

These require clinical judgment and informed consent:

- Migraine headaches
- Hypertension with resting diastolic blood pressure of 90 or greater, or a resting systolic blood pressure of 140 or greater on three or more visits, or an accurate measurement of 110 diastolic or more on a single visit
- Uterine leiomyoma (This condition does not seem to be a problem with the new low-dose formulations.)
- Elective surgery (The pill should be discontinued, if possible, 1 month prior to elective surgery to avoid an increased risk for postoperative thrombosis.)
- Epilepsy (The pill may increase the frequency of seizures.)
- Sickle cell disease or sickle C disease (but not sickle cell trait)
- Smoking in women over age 35
- Undiagnosed, abnormal vaginal bleeding
- Diabetes mellitus
- Long leg casts or major injury to lower leg
- Age: 45 years of age or older or 40 years or older if there is a second risk factor for the development of cardiovascular disease*

* This contraindication to combined birth control pills *may not* be a contraindication to progestin-only pills or may be *less* of a contraindication to them.

(*text continues on pg. 63*)

Table 3-2 Side Effects of Oral Contraception Due to Hormonal Imbalance

Estrogen Excess	Estrogen Deficiency	Progestin Excess	Progestin Deficiency	Androgen Excess
Skin Changes				
Choasma Hyperpigmentation Telangiectasia	Insignificant	Oily scalp Acne Hair loss	Insignificant	Acne Oily skin Hirsutism Pruritus
GI Changes				
Nausea	Insignificant	Increased appetite Decreased carbohydrate intolerance	Insignificant	Increased appetite
Weight Changes				
Cyclic weight gain Increased fat decomposition Edema	Insignificant	Noncyclic weight gain	Weight loss	Weight gain

Vascular Changes				
Headache Edema Leg cramps	Hot flushes	Headache between pill cycles Dilated leg veins Pelvic congestion	Insignificant	Insignificant
Psychological Effects				
Irritability	Irritability Nervousness Depression	Depression Fatigue Libido changes	Insignificant	Insignificant
Reproductive Tract Changes				
Menstruation				
Uterine cramps Heavy, frequent menses	Early and midcycle spotting Decreased menstrual flow No withdrawal bleeding	Shorter menstrual period	Late breakthrough bleeding and spotting Heavy menses with clotting Delayed onset of menses Dysmenorrhea	Insignificant
Uterus				
Growth of leiomyomas (fibroids) Cervical ectopy Leukorrhea	Pelvic relaxation Uterine prolapse	Insignificant	Insignificant	Insignificant

Table 3-2 Side Effects of Oral Contraception Due to Hormonal Imbalance (*continued*)

Estrogen Excess	Estrogen Deficiency	Progestin Excess	Progestin Deficiency	Androgen Excess
Vagina				
Insignificant	Dryness of mucosa Atrophic vaginitis Dyspareunia	*Candida* infection (yeast)	Insignificant	Insignificant
Breasts				
Suppression of lactation Cystic changes Tenderness Increased size (ductal and tissue), fluid retention	Diminished size	Increased size (alveolar tissue) Tenderness	Insignificant	Insignificant

- Heavy smoking (15 or more cigarettes a day) in women 30 years of age or older*
- Impaired liver function within the past year

Possible Contraindications
- Completion of term pregnancy within the past 14 to 20 days*
- Weight gain of 10 pounds or more while on the pill*
- Irregular menstrual cycles
- Profile suggestive of ovulation and infertility problems: late onset of menses or very irregular, painless menses
- Cardiac or renal disease (or history thereof)*
- Conditions likely to make patient unreliable in following instructions for pill use (mental retardation, major psychiatric problems, alcoholism or other drug abuse, pattern of taking oral medication incorrectly)
- Gallbladder disease or recent cholecystectomy
- Lactation*

Conditions Requiring Careful Observation
Pill use may be initiated by patients with the following problems with careful observation:

- Depression*
- Hypertension with resting diastolic blood pressure of 90 to 99 at a single visit*
- Chloasma or hair loss related to pregnancy (or history thereof)*
- Asthma*
- Epilepsy*
- Uterine leiomyomas*
- Acne
- Varicose veins*
- History of hepatitis, provided that liver function tests have been normal for at least 1 year

Effects of Oral Contraceptives on Nutrient Needs

See Table 3-3.

Danger Signals to Pill Users

Women using oral contraceptives who experience the following symptoms should be told to contact their physician or clinic immediately:

- Severe abdominal pain may indicate gallbladder disease, blood clot, hepatic adenoma, or pancreatitis.

* This contraindication to combined birth control pills *may not* be a contraindication to progestin-only pills or may be *less* of a contraindication to them.

(*text continues on pg. 66*)

Table 3-3 Effect of Oral Contraceptive Agents on Nutrient Needs

Nutrient	Need	Effect of Oral Contraceptive Agent	Dietary Sources
Vitamin B_6	Increased	Increased metabolism of the amino acid tryptophan; vitamin B_6 is required as a co-factor for several enzymatic reactions in the metabolic pathway for tryptophan.	Liver, meats, cabbage, banana, eggs, corn, whole wheat, fish, rolled oats, broccoli, brussel sprouts, sweet potatoes
Vitamin B_{12}	Increased	Possible enhanced tissue affinity for B_{12} resulting in a reduced serum concentration.	Animal protein foods including: beef, pork, lamb, liver, kidney, tuna, salmon, cheese, eggs, milk, yogurt, chicken
Riboflavin (vitamin B_2)	Increased	Possible interference with the metabolism of riboflavin.	Milk, cheese, eggs, meats, dark green leafy vegetables, lettuce, green peas, whole wheat, oats, rice
Folacin (folate, folic acid)	Increased	Possible increased plasma clearance and urinary excretion of folate.	Dark green leafy vegetables, lettuce, lima beans, cauliflower, liver, meats, eggs, nuts
Vitamin C (ascorbic acid)	Increased	Possible increase in the rate of vitamin C destruction.	Oranges, grapefruit, tomatoes, raw cabbage, dark green leafy vegetables, strawberries, green pepper.

Zinc	Increased	Reduced circulating zinc levels.	Wheat germ, beef, pork, lamb, liver, kidney, yellow cheeses, peanut butter, nuts
Iron	Decreased	Increased serum iron levels and iron-binding capacity and diminution of menstrual blood loss.	
Copper	Decreased	Increased serum copper and ceruloplasmin and no changes in urinary copper excretion.	

Adapted from Kerwin D: Effect of oral contraceptive agents on nutrient needs. In Hinton SN, Derwin DR (eds): Maternal Infant & Child Nutrition, Chapel Hill, Health Sciences Consortium, 1983.

- Severe chest pain or shortness of breath may indicate pulmonary embolism or myocardial infarction.
- Severe headache may indicate stroke, hypertension, or migraine headache.
- Eye problems—blurred vision, flashing lights, or blindness—may indicate stroke, hypertension, or other vascular problems.
- Severe pain in the calf or thigh may indicate a blood clot in the leg.

Self-Care Teaching: Oral Contraceptive Use

- Begin the first pack of pills in one of the following three ways:
  —Take the first pill from the pack on the first day of menstrual bleeding (day 1 of the cycle).
  —Start the first pack on the Sunday following your period, whether you are bleeding or not. This method ensures that you will have no menstrual periods on weekends.
  —Start the first pack of pills on the fifth day of your menstrual period.
- Use a back-up method of birth control, such as foam and condoms or a diaphragm, each time you have sex during the first month of pill-taking.
- Take the pill at approximately the same time each day to maintain the blood hormone level. Associate taking the pill with some routine activity, such as brushing teeth, getting ready for bed, or eating breakfast.
- If you miss a pill, take it as soon as you remember.
- If you miss a pill and don't remember until the next day, take two pills (yesterday's and today's). If this happens, use a back-up method of contraception until the pack of pills is finished.
- If you miss two pills in a row, take two pills as soon as you remember and two the next day. *Be sure* to use your back-up method of birth control until the pack of pills is finished.
- If you miss three pills, it is possible to ovulate and get pregnant. Begin to use a second method of birth control immediately and throw away the pills that are left in the pack. Begin a new pack on the Sunday after you missed three or more pills, even if you are bleeding. Continue to use your back-up method of birth control until you are two weeks into the new pack. If pills are frequently forgotten, especially for several days, it might be best to consider another birth control method.

  When a menstrual period is missed and the pills have been taken correctly, it is unlikely that pregnancy has occurred, and a new package of pills can be started at the regular time. Periods may occasionally be missed when you are using oral contraception. If you are concerned, call your health care provider for advice.

- If you have missed one or more pills and no menstrual cycle begins, stop taking the pill. Begin using another birth control method and obtain a pregnancy test.
- If you miss two periods after taking the pills correctly, a pregnancy test should be done.
- If pregnancy occurs while taking birth control pills, there is a slight risk of having an infant with birth defects. A few providers may recommend abortion, although many would not.
- Use of the pill may initially cause minor side effects, such as nausea, headache, breakthrough bleeding, breast tenderness, or bloating. These symptoms result from the hormones contained in the pill and usually disappear in 1 to 3 months. If they persist, a change of pill may be needed.
- If an illness causes several days of vomiting and diarrhea, use a back-up method of birth control until the next menstrual period.
- If you experience light bleeding (spotting) during two or more cycles, you may need a change of pill. Call your health care provider.
- If pregnancy is desired, the pill should be stopped. It is best to have several months of spontaneous menstrual cycles before becoming pregnant. This will ensure return of normal menses before pregnancy begins. An alternative method of birth control should be used during these 3 months.
- Never borrow pills or share yours with anyone. Women who have not been examined and taught pill use and danger signals may have contraindications to pill use unknown to the lender.
- If you are admitted to a hospital or see a physician for any reason, inform your health care providers that you are using oral contraceptives.
- Many physicians suggest to women taking birth control pills that they need a "rest period" from pill use. This practice has resulted in many unwanted pregnancies, and there is no evidence that this practice will decrease side effects or complications.
- If you smoke more than 15 cigarettes a day, be aware of the danger signals that accompany smoking and pill use.
- Concurrent use with other medications may reduce the effectiveness of the pill or the other drugs. Such drugs include anticonvulsives, phenobarbital, rifampin, antibiotics, antacids, sedatives, hypnotics, phenothiazines, tranquilizers, insulin or oral hypoglycemics, corticosteroids, and antihistamines.
- If *Candida* (yeast) vaginitis is a chronic problem, a pill with high progestin content may increase its incidence.

The Mini–Pill

The mini–pill, which contains only a progestin, was developed for women who experience extreme estrogen-related side-effects and in whom estrogen is contraindicated. Pregnancy rates for women using these pills are two to three times greater than the rates for the combination pill.

Advantages

- Can be used by women who have developed estrogen-related side-effects on the combination pill, such as chloasma, breast tenderness, nausea, and vomiting
- Is safer for women in whom estrogen is contraindicated, such as those with obesity, hypertension, or endocrine disorders or those with a history of thromboembolic or liver disease
- Can be used by women in the 35 to 40 age group who want oral contraception
- Decreases symptoms of dysmenorrhea
- May be used by postpartum lactating women. (The quantity of milk is not reduced, as it is with estrogen use, but the effect on the milk is unknown.)
- Are taken daily and therefore are less likely to be forgotten
- May reduce the risk of pelvic infection

Disadvantages

- Are less effective than the combination pill
- Produce side-effects (primarily alterations in the bleeding pattern, such as breakthrough bleeding, heavy irregular bleeding, and amenorrhea)
- Require use of a back-up method of contraception for the first 3 months
- Are associated with an increased incidence of monilia (yeast) vaginitis

Contraindications

- All the absolute contraindications for the combination pill
- Undiagnosed abnormal genital bleeding
- Irregular menstruation
- History of ectopic pregnancy
- History of reproductive cancer

Self-Care Teaching: Mini-Pill Use

- Begin taking the mini-pill on the first day of the next menstrual period.
- Take one pill a day continuously; never miss a pill or take a break from pill-taking.

- Take the pill at the same time each day to maintain hormonal level and prevent spotting.
- Be sure to use a second method of birth control for at least the first 3 months of pill-taking, and during midcycle after that.
- If a pill is missed, take it as soon as you remember, and take the next pill at the usual time. Use your back-up method of contraception until the next period.
- If two pills are missed, take one of the missed pills as well as the pill for that day as soon as you remember. Take the second missed pill the next day along with the regular pill for that day. Use a back-up method of contraception until the next period.
- If you have not had a period for 45 days, even though you have not missed a pill, get a pregnancy test.
- Menstrual cycles may change in length and amount of bleeding; spotting may occur; and missed cycles (without pregnancy) may be experienced.
- If severe abdominal pain occurs while you are on the pill, see your clinician immediately. Users of the mini-pill are at higher risk for ectopic pregnancy if a pregnancy should occur.
- Remember, it is important to perform breast self-examination monthly.
- Return for a check-up before the third package of pills is finished. At this time you will be given a 1-year supply, and yearly check-ups will be adequate. Return for care immediately if you experience any of the danger signals or feel that you are having problems with the pill.

Postpartum Use of Oral Contracepton

- Breastfeeding provides little contraceptive effect and should not be depended upon as a reliable method of controlling pregnancy.
- Breastfeeding women should not use oral contraceptives, especially those containing estrogen. The effect of these steroids on the infant is unknown.
- An alternative way to avoid pregnancy during this time is the use of foam and condoms.
- Women who are not breastfeeding should avoid pill use for 1 month after delivery. During this time the risk for thromboembolic disease is very high and estorgen ingestion is contraindicated.
- Following abortion it is safe to begin oral contraception immediately.

Intrauterine Device (IUD): Progestasert

The Progestasert is the only IUD that remains available in the United States (Fig. 3-1).

It is made of ethyl vinyl acetate in a "T" shape.

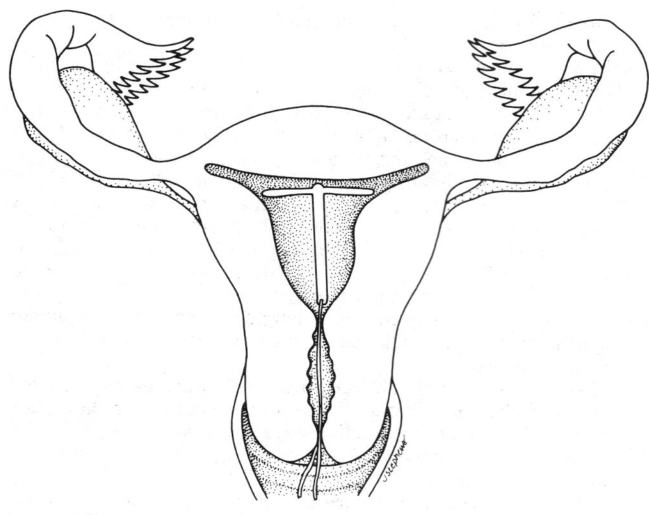

Progestasert

Figure 3-1 The Progestasert. The illustration shows placement within the uterus with the strings extending from the cervical os. (Childbirth Graphics)

It contains 38 mg of progesterone in a silicon oil base that releases the hormone at the rate of 65 μg/d.

Advantages

- Reduced blood loss during menses
- Lower incidence of anemia
- Decreased blood loss in women who experience heavy menses

Disadantages

- Increased number of days of nonmenstrual bleeding and spotting
- The need for yearly replacement.

Danger Signals in IUD Users

- Missed or late menstrual period
- Abdominal or pelvic pain
- Fever, chills
- Heavy bleeding, clots, spotting, heavy periods

- Strings absent or hard object felt in cervix
- Heavy, foul, or unusual vaginal discharge

Barrier Methods of Contraception

- Diaphragm
- Cervical cap
- Vaginal contraceptive sponge
- Vaginal spermicides: foam, creams, jellies, suppositories
- Condom

Users and Nonusers of Barrier Method Contraception

Women most inclined to use barrier methods are those who:

- Are postpartum or lactating
- Have infrequent intercourse
- Forget to take pills
- Are awaiting sterilization
- Are unable to get medical care
- Have many sexual partners, increasing their risk of sexually transmitted disease
- Want to increase IUD effectiveness
- Want an interim method before attempting pregnancy
- Have male partners with recent vasectomies
- Are over age 35
- Are premenopausal

Women who dislike barrier methods are those who:

- Want more effective contraception
- Do not want to insert a device just prior to intercourse
- Find them greasy or messy or dislike the sensation of burning or itching experienced with some products
- Do not want to wait for or interrupt intercourse
- Have a male partner who does not like the method
- Need a contraceptive that can be used without the partner's knowledge
- Are uncomfortable about touching themselves or inserting devices or spermicidal preparations into the vagina

Diaphragm

Advantages
- No interference with breastfeeding
- Ability to insert the device 2 to 6 hours prior to intercourse
- Avoidance of daily pill taking

- No interference in the metabolic and physiologic processes of the body
- The noncontraceptive benefits of diaphragm use include some protection against both sexually transmitted disease and the development of cervical dysplasia.

Side Effects and Complications

Few serious or life-threatening side-effects or complications arise from diaphragm use. Side-effects that might occur include:

- Itching, burning, or swelling of the vaginal tissue as a result of allergy to latex, rubber, or spermicidal jelly or cream
- Bladder irritation from a poorly fitted diaphragm. When too large a diaphragm is worn for a number of hours, its rim can exert substantial pressure on the bladder or urethra, causing discomfort and, possibly, recurrent infection. It can also cause erosion and tenderness of the vaginal wall.
- Interference with bowel movements or size of stool and hemorrhoids may occur when posterior pressure is exerted on the descending colon through the vaginal wall by a too large diaphragm
- Pain from unhealed vaginal tissue or episiotomy when a diaphragm is fitted too soon after a full-term delivery
- Toxic shock syndrome, which has been reported as occurring after diaphragm use. Its signs are temperature elevation of 101°F or more, diarrhea, vomiting, muscle aches, and a sunburnlike rash.

Contraindications

- Allergies to rubber or spermicide
- History of recurrent urinary tract infection
- Genital tract abnormalities resulting from weak musculature, such as uterine prolapse, cystocele, rectocele, and decreased vaginal tone, most of which occur in multiparous women. (Some women with these problems can use an arching spring diaphragm.)
- Fixed retroflexed or retroverted uterus
- Lack of time or trained personnel to fit the diaphragm and instruct the patient in its use
- Past history of toxic shock syndrome
- Inability of the woman to learn to insert and remove the diaphragm
- Lack of facilities and privacy for insertion, hygiene, or storage
- Tight vaginal musculature that impedes diaphragm insertion
- A notch behind the pubic bone too shallow to support the diaphragm rim

Cervical Cap

- Available only to women enrolled in FDA projects researching its safety and effectiveness.
- A soft, thimble-shaped rubber device that fits tightly over the cervix and blocks the passage of sperm (Fig. 3-2). It is deeper and smaller in diameter than the diaphragm and is held in place by suction.
- The cap must be half-filled with spermicidal jelly to improve its effectiveness.
- The cervical cap must be fitted by specially trained personnel.
- Placement and removal of the cervical cap may be more difficult than placement and removal of the diaphragm.
- Its effectiveness is thought to be about that of the diaphragm.

Contraindications

- Lack of trained personnel to fit and teach its use
- Allergy to rubber or spermicide
- Anatomic abnormalities of the cervix or vagina
- Inability of the woman to learn the technique of insertion
- Cervical or vaginal infections
- Delivery of a full-term infant within the previous 6 weeks
- Abnormal Pap smear
- History of toxic shock syndrome

Side-Effects and Complications

- Discomfort caused by the device to either partner
- Vaginal lacerations or abrasions

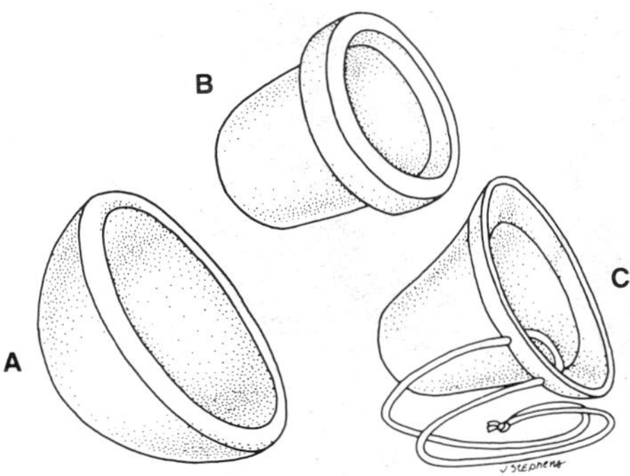

Figure 3-2 Three types of cervical caps. (A) Vimule cap; (B) Prentif cavity rim cervical cap; (C) Dumas cap. (Childbirth Graphics)

Vaginal Contraceptive Sponge

Natural collagen and synthetic sponges incorporating spermicide were approved by the Food and Drug Administration (FDA) in 1983 for use in the United States. The Today Vaginal Contraceptive Sponge is available in one size only and may be purchased over the counter without prescription. The sponge is small, pillow-shaped, and made of polyurethane that contains 1 g of spermicide. In addition to its spermicidal properties, the sponge acts as a cervical barrier and traps sperm within it. On one side the sponge has a concave depression into which the cervix fits; on the reverse, a loop is attached to expedite its removal (Fig. 3-3).

The sponge provides protection for 24 hours. Prior to insertion it is moistened with water. Repeated intercourse may occur during

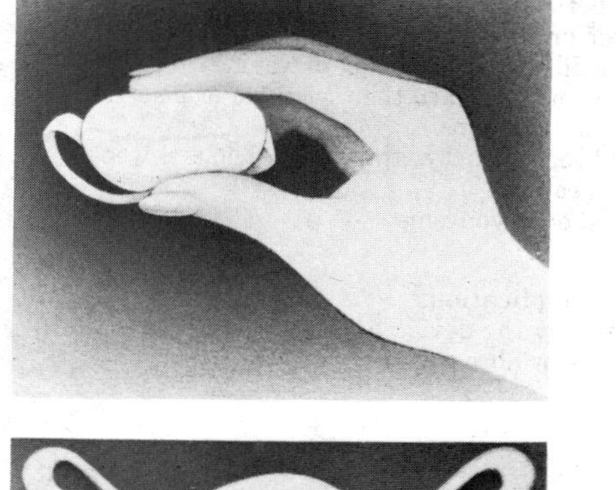

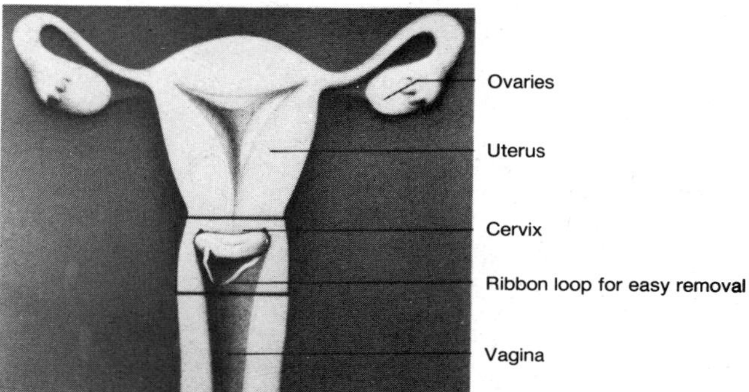

Figure 3-3 The contraceptive sponge is inserted into the deepest part of the vagina, just below the cervix. (Courtesy of *Today*)

this period without further precautions. After 24 hours the sponge is removed and discarded.

Its effectiveness is thought to be similar to but probably lower than that of the diaphragm.

Contraindications

- Allergy to spermicide or polyurethane
- Abnormalities of pelvic structures that would interfere with its placement, retention, or removal
- Inability of the woman to insert or remove the device
- Inability to remember to use the sponge
- History of toxic shock syndrome
- Vaginal colonization of *Staphylococcus aureus*

Side-Effects and Complications

- Redness, irritation, and itching of the vulva resulting from allergy to spermicide
- Tearing of the device during insertion, removal, or intercourse
- Dryness of the vagina resulting from absorption of vaginal secretions by the sponge

Vaginal Spermicides

These preparations all contain an inert vehicle that works in two ways: (1) by physically blocking the passage of sperm into the cervix, and (2) by releasing spermicides, which kill the sperm. They are being viewed more favorably as a contraceptive method in part because of their safety and their availability without a prescription. Their effectiveness has been estimated at 80% to 95%, depending on the consistency of their use and their placement deep within the vagina.

Contraceptive Foam

Sold in drugstores without a prescription, spermicidal foam, when used as directed, blocks the entrance of sperm into the cervix and kills sperm through the action of its spermicide. It is an interim or back-up method in conjunction with a condom and is a protective measure against sexually transmitted disease.

Self-Care Teaching: Foam Use

- The foam must be used every time you have sex.
- Read the instructions on the can of foam.
- The foam may be inserted 30 minutes before intercourse, but it will be more effective if used just before it. If after 30 minutes intercourse has not occurred, insert another applicator of foam.

- Shake the can of foam vigorously to ensure complete mixing and foaming action before use.
- Place the applicator on the can and fill it by applying pressure to the top of the can. Use one or two applicators as indicated on the label.
- Lie on your back with your knees bent and spread apart. With your fingers, spread the lips of the vagina and carefully insert the applicator into the vagina as far back as possible.
- Push the plunger to insert the foam and then remove the applicator from the vagina. Repeat this process if two applications are specified. Wash the applicator with soap and water.
- If douching is desired wait at least 8 hours after the last intercourse for optimum spermicidal effect.
- To avoid running out of foam, have a spare can available.

Spermicidal Creams, Jellies, and Suppositories
These products are less than adequate for reliable contraception. They may be purchased over the counter, and their labels should be read carefully to avoid confusion between spermicidal and hygienic products. The use of foam is recommended over these products, since its effectiveness rates are generally higher.

Condom

The major form of male barrier contraceptive is the condom (rubber). The condom ranks second only to the pill in popularity as a contraceptive method in the United States.

The majority of condoms are made of latex or processed collagenous sheaths. The latter are superior in preserving sensitivity and are reusable. A variety of condoms are now on the market. Newer types are thinner and may be prelubricated. They are also available in bright colors, and some have erotic ribbings. The FDA has stringent standards of quality for condom manufacture. Condom effectiveness is reported to be between 97% and 98%. If used in conjunction with a vaginal barrier method, the combined effectiveness approaches that of the pill.

Noncontraceptive Benefits
- Prevention of vaginal infections, the spreading of sexually transmitted disease and, possibly, pelvic inflammatory disease
- An increase in comfort and sexual satisfaction with lubricated condoms
- Inclusion of the condom in the sexual foreplay when the woman positions it on the male
- Reduction of antibody titers in couples where the woman is producing antibodies against her partner's sperm

---

Self-Care Teaching: Condom Use

- Use the condom each time you have sex.
- Carry a condom for "emergency" situations.
- Handle the condom carefully to avoid tearing.
- Apply the condom to the erect penis (either partner may do this) before the penis penetrates the vagina.
- Unroll the condom to its full length over the penis, leaving a half-inch empty space at the bottom, or purchase condoms with nipple tips.
- Use a lubricant, such as contraceptive cream, when the vagina is dry to prevent friction, pain, or the tearing of the condom.
- When withdrawing the penis, hold the rim of the condom to avoid spilling sperm in or near the vagina.
- Withdraw the penis before erection is lost to prevent the condom from slipping off in the vagina.
- Store condoms in a cool, dry place.

Permanent Contraception: Surgical Sterilization

Sterilization is a permanent method of contraception available to both men and women, who may choose it for any of the following reasons:

- Dissatisfaction with reversible contraceptive methods
- Family has been completed
- Need for 10 to 20 years of pregnancy protection

Informed Consent

Prior to a sterilization procedure, the man or woman must be fully informed regarding:

- The irreversible nature of the procedure
- Performance of the procedure
- Minor or major risks and possible side-effects
- Alternative birth control methods
- Possible positive benefits
- Their right to ask questions and to change their mind
- Signing of a medical permission document and the informed consent form.

Female Sterilization

Tubal ligation blocks the fallopian tubes and prevents the migration of the ovum into the uterus. A variety of methods are used, including ligation, coagulation, and the application of clips, rings, or bands. All of these are accomplished by entering the pelvis through the abdominal wall or the posterior vaginal cul–de–sac.

Abdominal Tubal Ligations
Mini-laparotomy: Mini-laparotomy can be done under local anesthesia through an abdominal incision. The procedure takes up to 20 minutes and can be performed postpartally. Recovery is swift, and the woman is discharged within a few hours.

Laparoscopic Tubal Ligation: Under general anesthesia a laparoscope is inserted into the pelvis to allow visualization of the organs. The tubes are either occuled by cautery, ligated, or clamped with bands or clips. Patient recovery is rapid, and there is a low rate of complications.

Vaginal Tubal Ligations
Colpotomy: Colpotomy is performed as an inpatient or outpatient procedure on women of high parity. Using general or local anesthesia, the surgeon makes an incision through the posterior fornix to provide access to the fallopian tubes for cautery. The procedure takes about one-half hour.

Culdoscopy: Access to the fallopian tubes through the posterior cul–de–sac occurs by means of an endoscope. Culdoscopy and colpotomy have generally been replaced by the mini-laparotomy, which is safer and more reliable.

Male Sterilization: Vasectomy

Bilateral partial vasectomy is an uncomplicated operative procedure and is the simplest and safest method of surgical sterilization. Vasectomy produces sterility by interrupting the vas deferens and preventing sperm from being ejaculated in the semen.

Local anesthesia is used, and the procedure takes less than 30 minutes in a physician's office or clinic. The patient must be informed that he will not become immediately sterile, since the vas contains sperm for 1 to 3 months. Pregnancy can occur during this time, so a contraceptive method must be used. After 3 months a semen specimen is examined. If it is free of sperm, sterilization is complete.

Reversibility depends to a large extent on the type of procedure performed. Only 18% to 60% of reanastomoses are successful.

NATURAL FAMILY PLANNING

Increasing numbers of couples are turning to less intrusive and more personal methods of contraception known collectively as natural family planning. This group is motivated, often for religious reasons, to spend time and effort learning to assess and maintain control of their own fertility. All natural family planning methods require regular abstinence from sexual intercourse for a specific number of days. The methods do not depend on regular menstrual cycles but rely on signs and symptoms of fertility.

Currently four techniques are used in natural family planning (referred to as "periodic abstinence" by some):

- Calendar rhythm method
- Temperature, thermal, or basal body temperature method
- Cervical mucus or ovulation method
- Sympto–thermal method

These terms are used to describe specific techniques for identifying or predicting the fertile period.

Learning natural family-planning techniques is a complex and time consuming effort that requires a high degree of self-awareness, dedication, and motivation. These techniques are briefly described in the text *Comprehensive Maternity Nursing* and are beyond the scope of this clinical manual.

ELECTIVE ABORTION (THERAPEUTIC ABORTION)

Common Reasons for Unwanted Pregnancies

- Lack of access to birth control
- Lack of knowledge of where to seek care or fear of doing so
- Failure of the contraceptive method
- Failure to use a back-up method during early use of a new method or after missing pills
- Use of less effective contraceptive methods, such as douching, withdrawal, rhythm method
- Late or no return visits to the health care setting to obtain more pills or have IUD replaced or diaphragm refitted
- Lack of funds to pay for a contraceptive method
- Psychosocial conflicts:
    - Denial that pregnancy can occur (most common among teenagers)
    - Belief that sex must be completely spontaneous

- Ambivalence regarding pregnancy
- Desire for independence (among teenagers)
- Attempt to involve partner in marriage or relationship through pregnancy
- Prior pregnancy that was aborted because of peer or family pressure
- Desire to confirm femininity
- Thrill of risk taking
- Identity conflicts

Methods

Menstrual Extraction (5 to 7 weeks)

Vacuum extraction of the uterine contents 5 to 7 weeks after the last menstrual period is rarely performed. With sophisticated pregnancy testing this procedure has become obsolete, and early vacuum has replaced this procedure.

Early Vacuum Abortion (up to 12 weeks)

Also called suction curettage, early vacuum abortion now accounts for 80% of abortions performed in the United States. It is performed under local or general anesthesia, and the uterine contents are removed by suction after cervical dilation.

Dilation and Evacuation (13 to 24 weeks)

This procedure uses vacuum curettage and curette scraping as in early vacuum abortion. Since the products of conception are larger, greater cervical dilation and use of additional instrumentation are needed. This method is safer for the mother than amniocentesis but is more stressful to the health care staff.

Amniocentesis (15 to 24 weeks)

After 15 weeks gestation amniocentesis is performed by inserting an 18-guage needle through the abdomen into the amniotic sac. Prostaglandin is infused into the sac to initiate uterine contractions. Contractions begin within 12 to 48 hours and end when the fetus is born.

Self-Care Teaching: After Abortion

- Normal activities may be resumed, but avoid strenous work or exercise for a few days.
- Resume normal eating and drinking habits.
- Bleeding and cramping may occur for a week or two. If either becomes severe, seek medical advice. Light bleeding and spotting are normal for about a month.
- Menstruation should resume in 4 to 6 weeks.
- Use a method of birth control if you have sex before menstruation resumes. It is possible to get pregnant during this period.
- Do not use tampons for the first week after the abortion to avoid possible infection. Use sanitary pads instead.
- Refrain from intercourse for 1 week after abortion. You are vulnerable to infection until the uterine lining heals.
- Refrain from douching 1 week to prevent infection.
- Take your temperature twice a day to detect possible infection. If it reaches 100°F or more, seek medical help.
- Keep your follow-up appointment in two weeks. It is important to ensure your full recovery.

NOTES

4
Adaptations of Pregnancy and Fetal Development

PHYSIOLOGIC ADAPTATIONS DURING PREGNANCY

The period from conception to delivery lasts about 40 weeks. During these weeks the mother's body undergoes physiological changes of such magnitude and complexity that many are still not well understood. Many of these changes are orchestrated by the female hormones as well as the hormones active during pregnancy. Body changes are so dramatic that they would be considered pathologic in the nonpregnant woman. These changes are the body's adaptive response to the growing fetus's requirements for nutrients, waste removal, protection from harm, and space in which to grow.

Nursing Objectives in Assessing Adaptations to Pregnancy

- To identify body changes during pregnancy that result from normal physiologic change
- To assess the patient's physical and emotional complaints by history taking and physical examination.
- To be alert to signs or symptoms of possible pathology and to seek consultation
- To identify and be sensitive to patient concerns about family or other problems that may affect her pregnancy
- To follow up on patient outcomes by chart review or discussion with the primary care provider

---

Physiologic/Biologic Adaptations of the Reproductive System

Major physiologic/biologic adaptations of the reproductive system during pregnancy are outlined in Table 4-1 and are illustrated in Figures 4-1 and 4-2.

(*text continues on pg. 88*)

Table 4-1 Physiologic/Biologic Adaptations of the Reproductive System During Pregnancy

Organ/System	Adaptation	Stimulation	Clinical Significance
Uterus	• Growth: Weight increases from 70 g to 900 to 1200 g at term Volume increases from 10 ml to 2 to 10 Liter at term (1000× increase in size) See Figure 4-1.	• Estrogen and progesterone	• Stimulates uterine growth and compliance • Progesterone prepares implantation site and inhibits myometrial contractility • Palpation of uterus —symphysis at 3 months —umbilicus at 5 months —xiphoid process at 9 months • Observation of fetal movement
	• Position: Lifts into the pelvis at 12 weeks; Dextrorotates to the right	• Pressure from rectosigmoid	• Causes pressure on the right ureter • Weight of third trimester uterus on the vena cava and aorta may cause supine hypotensive syndrome.

(continued)

Table 4-1 Physiologic/Biologic Adaptations of the Reproductive System During Pregnancy (*continued*)

Organ/System	Adaptation	Stimulation	Clinical Significance
Uterus	• Maintains longitudinal position in line with the pelvic axis (Figure 4-2) • Anterior support by abdominal wall		• Palpation of fetal growth • Loss of center of gravity as uterus enlarges • Diastasis recti
	• Contractility: Until midpregnancy, uterus less sensitive to contractions Latter half of gestation, uterus more susceptible to contractions	• Oxytocin	• Causes uterine myometrium to contract • Early contractions may cause abortion • May cause risk of preterm birth • Initiates labor at term • Causes ripening, dilatation, and effacement of cervix at term

Braxton Hicks Contractions	• Irregular, sporadic, and nonrhythmic contractions that continue throughout pregnancy	• Estrogen and stretching and distention of myometrium	• Patent feels sensation of painless uterine tightening and pressure • Can be palpated by examiner • May be mistaken for labor in the third trimester
Endometrium	• Proliferation of the uterine lining in preparation for ovum implantation	• Estrogen	• If inadequate, proliferation of the lining does not occur
	• Storage of glycogen to nourish the blastocyst, should pregnancy occur	• Progesterone	• When inadequate, implantation will not occur or early abortion may result
Cervix	• Increased vascularity, edema, softness • Hypertrophy of cervical glands	• Estrogen	• Chadwick's sign, Goodell's sign • Forms a mucous plug that acts as a barrier to protect the fetus from mechanical or bacterial invasion. In early labor, it separates, its blood vessels are severed, and it is expelled as the "bloody show."

(*continued*)

Table 4-1 Physiologic/Biologic Adaptations of the Reproductive System During Pregnancy (*continued*)

Organ/System	Adaptation	Stimulation	Clinical Significance
Ovaries	• Formation of the corpus luteum of pregnancy	• Progesterone	• Secures implantation of the blastocyst and development of the placenta
		• HCG	• By the eighth gestational day begins to provide nutrition and hormones to sustain the corpus luteum for 7 to 10 weeks until the placenta takes over • HCG may remain in postpartum circulation for 3 days
Fallopian Tubes	• Facilitates fertilization of the ovum by the sperm	• Estrogen and progesterone	• Fluid in the oviduct conveys signals that condition events of sperm capacitation and cleavage in the gametes.
	• Controls timing of egg transport into the uterus		• Adequate preparation of the endometrium for egg implantation

Vagina	• Becomes vascularized and congested • Increased secretions that are thick, white, and acidic	• Estrogen	• Proliferation of cells causes walls to become thickened, pliable, and distensible in preparation for passage of the fetal head. • Acidity of the vagina maintained by lactic acid produced by lactobacilli favorable to sperm survival. Acidity controls growth of pathogenic bacteria in the vagina (*p*H 3.5 to 5.0)
Breasts	• Increased size and nodularity, sensitivity • Ductal system growth intense for first 3 months • Later pregnancy, alveolar cells become secretory	• Estrogen and progesterone	• Breasts enlarge; nipple larger, darker, erect; areolae darken; glands of Montgomery enlarge • Preparation for lactation • Production of colostrum • Continued breast enlargement

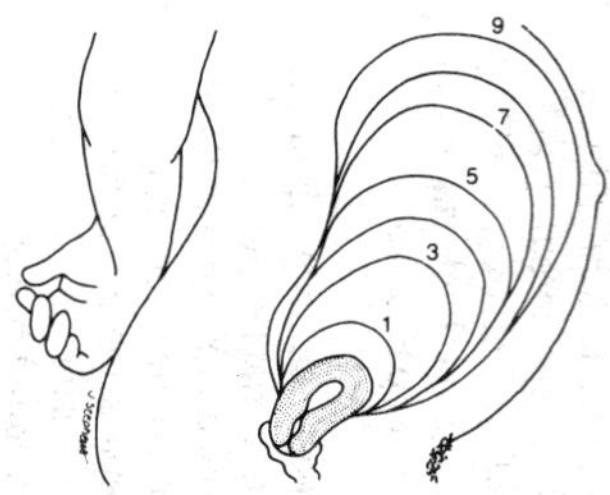

Figure 4-1 Uterine growth during successive months of pregnancy. (Childbirth Graphics)

Physiologic Adaptations of Body Systems

During pregnancy the cardiovascular system exhibits the most profound changes of all the body's systems. The mother's circulatory system has the steadily increasing burden of delivering nutrients to the fetus as well as excreting its wastes. As pregnancy progresses, the work of maintaining the fetus adds to the metabolic burden of the mother's body.

Major physiologic adaptations of body systems are discussed in Table 4-2.

(*text continues on pg. 98*)

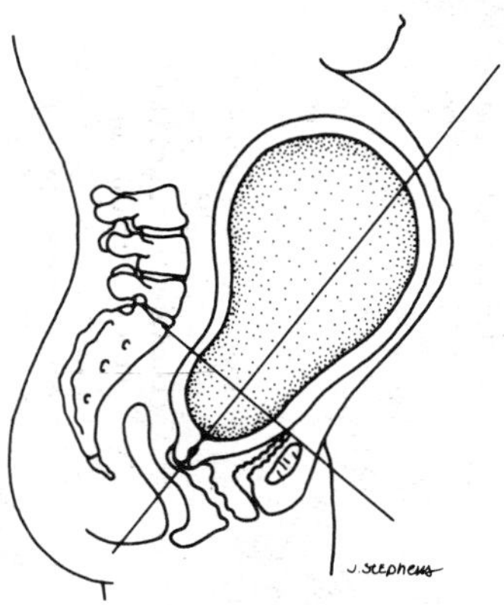

Figure 4-2 Relationship of the axis of the pregnant uterus to the pelvic axis, showing anterior support of the uterus by the abdominal wall. (Childbirth Graphics)

Table 4-2 Physiologic Adaptations of Body Systems During Pregnancy

Physiologic Changes	Clinical Significance
Cardiovascular Changes	
Mechanical Changes	
• Cardiac volume increases by 10% (to 75 ml).	• Size of the heart on x-ray films increases
• Elevation of the diaphragm from pressure of the uterus displaces the heart to the left and upward.	• Changes (murmurs) in cardiac sounds that would be considered abnormal in the nonpregnant state occur: Pulmonic systolic murmurs are common. Apical systolic murmurs are heard in 60% of pregnant women.
• Blood viscosity is lowered and torsion of the great vessels occurs because of the enlarged uterus.	• Exaggerated splitting of first heart sound and loud third sound may be heard. • Diastolic murmurs are abnormal (18% of women have soft, transient murmurs).
Blood Volume Changes	
• Plasma volume increases by by 50% (600 to 1250 ml) peaking at 30 to 40 weeks.	• There is significant hydration of maternal tissues.
• Total plasma albumin decreases from a nonpregnant value of between 4.0 and 4.5 g/dl to pregnant value of between 3.0 and 3.5 g/dl.	• Physiologic anemia from hemodilution occurs. • Vessel walls are more permeable.
Cardiac Output Changes	
• Heart rate increases.	• Pulse increases 10 to 15 beats/minute, reaching maximum in the third trimester. • Kidney filtration increases. • Oxygen transport increases.
• Cardiac output increases. The nonpregnant heart pumps 5.0 to 5.5 liter/	

(continued)

Table 4-2 Physiologic Adaptations of Body Systems During Pregnancy (*continued*)

Physiologic Changes	Clinical Significance
Cardiovascular Changes	
Cardiac Output Changes	
minute. This rate is increased 30% to 50% by the end of the first trimester. It increases a further 10% during the last two trimesters when the patient is in the lateral recumbent position.	
• The distribution of cardiac output changes.	• Maternal–placental circulation in late pregnancy receives blood at a rate of 1,000 ml/minute. This is 10% of cardiac output. • The following factors decrease uterine blood flow: Uterine contractions Hypertonus, hypertension, hypotension Strenous exercise Smoking Pathologic states: anemia, placental problems, infarcts, abruption, preeclampsia • The following factors increase blood flow: Bed rest Lateral recumbent position
• The increase in red cell volume (erythrocytes) is less than one third the increase in plasma volume.	• Packed cell volume (hematocrit) and hemoglobin values fall.
• The production of red cells accelerates.	• The reticulocyte count increases. With a regular diet (no iron supplementation), red cell volume increases 18% to 250 ml. With therapeutic iron supplementation, it increases 30% to 400 to 450 ml.

Table 4-2 Physiologic Adaptations of Body Systems During Pregnancy (*continued*)

Physiologic Changes	Clinical Significance
Cardiovascular changes	
Cardiac Output Changes	
	• Oral supplementation of 60 to 80 mg/day of elemental iron from early pregnancy allows near maximum red cell volume expansion but does not maintain or restore iron stores. Therefore, women with iron stores should receive 30 to 60 mg/day of elemental iron, and those without stores should receive a therapeutic amount of 120 to 240 mg/day.
• Of the red cells added to the maternal circulation, 50% (about 600 ml) are lost during delivery and postpartum.	• A total of 800 mg of iron is needed during pregnancy to meet maternal and fetal demands (200 mg is excreted during pregnancy).
Peripheral Circulatory Changes	
• Total peripheral resistance decreases.	• Venous return to the heart increases.
• Uteroplacental circulation is a low-resistence system that works as an arteriovenous shunt, decreasing total body vascular resistance by bypassing systemic circulation.	
• The uterus presses on pelvic veins and inferior vena cava	• Stagnation of blood in lower extremities may occur.
• Blood flow to the skin increases.	• Dissipation of fetal heat precedes feelings of warmth in the mother • Vascular dilation of nasal mucous membranes may cause nose bleeds. • Increased blood flow to the skin of the hands may cause erythema.

(*continued*)

Table 4-2 Physiologic Adaptations of Body Systems During Pregnancy (*continued*)

Physiologic Changes	Clinical Significance
Cardiovascular Changes	
Blood Pressure Changes	
• Systolic and diastolic pressure is decreased during the first half of pregnancy (5 to 10 mm Hg) and then rises to a nonpregnant level.	• Any rise of 30 mm Hg systolic pressure above the norm is an abnormal finding. • Brachial artery blood pressure varies with the patient's position: Highest: sitting Intermediate: supine Lowest: lateral recumbent
• Compression of the interior vena cava and aorta in third-trimester pregnant women who lie on their backs may cause a decrease in cardiac output. Turn patient to left side.	• Supine hypotensive syndrome may occur. Faintness may result from an 8% to 30% decrease in systolic blood pressure. Bradycardia may ensue, and the cardiac rate may be decreased by 50%. This can cause a decrease in uterine arterial pressure, which may be deleterious to the fetus if it occurs with hemorrhage or conduction anesthesia during delivery.
Respiratory Changes	
Anatomic Changes	
• Changes that improve gaseous exchange occur. The lower ribs flare to increase space long before mechanical pressure occurs. They may not return to original position after delivery. The level of the diaphragm rises 4 cm, and the transverse diameter of the chest increases 2 cm.	• The movement of tidal air (the volume of air with each breath) increases. • More complex expiration is possible.

Table 4-2 Physiologic Adaptations of Body Systems During Pregnancy (*continued*)

Physiologic Changes	Clinical Significance
Respiratory Changes	
Hormonal Influences	
• Estrogen levels increase.	• Estrogen causes decreased pulmonary resistance by increasing the pliability of connective tissue.
• Progesterone levels increase.	• Progesterone causes decreased pulmonary resistance by relaxing smooth muscle. • Minute ventilation increases 37%. • Hyperventilation and respiratory alkalosis may occur.
• Respiratory center in the brain is sensitive to progesterone, which maintains low serum CO_2 levels. Fetal plasma CO_2 level exceeds that of maternal plasma by 4 to 8 mm Hg.	• This permits easy passage of CO_2 from fetal to maternal circulation. • Dyspnea may occur as a consequence of low CO_2 levels. Its immediate cause is not necessarily related to exercise.
• Vocal cords increase in size because of increased circulation due to the influence of progesterone.	• The voice becomes deeper.
Urinary Tract Changes	
Mechanical Changes	
• The uterus enlarges, causing the bladder to be compressed against the pelvis.	• Bladder capacity is reduced, causing more frequent urination.
• The enlarged, dextrorotated uterus compresses the ureters as they pass over the pelvic brim, especially on the right side. (The sigmoid colon cushions the left ureter.)	• Dilation of the ureters and renal pelves occurs. They may contain as much as 200 ml of urine, causing stagnation and increased susceptibility to urinary tract infection (2% of pregnant women suffer from pyelonephritis).

(*continued*)

Table 4-2 Physiologic Adaptations of Body Systems During Pregnancy (*continued*)

Physiologic Changes	Clinical Significance
Urinary Tract Changes	
Mechanical Changes	
• Vesicoureteral reflux may occur.	• This may cause changes in 24-hour urine collections (for HCG or estriol testing).
• Dilation of the ovarian vein complex over the right ureter occurs.	• Blood drainage decreases.
• Base of the bladder is pushed forward and upward from the engaged presenting part of the fetus.	• Increased edema and possible trauma may occur. • The possibility of infection is increased.
Circulatory Changes	
• Renal blood flow increases up to the third trimester.	• Glomerular filtration rate increases 50% (greater in lateral recumbent position and less when standing or sitting). • Renal threshold for glucose is lowered (tubules reach maximum of readsorption); glucose is spilled in the urine.
Hormonal Influences	
• Under the influence of estrogen, total water retention is 6 to 8 liters in late pregnancy, distributed among the mother, fetus, placenta, and amniotic fluid.	• Physiologic edema may occur.
• Progesterone increases kidney size.	• Sodium and electrolyte loss in the urine (natriuresis) may occur.
• Aldosterone secretion from the adrenals and estrogen secretion from the placenta balance progesterone, causing dilation of ureters and	• Readsorption of sodium chloride and water by renal tubules occurs. • Volume of urine for secretion does not increase.

Table 4-2 Physiologic Adaptations of Body Systems During Pregnancy (*continued*)

Physiologic Changes	Clinical Significance
Urinary Tract Changes	
Hormonal Influences	
relaxation of bladder and trigone.	• Urine secretion in late pregnancy decreases; fluid retention increases. • Bladder becomes edematous and easily traumatized.
Postural Effects	
• Posture affects blood and renal function.	• When the patient sits or stands a decrease occurs in: —Renal blood flow and glomerular filtration rate from pooling of blood in pelvis and legs —Urine volume and secretion —Cardiac output, causing compensatory renal vasoconstriction • Water accumulates in the body during the day, causing dependent edema. • When the patient is in the lateral position at night, the effect of gravity is removed, distributing fluid throughout the body with the following effects: Increased kidney filtration, causing nocturia Increased excretion of water and salt
Changes in Nutrient Value of Urine	
• The proportion of nutrients in pregnant urine is high.	• There is increased excretion of folates, glucose, lactose, amino acids, vitamin B_{12} and ascorbic acid. • Higher nutrient content of urine favors rapid growth

(*continued*)

Table 4-2 Physiologic Adaptations of Body Systems During Pregnancy (*continued*)

Physiologic Changes	Clinical Significance
Urinary Tract Changes	
Changes in Nutrient Value of Urine	
	of urinary bacteria with greater risk of urinary tract infection.
Gastrointestinal (GI) Changes	
Mechanical Changes	
• Enlarging uterus puts increasing pressure on the stomach and intestines. • Stomach and intestines are displaced; the appendix is moved upward and laterally. • Venous pressure increases below the enlarged uterus.	• Hiatal hernia from partial rupture of the stomach through the diaphragm may occur. • Constipation and heartburn (pyrosis) are common. • Hemorrhoids and varicosities may occur.
Hormonal Influences	
• Tone and mobility of the GI tract are lowered. Gastric emptying time decreases.	• Reflux esophagitis, constipation, and nausea may occur.
• Water absorption from the colon increases.	• Constipation may occur.
• Cholestasis (suppression of bile flow) may occur.	• Pruritus (generalized itching of the skin) results from increased retention of bile salts. • Jaundice may occur.
• Gastric secretion of hydrochloric acid and pepsin decreases (usually after the first trimester).	• Indigestion may occur. • Peptic ulcers improve because of decreased secretory response to histamines.
• Estrogen affects adhesiveness of fibers in collagenous tissue	• Epulis may occur. Swollen, spongy gums bleed easily; condition regresses spontaneously after delivery.
• Eating disorders of unknown etiology occur.	• Pica, a craving for substances that may or may not be foods, such as clay, laundry starch, soap, toothpaste, plaster, occurs in some women.

Table 4-2 Physiologic Adaptations of Body Systems During Pregnancy (*continued*)

Physiologic Changes	Clinical Significance
Gastrointestinal (GI) Changes	
Hormonal Influences	
• Saliva production increases (etiology unknown).	• Ptyalism is a problem for some women. However, some feel that nauseated women find it difficult to swallow saliva, making it appear excessive.
• Dental caries do not increase during pregnancy.	• Routine dental care is needed during pregnancy.
Metabolic Changes	
• Pregnancy has a profound effect on carbohydrate metabolism. Carbohydrates in the form of glucose are the primary energy source for the brain and fetoplacental unit.	• Fasting plasma glucose levels drop during pregnancy. • Plasma insulin levels show little change until the third trimester, when they rise about 30%.
• Lipid metabolism in pregnancy causes fat stores to accumulate for periods of fetal growth and lactation.	• About 3.5 kg of extra fat is stored by 30 weeks of gestation.
• Protein is used by the fetus for growth.	• Protein is probably not stored during pregnancy. If inadequate protein is ingested, the pregnant woman's muscle mass may be enlisted as a protein reserve.
Musculoskeletal Changes	
Hormonal and Mechanical Influences	
• Joints relax under the influence of relaxin.	• Mobility and pliability of sacroiliac, sacrococcygeal, and public joints increases in preparation for delivery.
• Weight of the enlarging uterus increases.	• Round ligament pain may occur.
• Postural changes occur.	• Center of gravity shifts, and some women experience backache. Leaning back-

(*continued*)

Table 4-2 Physiologic Adaptations of Body Systems During Pregnancy (*continued*)

Physiologic Changes	Clinical Significance
Musculoskeletal Changes	
Hormonal and Mechanical Influences	
	ward to compensate may cause lordosis and back strain. • Spasm of the uterosacral ligaments may occur. • Women may experience aching or numbness of upper extremities as a result of anterior slumping of the shoulders and chest.
• Diastasis recti may occur.	• Uterus may partially herniate.
Skin Changes	
Hormonal Influence	
• Estrogen has decided effects on the skin.	• In many women the influence of estrogen produces increased pigmentation (chloasma, linea nigra) stretch marks, spider angiomas, and palmar erythema.

Hormonal Influences in Pregnancy

In nonpregnant women the steroid hormones estrogen and progesterone are produced by the ovaries. In pregnancy this mechanism is shut down. Instead, these hormones are synthesized in the maternal–fetal–placental unit. Activated at the moment of conception, this process assures the fetus a mechanism by which it can control its own environment. See Table 4-3.

Functions of the Lactation Hormones

Estrogen and Progesterone

- Growth of the ductal and lobulo-alveolar systems
- Inhibition of milk production during pregnancy
- Initiation of milk production facilitated by decreased estrogen and progesterone secretion after loss of the placenta

(*text continues on pg. 106*)

Table 4-3 Hormonal Influences in Pregnancy

Site of Production	Actions	Clinical Implications
Estrogen (Primarily estriol E_3) (Increases 1000-fold during pregnancy)		
Ovary Adrenal cortex Fetoplacental unit (after the seventh week of gestation, a 50% increase in section is ascribed to the placenta) Fetal liver and adrenals (secreted with precursors)	• Growth and function of the uterus Hypertrophy of the uterine musculature Proliferation of the endometrium Increased blood supply to the uteroplacental unit	• Index of fetal well-being provided by measurement of estriol in urine or amniotic fluid. Uterine size as assessed by McDonald's measurements should reflect appropriate or inappropriate fetal growth.
	• Development of ducts, alveoli, nipples of the breasts • Enlargement of external genitalia	• Increased breast size and tenderness
	• Increased pliability of connective tissue (tissues become hygroscopic and softer) Relaxation of pelvic joints and ligaments Stretching capacity of the cervix	• Lordosis, backache • Tenderness of the symphysis pubis • Cervical dilatation

(continued)

Table 4-3 Hormonal Influences in Pregnancy (*continued*)

Site of Production	Actions	Clinical Implications
Estrogen		
	• Decreased gastric secretion of hydrochloric acid and pepsin	• Indigestion, nausea, heartburn, decreased absorption of fat
	• Increased pigmentation of skin (increased melanocyte-stimulating hormone to pituitary)	• Hyperpigmentation: chloasma, darkened genitalia and areolae, linea nigra
	• Sodium and water retention	• Edema, increased plasma volume (physiologic anemia)
	• 50% increase in clotting potential of blood fibrinogen (factor I)	• Increased sedimentation rate
		• Palmar erythema, vascular spiders (angiomas)
	• Increased production of estriol in the late third trimester (may stimulate prostaglandin production)	• Enhancement of rhythmic uterine contractions; increased vascularity and responsiveness to oxytocin stimulation
	• Psychological changes	• Emotional lability, possibly changes in libido
Progesterone (Increases tenfold in pregnancy)		
Corpus luteum of the ovary for the first 7 weeks of pregnancy; then maternal-fetal unit	• Development of decidual cells in the endometrium	• Meets early nutritional needs of the embryo by deposition of glycogen
	• Possible role in suppression of the	

maternal immunologic response to the fetus	
• Decrease in contractility of gravid uterus	• Prevention of premature labor
• Development of lobulo-alveolar system of the breasts (secretory character)	• Breast tenderness
• Apparent resetting of three hypothalamic centers, causing	• Changes in fat storage, respiration and sensation:
Extensive fat storage to protect mother and fetus during starvation or strenous physical exertion	Average storage of 3.5 kg of body fat (7.7 pounds)
Stimulation of the respiratory center; decrease in pCO_2 to facilitate transfer of CO_2 from fetal to maternal blood	• Decreased alveolar and arterial pCO_2 in mother; hyperventilation
Increase of 0.5°F in basal body temperature until mid-pregnancy; then return to normal	• Sensation of being overly warm; increased perspiration
• Stimulation of natriuresis	• Secretion of aldosterone (sodium saver) to maintain water and electrolyte balance
• Relaxation of smooth muscle	• Nausea, reflux esophagitis, indigestion

(*continued*)

Table 4-3 Hormonal Influences in Pregnancy (*continued*)

Site of Production	Actions	Clinical Implications
Progesterone		
(Increases tenfold in pregnancy)	• Decrease in stomach motility, colonic activity	• Delayed emptying with readsorption of water from the bowel, resulting in constipation and hemorrhoids
	• Decrease in tone of bladder and ureter; dilatation throughout the system	• Stasis of urine, urinary tract infections
Human Chorionic Gonadotropin (HCG)		
Placenta, secreted by the syncytiotrophoblasts (appears as early as 8 days after conception; peaks at 60 to 90 days, when corpus luteum function is no longer needed to maintain the pregnancy. (Peak secretion is 50,000 to 100,000 mIU/ml/day; it drops to 25,000 to 50,000 mIU/ml after 4 months of gestation.)	• Maintenance of the function of the corpus luteum in early pregnancy • Possible use in regulating steroid production in the fetus	• Possible relationship with nausea • Use in pregnancy testing (negative test after 16 to 20 weeks) • Use in testing for multiple pregnancies (amount increases) • Indication of threatened abortion (amount decreases) • Use in diagnosis of trophoblastic disease and ectopic pregnancy (measured by the subunit HCG radioimmunoassay; no cross reaction with luteinizing hormone)

Human Placental Lactogen (HPL)		
Placenta, syncytiotrophoblasts (detected in the serum of pregnant women at 6 weeks of gestation; reaches 6,000 ng/ml at term)	• Action similar to that of growth hormones • Anti-insulin effect; sparing of maternal glucose • Maintenance of adequate supply of nutrients for the fetus when the mother is fasting (amount of HPL secreted correlates with fetal and placental weight)	• Increased availability of glucose for fetal use • Increased protein synthesis • Increased circulating fatty acids to meet increased metabolic needs; conservation of glucose and amino acids for use by the fetus • Avoidance of ketosis that might be caused by inadequate maternal glucose intake and that might impair fetal brain development
	• Possible effect on the increased incorporation of iron into erythrocytes (currently under study) • Stimulation of breast development, casein synthesis, and milk production	• Association between high levels of HPL and multiple pregnancies
Prostaglandin		
Maternal-placental-fetal unit (widely distributed in all cells of the body)	• Uncertain role in pregnancy: prostaglandin F_2 found in amniotic fluid, decidua, and maternal venous blood before labor	• Possible oxytocic effect on the uterine muscle • Prostaglandin E used vaginally or in amniocentesis for second trimester abortions and in labor induction

(*continued*)

Table 4-3 Hormonal Influences in Pregnancy (*continued*)

Site of Production	Actions	Clinical Implications
Progesterone		
	• Synthesis inhibited by anti-inflammatory drugs such as aspirin and indomethacin	• Possible function in increasing length of gestation • Use of indomethacin to halt premature labor
Prolactin		
Fetal pituitary, maternal pituitary, uterus (elevated blood levels at 8 weeks of gestation, reaching a peak of 200 ng/ml at term)	• Sustaining milk protein, casein, fatty acids, lactose, and volume of milk secretion during lactation	• Necessity of suckling response for release of prolactin
Thyroxine		
Thyroid gland, with stimulation from adenohypophysis (T_3 decreases until the end of the first trimester, then stabilizes; returns to normal 12 to 13 weeks postpartum; T_4 increases during pregnancy)	• Thyroid enlargement with a 20% increase in function from tissue hyperplasia and increased vascularity	• Increase of 25% in basal metabolic rate resulting from metabolic activity of the fetoplacental unit • Increase of protein-bound iodine from 3.6 to 8.8 to 10 to 12 units/dl during pregnancy

		• Palpitations, tachycardia, emotional lability, heat intolerance, fatigue, perspiration
Oxytocin		
Hypothalamus to pituitary for release	• Stimulates milk let-down and ejection • Stimulates uterine contractions (is not responsible for initial labor but increases the intensity of contractions) • Ferguson's reflex—release of oxytocin by cervical and vaginal distention during labor	• Lactation • Uterine involution • Role in onset of labor unknown

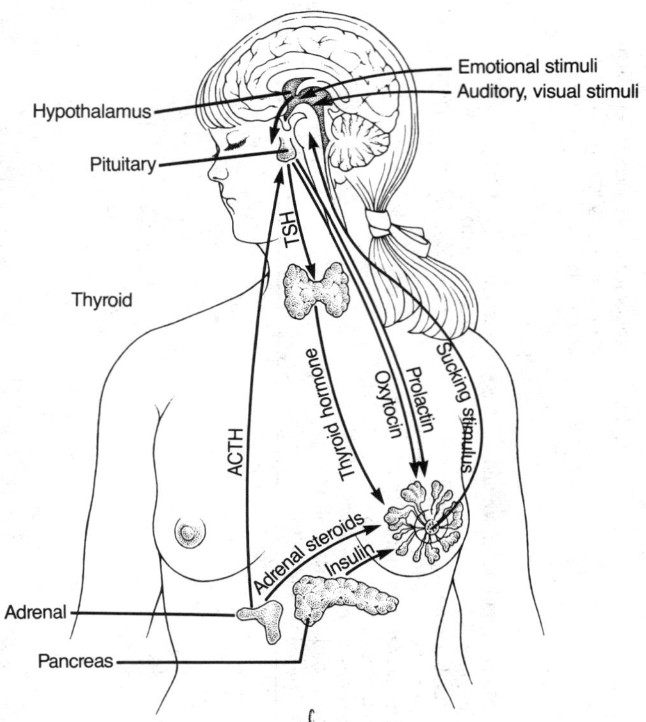

Figure 4-3 Neurohormonal pathways influencing lactation and milk ejection. (Redrawn from Hytten FE, Leitch I: The Physiology of Human Pregnancy, 2nd ed. Oxford, Blackwell Scientific Publications, 1971)

Prolactin

- Is an essential hormone required for successful lactation
- Promotes final maturation of the lobulo-alveolar system
- Is responsible for the production of milk sugar (lactose) and the content of water and electrolytes in the milk
- Is released when the infant's suckling causes inhibition of the prolactin inhibiting factor (PIF) from the hypothalamus

Insulin

- Synthesizes and metabolizes nutrients for the mother and baby during lactation in the following ways:

- Promotes glucose uptake from the maternal bloodstream
- Induces synthesis of enzymes needed for carbohydrate metabolism
- Helps stimulate the production of proteins and lipids in the active mammary gland

Glucocorticoids
- Regulate water transport across the cell membranes in pregnancy and during lactation

Parathyroid Hormone
- Limits the calcium content of the mother's milk
- Adjusts the iron content of milk to the needs of the infant
- Protects the mother against hypocalcemia and excessive calcium depletion

Thyroid Hormone
- Regulates the metabolic processes of the mother by:
  - Stimulating appetite
  - Enhancing absorption of nutrients
  - Maintaining glucose and prolactin concentration in the maternal plasma

Oxytocin
- Causes ejection of milk from the nipples after stimulation from the myoepithelial cells (Fig. 4-3)
- Causes uterine contractions during breastfeeding

Clinical Applications of Prostaglandins and Prostaglandin Inhibitors

Prostaglandins
Established applications:

- Termination of first- and second-trimester pregnancies
- Termination of molar pregnancy in case of fetal death or missed abortion
- Menstrual induction
- Preoperative cervical dilation in the first and second trimesters of pregnancy
- Termination of third-trimester pregnancy with fetal anomaly
- Management of third-stage labor and prevention of postpartum hemorrhage

*From Schulman H: Prostaglandins. In Fuchs F, Klopper A (eds): Endocrinology of Pregnancy, p 242. Philadelphia, Harper & Row, 1983

- Management of third-stage labor and prevention of postpartum hemorrhage
- Induction and acceleration of labor at term
- Preinduction cervical softening and dilation at term
- Maintenance of patency in ductus arteriosus in neonatal congenital heart disease

Potential applications:

- Treatment of toxemia of pregnancy
- Treatment of disseminated intravascular coagulation
- Treatment of male infertility

Prostaglandin Inhibitors
Established applications:

- Prevention of premature labor
- Treatment of dysmenorrhea
- Closure of ductus arteriosus

Potential applications:

- Prevention of spontaneous abortion
- Ovulation block
- Male contraception

PRECONCEPTION HEALTH SCREENING

Couples desiring to prepare themselves for pregnancy can do so by improving their preconception health. By anticipating conception and seeking health care, they are increasing their probability of delivering a normal, healthy infant.

Assessment

- Complete medical history on both partners that includes:
  - Pre-existing medical conditions and surgical procedures
  - Contraceptive use
  - Family history on both sides to determine sickle cell disease or trait, diabetes, RH factors, Tay-Sachs disease, trisomy 21, and other genetic disease
  - Immunization status of the women (especially regarding rubella)
  - History of herpes infection
- Complete physical examination of the woman that focuses on the reproductive system and assesses for abnormal discharge, infection, diethylstilbestrol (DES) exposure, lesions, structural abnormalities, past surgery
- A urologic examination of the male partner to assess infection;

lesions, masses, cysts, and hernia; undescended testicles or small testes; and sperm count (normal 20 million/ml)
- Blood tests: rubella titer, complete blood cell count (CBC), hemoglobin electrophoresis (to rule out hemoglobinopathies), glucose screening, toxoplasmosis and cytomegalovirus titers, and VDRL
- Cervical cultures: Pap smear, gonorrhea smear, chylamydia culture, herpes, if indicated
- Urinalysis

Nursing Intervention

Health Teaching

- Maintain a menstrual calendar.
- Discontinue birth control pills 3 months prior to conception.
- Remove IUD 1 month prior to conception.
- Discontinue use of contraceptive foam or gel.
- Use condoms in the interim.
- Avoid use of alcohol, recreational drugs, and cigarettes.
- Optimize nutrition and lose or gain weight as indicated.
- Avoid x-rays or confine them to the first half of the menstrual cycle; wear lead apron.
- Know symptoms of pregnancy; after one missed period a pregnancy test should be done.

Referral for Genetic Counseling

See Figure 4-4.

PREGNANCY DIAGNOSIS

Nursing Objectives in Pregnancy Diagnosis

- To be sensitive to the fact that women seeking pregnancy diagnosis may not be pleased with positive outcome
- To be prepared to refer women who are ambivalent about continuing a pregnancy for pregnancy counseling
- To support women who desire pregnancy and to explain the value of early prenatal care
- To support women who desire pregnancy but have not become pregnant. When no pregnancy occurs after 1 year of consistently unprotected intercourse, discuss the possibility of seeking a fertility workup.

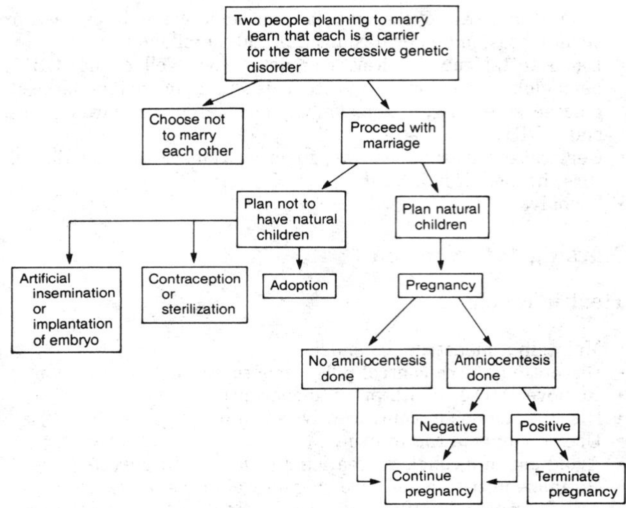

Figure 4-4 Flow chart for decision making in premarital screening.

Possible Nursing Diagnoses Related to Pregnancy Diagnosis

- Knowledge deficit related to prenatal care
- Knowledge deficit related to neonatal care
- Alteration in comfort (nausea) related to pregnancy
- Alteration in family processes related to couple's desire for, ambivalent feelings toward, or lack of desire for a baby
- Alteration in nutrition (less than body requirements) related to morning sickness
- Noncompliance related to age of client (adolescent)

Assessment: Methods of Pregnancy Diagnosis

Clinical Changes of Pregnancy

Presumptive Evidence of Pregnancy in Sexually Active Women
- Abrupt cessation of menses
- Nausea and vomiting
- Urinary frequency

- Breast tenderness
- Fatigue

Probable Signs of Pregnancy in Sexually Active Women

- Abdominal enlargement
- Ballottement of the fetus
- Softening of the lower uterine segment (Hegar's sign)
- Chadwick's sign (purplish hue of vagina and cervix)
- Sensation of fetal movement

Positive Signs of Pregnancy

- Fetal heart beat
- Fetal movement
- Ultrasound diagnosis

Pregnancy Tests (Detection of Human Chorionic Gonadotropin [HCG] in Blood or Urine)

- Immunologic:
  - Slide urinary
  - Tube urinary
- Radioimmunoassay (RIA beta-subunit HCG blood test)
- Radioreceptor (RRA)
- Home pregnancy tests (tube immunologic)

Ultrasound Diagnosis of Pregnancy

- Real-time scanner demonstrates:
  - Gestational sac in the uterus as early as 6 weeks from the last menstrual period (LMP)
  - Fetal heart movement at 10 weeks
  - Fetal movement at 12 weeks
  - Fetal head and thorax at 14 weeks

FETAL DEVELOPMENT

Periods of Fetal Growth

Weeks 1 to 3

Pre-embryonic (Zygote)	Fertilization of the ovum and development of the conceptus until the formation of the three layers of the embryonic disc

Weeks 4 to 8

Embryonic	Rapid growth, tissue differentiation, and formation of all major body organs

Weeks 9 to 40

Fetal	Growth and development of major body organs and differentiation of organ systems

---

Period I: The Pre-embryonic Period (First to Third Weeks of Life)

First Week

- Fertilization and formation of the zygote (30 hours)
- Cleavage of the zygote into 12 to 16 blastomeres—the morula (days 2 and 3)
- Formation of the blastocyst (day 4)
- Attachment of the blastocyst (days 5 to 8)

Second Week

- Formation of the inner cytotrophoblast and outer syncytiotrophoblastic layers (days 7 and 8)
- Trophoblasts invade maternal endometrium and sinusoids (day 8)
- Appearance of the amniotic cavity (day 8)
- Formation of lacunar networks (day 9)
- Establishment of primitive uteroplacental circulation (day 11)
- Formation of primitive chorionic villi (day 13)
- Decidualization of the uterine lining (day 14)
- Development of prochordal plate (day 14)

Third Week

- Formation of blood vessels within the chorionic villi (day 13)
- Gastrulation or conversion of the bilaminar embryonic disc into the three-layered trilaminar disc (day 14)
- Continued development of the chorion with formation of tertiary chorionic villi (days 15 to 20)
- Development of the neural tube (day 18)
- Formation of somites (day 21)
- Beginning of blood circulation (day 24)

Period II: The Embryonic Period (Fourth to Eighth Weeks of Life)

During this short, 4-week period, embryonic development is extremely rapid. All major internal and external organs and organ systems are formed, a process known as organogenesis. The embryo changes in shape, and major features of the external body are recognizable by 8 weeks (morphogenesis). This stage of growth and development holds the potential for major congenital malformations if the embryo is exposed to teratogens such as drugs, chemicals, viruses, and other substances.

Weeks 4 to 8

- Conversion of the first trilaminar embryonic disc into a C-shaped cylindrical embryo
- Formation of the head, tail, and lateral folds
- Formation of the primitive gut by incorporation of the yolk sac into the embryo
- Acquisition of an epithelial covering by the umbilicus through the expansion of the amnion
- Establishment of ventral position of the heart and development of the brain in the cranial region of the embryo
- Differentiation of the three germ layers into various tissues and layers that will become established as the major organ systems
- Appearance of the brain, limbs, ears, eyes, and nose
- Development of human appearance by the embryo

See Figure 4-5

Period III: The Fetal Period (9th to 40th Weeks of Life)

When the basic organ structures of the embryo have been established and it is recognizable as a human being, it is called a fetus. During the fetal period, from 9 to 40 weeks, there is further growth and differentiation of the tissues and organs that began their development during the embryonic period. Growth is considerable: The fetus's crown-rump length (CRL) goes from approximately 30 mm to 300 mm. Body proportions change, and the fetus's tiny organs begin to function and to supply a portion of its metabolic needs (Fig. 4-6).

Major Events of Fetal Period

Weeks 9 to 12

- Size of fetal head is half that of the fetal body.
- CRL doubles between 9 and 12 weeks.
- Eyelids remain fused.
- Upper limbs develop to normal proportions while lower limbs remain less developed.
- Male and female genitalia are recognizable by 12 weeks.

(*text continues on pg. 117*)

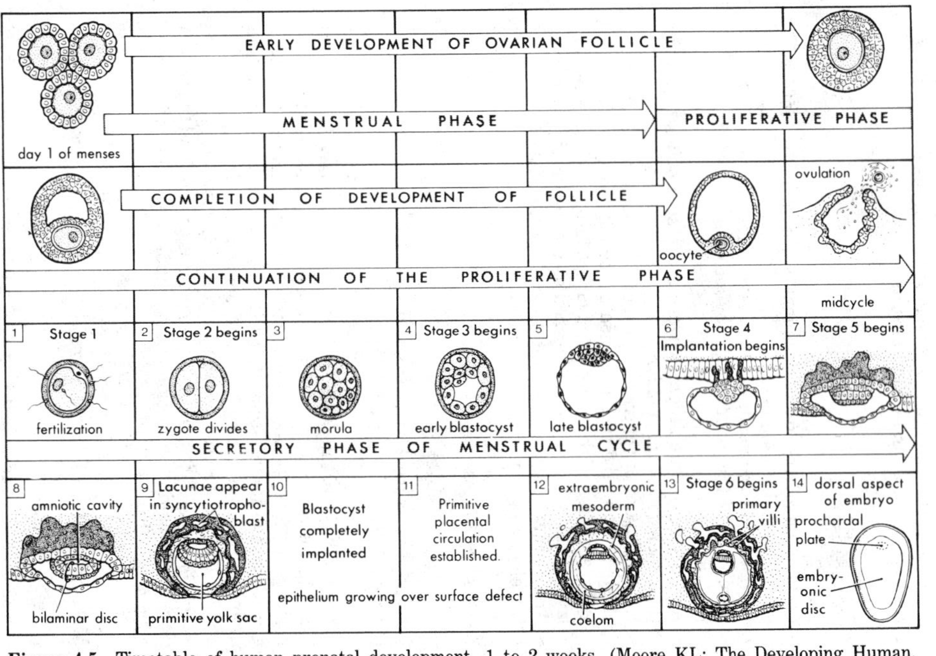

Figure 4-5 Timetable of human prenatal development, 1 to 2 weeks. (Moore KL: The Developing Human. Philadelphia, WB Saunders, 1982)

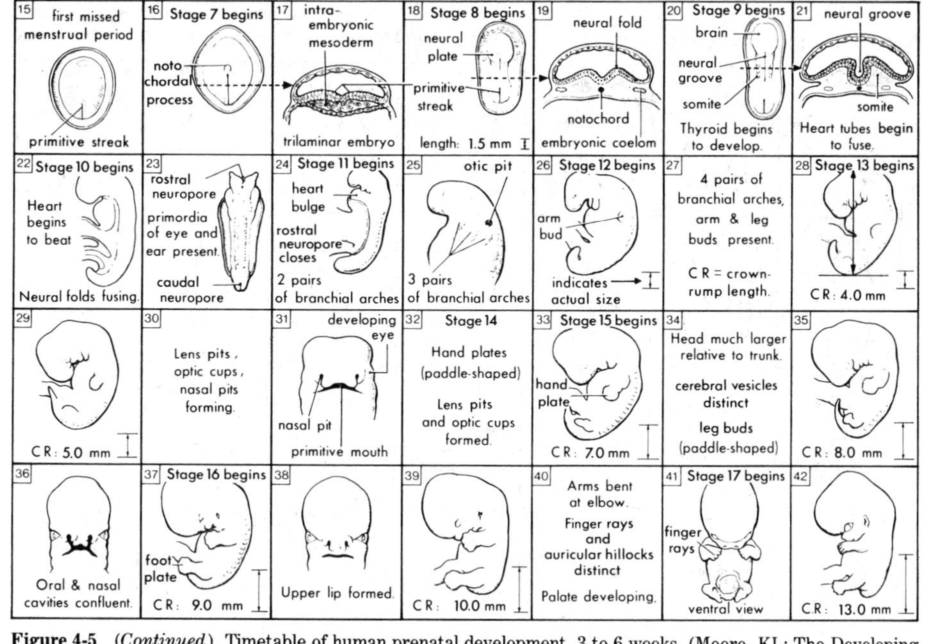

Figure 4-5 (*Continued*). Timetable of human prenatal development, 3 to 6 weeks. (Moore, KL: The Developing Human. Philadelphia; WB Saunders, 1982)

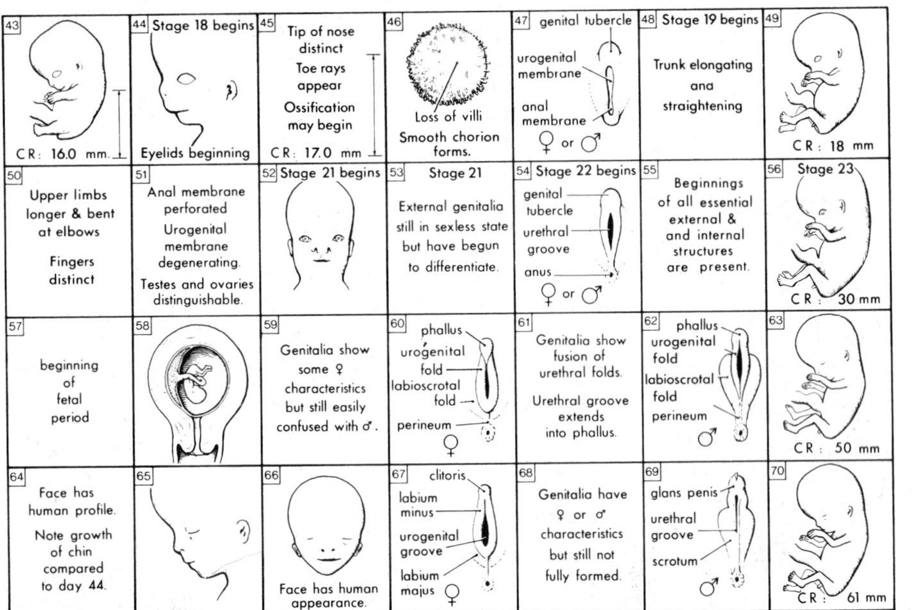

Figure 4-5 (*Continued.*) Timetable of human prenatal development, 7 to 10 weeks. (Moore KL: The Developing Human. Philadelphia, WB Saunders, 1982)

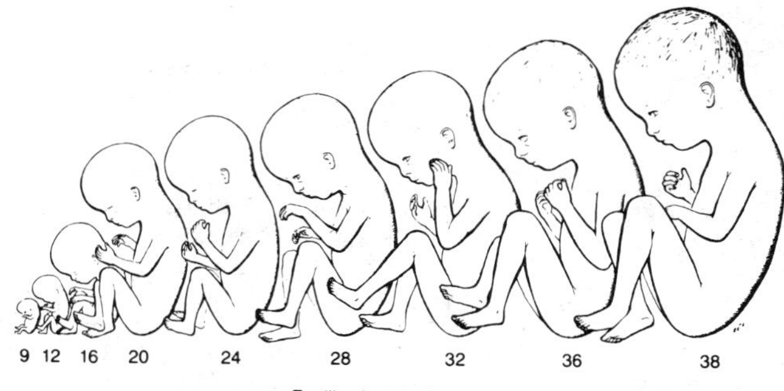

Figure 4-6 Head hair begins to appear at about 20 weeks. Eyebrows and eyelashes are usually recognizable by 24 weeks, and the eyes reopen by 26 weeks. Fetuses born prematurely (22 weeks or more) may survive, but intensive care is required. The mean duration of pregnancy is 266 days (38 weeks) from fertilization, with a standard deviation of 12 days. In clinical practice, it is customary to refer to full term as 40 weeks from the first day of the last menstrual period (LMP), assuming that conception occurs 2 weeks after the onset of menses. Thus, when a provider refers to a pregnancy of 20 weeks, the actual age of the fetus is only 18 weeks. (Moore KL: The Developing Human, Philadelphia, WB Saunders, 1982)

- Production of red blood cells is transferred from the liver to the spleen at 12 weeks.

Weeks 13 to 16

- Rapid fetal growth occurs.
- Fetus doubles in size.
- Lanugo begins to grow.
- Fingernails are formed.
- Kidneys begin to secrete urine.
- Fetus begins to swallow amniotic fluid.
- Fetus appears human.
- Placenta is fully formed.

Weeks 17 to 23

- Fetal growth slows.
- Lower limbs become fully formed.
- Fetal body is covered with lanugo.
- Vernix caseosa covers the body to protect the skin from amniotic fluid.
- Fetal movement is first felt by the mother around 20 weeks.
- Fetal heartbeat is first heard with a fetoscope.
- Brown fat forms.

Weeks 24 to 27

- Skin growth is rapid, and skin appears red and wrinkled.
- The eyes open, and eyelashes and eyebrows are formed.
- The fetus becomes viable at 24 weeks.

Weeks 28 to 31

- Subcutaneous fat is deposited.
- If the fetus is born at this time, respiratory distress syndrome may occur, because of immature lungs.

Weeks 32 to 36

- Weight gain is steady.
- Lanugo has disappeared from the body but remains on the head.
- Fingernails are growing.
- The fetus has a good chance of survival if born during these weeks.

Weeks 37 to 40

- Subcutaneous fat increases steadily, and fetal contours become rounded.
- Fingernails and toenails are fully formed and extend beyond the ends of the fingers and toes.
- Both testes have descended in the male.
- The skull is fully developed and is larger than any other part of the body.

TERATOGENS

See Figure 4-7 and Appendix C.

Infectious Agents During Pregnancy

See Table 4-4.

Effects of Fetal Alcohol Syndrome on the Infant

- Eyes: shortened palpebral fissures, ptosis, strabismus, myopia, microphthalmia (abnormally small eye size), tourtuosity of the arterial and venous retinal vasculature
- Nose: short and upturned nose: low, broad bridge; hypoplastic philtrum (flat or absent groove above upper lip); greater than normal distance from upper lip to nose
- Ears: large, low-set ears rotated posteriorly
- Jaw: underdeveloped upper and lower jawbones

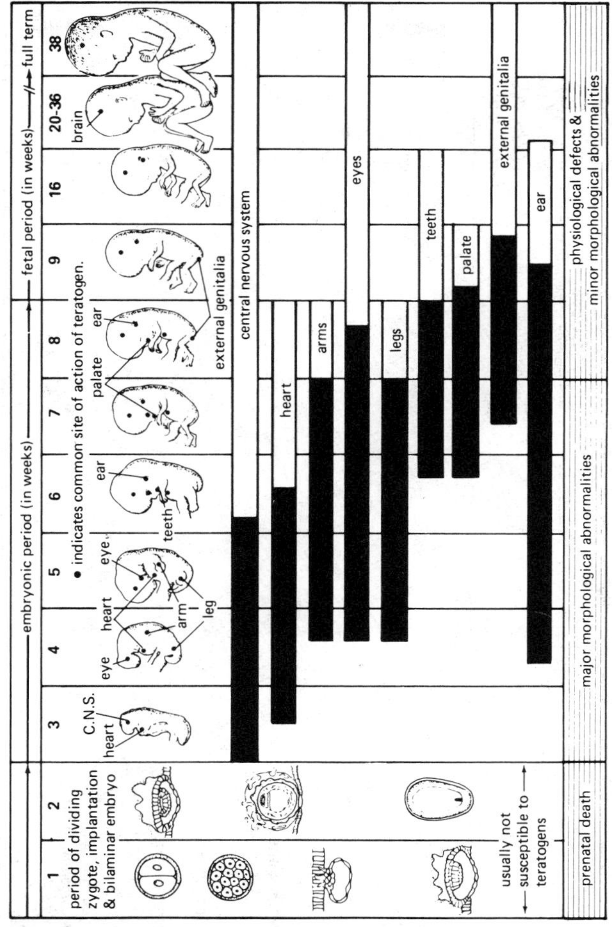

Figure 4-7 Fetal development and relative sensitivity to teratogenesis. The dark areas represent the most susceptible interval for teratogenesis. (Moore KL: The Developing Human. Philadelphia, WB Saunders, 1982)

Table 4–4 Harmful Effects of Selected Infectious Agents During Pregnancy

Agent	Effect		
	Increased Reproductive Loss	*Congenital Malformations*	*Prematurity of Growth Retardation*
Viral			
Cytomegaloviruses	+	+	+
Rubella (3-day measles)	+	+	+
Chicken pox (*Varicella-zoster*)	0	+	+
Herpes simplex 1 and 2	+	+	+
Mumps	+	?	0
Polio	+	0	+?
Rubeola (measles)	+	?	+
Venezuelan equine encephalitis	+	+	0
Coxsackie B	+	?	0
Bacterial			
Syphilis (*Treponema pallidum*)	+	+	?
Tuberculosis	+	0?	+
Listeriosis (*Listeria monocytogenes*)	+	0	+?
Parasitic			
Malaria (*Plasmodium*)	+	0	+
Toxoplasmosis (*Toxoplasma gondii*)	+	+	+
Chagas disease (*Trypanosoma cruzi*)	+	0	?
Fungal			
Valley fever (*Coccidioides immitis*)	+	0	+

+ = established, 0 = no present evidence, ? = possible, not established.
Note: Smallpox and vaccinia virus have not been included because of the eradication of smallpox.
(Cohen F: Clinical Genetics in Nursing Practice. Philadelphia, JB Lippincott, 1984)

Table 4-5 Reported Action of Marijuana on Reproductive Systems

Females	Males
Decreases levels of follicle-stimulating hormone (FSH), luteinizing hormone (LH), and prolactin (PRL)	Decreases FSH, LH, and PRL levels
Inhibits ovulation	Decreases testosterone levels (tolerance develops)
Disrupts menstrual cycle (tolerance develops)	Inhibits spermatogenesis and sperm motility
Crosses placenta and may affect fetal growth and development	Alters sperm function
Passes readily into milk	

(From Asch RH, Smith CG: Effects of marijuana on reproduction. Contemp Ob/Gyn October 1982, p. 217. Copyright 1983 Medical Economics Company. Reprinted by permission.)

Cardiovascular Abnormalities

- Ventricular septal defect, tetralogy of Fallot, patent ductus arteriosus, great vessel defects

Urogenital Abnormalities

- Hydronephrosis, kidney hypoplasia, renal agenesis (absence of one or both kidneys), undescended testicles, clitoral hypertrophy, labial hypoplasia

Skeletal Deformities

- Microcephaly, hypoplastic nails (defective development), shortened fingers or toes, cervical spinal fusion, clinodactyly (permanent deflection of one or more fingers), aberrant palmar creases, numerous less common deformities

Central Nervous System (CNS) Disorders

- Mental retardation, hyperactivity (impulsivity and difficulty focusing attention), sleep disturbances, developmental delay, decreased muscle tone, weak sucking

Growth Deficiency

- Intrauterine growth retardation (IUGR), failure to thrive

Effects of Tobacco Smoking on the Fetus

Smoking is associated with a lowered birth rate and may have harmful effects on the fetal CNS during the third trimester. Besides being associated with sudden infant death syndrome (SIDS) in the postpartal period, it is also associated with the following:

- Spontaneous abortion
- Stillbirth

Effects of Marijuana

See Table 4-5.

NOTES

5
Nutritional Aspects of Pregnancy and the Fourth Trimester

Nursing Objectives in Nutritional Care During Pregnancy and the Fourth Trimester

- To assess maternal nutritional status through a comprehensive health history, dietary history, and interpretation of selected laboratory studies
- To identify nutritional needs and to plan nutritional care to meet those needs
- To teach pregnant women about the importance of good nutrition during pregnancy to prevent maternal complications and to ensure normal fetal growth and development
- To assist pregnant women to maintain or improve their own nutritional status
- To assess the current knowledge of both breastfeeding and formula-feeding mothers regarding their nutritional needs during the fourth trimester

Possible Nursing Diagnoses Related to Nutritional Care in Pregnancy and the Fourth Trimester

- Nutritional intake less than body requirements related to nausea or lack of knowledge about nutritional requirements during pregnancy
- Nutritional intake more than body requirements related to decreased appetite or lack of knowledge about nutritional requirements during pregnancy
- Constipation related to decreased peristalsis and iron supplementation during pregnancy
- Alterations in health maintenance related to changing dietary patterns secondary to infant demands

Table 5-1 Energy Requirements During Pregnancy

Age in Years	Recommended Ratio kcal/kg Body Wt	Nonpregnant Requirement (kcal/day)	Pregnant Requirement (kcal/day)
11–15	50	2200	2500
15–22	40	2100	2400
23–50	36	2000	2300

(Adapted from National Research Council: Recommended Dietary Allowances, 9th ed. Washington, DC, National Academy of Sciences, 1980)

- Nutritional intake less than body requirements related to breastfeeding
- Nutritional intake more than body requirements related to ingestion of excess calories

PREGNANCY NUTRITIONAL REQUIREMENTS

Energy Requirements

The total energy cost of pregnancy is 80,000 kcal. When divided over the length of pregnancy, the energy cost is 300 calories per day over nonpregnant needs. Because caloric needs differ among women, individual caloric needs are calculated by allowing a minimum of 36 kcal/kg of pregnant body weight. Pregnant adolescents' energy needs may reach 50 kcal/kg/day, depending on activity levels and growth rate. Table 5-1 summarizes energy requirements during pregnancy.

Table 5-2 Protein Requirements During Pregnancy

Age in Years	Recommended Ratio g/kg Body Wt	Nonpregnant Requirement (g/day)	Pregnant Requirement (g/day)
11–15	1.7	46	76
15–18	1.5	46	76
19–50	1.3	44	74

(Adapted from National Research Council: Recommended Dietary Allowances, 9th ed. Washington, DC, National Academy of Science, 1980)

Protein Requirements

Adult women need an additional 30 g/day of protein or a total allowance of 1.3 g/kg/day of protein above nonpregnant needs, as shown in Table 5-2.

Vitamin Requirements

Generally requirements for all vitamins are increased during pregnancy (Tables 5-3 and 5-4). One vitamin that requires special attention in pregnancy is folic acid (folacin). Folacin promotes fetal growth and prevents pregnancy-related anemias. The recommended dietary allowance (RDA) for folacin is doubled during gestation from 400 μg/day to 800 μg/day. Supplementation of this vitamin during pregnancy at 400 to 800 μg/day is recommended for women considered at risk because of poverty, poor dietary habits, frequent or multiple pregnancies, chronic hemolytic anemia, or anticoagulant drug therapy.

Mineral Requirements

See Table 5-5.

Assessment

- Health history
  - Lactose intolerance
- Findings of physical examination

See Table 5-6.

- Findings of laboratory tests

See Table 5-7.

- Dietary history
  - Cultural/religious dietary patterns
  - Food preferences and tolerances
  - 24-hour dietary recall
- Caffeine, alcohol, and tobacco use
- Common discomforts of pregnancy affecting nutritional status: nausea, vomiting, heartburn, constipation
- Ongoing nutritional assessment: weight gain

Table 5-3 Recommended Intake of Fat-Soluble Vitamins

Age in Years	Nonpregnant Intake			Pregnant Intake		
	*Vitamin A (μg RE)**	*Vitamin D (μg)*	*Vitamin E (mg TE)†*	*Vitamin A (μg RE)*	*Vitamin D (μg)*	*Vitamin E (mg TE)*
11–14	800	10.0	8	1000	15.0	10
15–18	800	10.0	8	1000	15.0	10
19–22	800	7.5	8	1000	12.5	10
23–50	800	5.0	8	1000	10.0	10

* RE = retinol equivalents.
800 = 4000 IU (international units)
1000 = 5000 IU (international units)
† TE = tocopherol equivalents
(Adapted from National Research Council: Recommended Dietary Allowances, 9th ed. Washington, DC. National Academy of Science, 1980)

Table 5-4 Recommended Intake of Water-Soluble Vitamins

	Age in Years			
Vitamin	*11–14*	*15–18*	*19–22*	*23–50*
Nonpregnant Intake				
Vitamin C (mg)	50.0	60.0	60.0	60.0
Thiamin (mg)	1.1	1.1	1.1	1.0
Riboflavin (mg)	1.3	1.3	1.3	1.2
Niacin (mg)	15.0	14.0	14.0	13.0
Vitamin B-6 (mg)	1.8	2.0	2.0	2.0
Folacin (mg)	400.0	400.0	400.0	400.0
Vitamin B-12 (mcg)	3.0	3.0	3.0	3.0
Pregnant Intake				
Vitamin C (mg)	70.0	80.0	80.0	80.0
Thiamin (mg)	1.5	1.5	1.5	1.4
Riboflavin (mg)	1.6	1.6	1.6	1.5
Niacin (mg)	17.0	16.0	16.0	15.0
Vitamin B-6 (mg)	2.4	2.6	2.6	2.6
Folacin (mcg)	800.0	800.0	800.0	800.0
Vitamin B-12 (mcg)	4.0	4.0	4.0	4.0

(Adapted from National Research Council: Recommended Dietary Allowances, 9th ed. Washington, DC, National Academy of Science, 1980)

Identifying Nutritional Risk Factors

Predisposing Factors for Nutrition Risk

- Adolescence (age 15 years or younger)
- History of three or more pregnancies during past 2 years
- Poverty
- Food faddism, history of unusual or restrictive diets
- Heavy use of tobacco, alcohol, or drugs
- Maintenance of a therapeutic diet for chronic illness
- Prepregnancy weight less than 85% or more than 120% of standard weight for height

Patients should be observed for the following risk factors as prenatal care progresses:

- Low or deficient hemoglobin/hematocrit (low = Hgb: 11.0 g/Hct: 33; deficient = Hgb: 10.0 g/Hct: 30)
- Inadequate weight gain (any weight loss during pregnancy or gain of less than 2 lb/month)

(*text continues on pg. 132*)

Table 5-5 Recommended Intake of Minerals

	Age in Years			
Mineral	*11–14*	*15–18*	*19–22*	*23–50*
Nonpregnant Intake				
Calcium (mg)	1200	1200	800	800
Phosphorus (mg)	1200	1200	800	800
Magnesium (mg)	300	300	300	300
Iron (mg)	18	18	18	18
Zinc (mg)	15	15	15	15
Iodine (mg)	150	150	150	150
Pregnant Intake				
Calcium (mg)	1600	1600	1200	1200
Phosphorus (mg)	1600	1600	1200	1200
Magnesium (mg)	450	450	450	450
Iron (mg)*	18	18	18	18
Zinc (mg)	20	20	20	20
Iodine (mg)	175	175	175	175

* An additional 30 to 60 mg of supplemental iron is needed daily in addition to dietary sources.

(Adapted from National Research Council: Recommended Dietary Allowances, 9th ed. Washington, DC. National Academy of Science, 1980)

Table 5-6 Indicators of Nutrient Deficiency on Physical Examination

Physical Finding	Nutrient Deficit
Significant nondependent edema	Protein
Filiform papillary atrophy of the tongue	Iron/folate
Diffusely enlarged and visible thyroid gland (goiter)	Iodine
Follicular hyperkeratosis of upper arms	Vitamin A
Diffusely swollen red interdental papillae of gums in a clean mouth	Vitamin C
Angular fissures and cheilosis of lips	Riboflavin

Table 5-7 Laboratory Values Reflecting Nutritional Status in Pregnancy

Laboratory Test	Normal Range		Findings in Deficiency
	Nonpregnant	*Pregnant*	
Hgb/Hct	>12/36	>11/33*	<11/33*
Serum folic acid	5 to 21 ng per ml	3 to 15 ng per ml	<3 ng per ml
Serum Fe/Fe binding capacity	>50/250–400 ng per 100 ml	>40/300–450 mcg per 100 ml	<40/450 ng per 100 ml
Urinary acetone	Negative	Faint positive in A.M.	Positive
Fasting blood sugar	70–100 mg per 100 ml	65–100 mg per 100 ml	<65 mg per 100 ml
2-hour postprandial blood sugar	<110 mg per 100 ml	<120 mg per 100 ml	—
Serum protein, total	6.5–8.5 g per 100 ml	6–8 g per 100 ml	<6 g per 100 ml*
Serum albumin	3.5–5 g per 100 ml	3–4.5 g per 100 ml	<3.5 g per 100 ml*
Blood urea nitrogen	10–25 mg per 100 ml	5–15 mg per 100 ml	<5 mg per 100 ml
Urine urea nitrogen/total nitrogen ratio	>60	>60	<60
Cholesterol	120–290 mg per 100 ml	200–335 mg per 100 ml	—
Serum vitamin A	20–60 ng per 100 ml*	20–60 ng per 100 ml	<20 ng per 100 ml
Serum carotene	50–300 ng per 100 ml	80–325 ng per 100 ml	<80 ng per 100 ml*

(continued)

Table 5-7 Laboratory Values Reflecting Nutritional Status in Pregnancy (*continued*)

Laboratory Test	Normal Range		Findings in Deficiency
	Nonpregnant	*Pregnant*	
Serum calcium	4.6–5.5 mEq per liter	4.2–5.2 mEq per liter	<4.2 mEq per liter or normal
Serum phosphate	2.5–4.8 mg per 100 ml	2.3–4.6 mg per 100 ml	No change
Alkaline phosphatase	35–48 IU per liter	35–150 IU per liter	No change
Serum ascorbic acid	0.2–2.0 mg per 100 ml*	0.2–1.5 mg per 100 ml*	<0.2 mg per 100 ml*
Prothrombin time	12–15 sec	12–15 sec	Prolonged
Blood thiamine	1.6–4.0 ng per 100 ml	—	Decreased
Urinary thiamine	>55 ng per g creatinine	—	<50
Blood lactic acid	5–20 mg per 100 ml	—	Increased
Urinary riboflavin	>80 mg per g creatinine	—	<90*
N-methyl nicotinamide	1.6–4.3 mg per g creatinine	2.5–6 mg per g creatinine	<2.5 mg per g creatinine*

Kynurenic acid excretion	3 mg per 24 hr	—	Increased
Xanthurenic acid excretion	3 mg per 24 hr	—	Increased
FIGLU (Forminoglutamic acid) excretion (after 15 g L-histidine)	<3 mg per 24 hr	—	Increased
	1–4 mg per 24 hr	—	Increased
Serum vitamin B-12	330–1025 pg per ml	Decreased	Decreased
Methylmalonic aicd	<10 mg per 24 hr	—	Increased
Serum calcium	4.6–5.5 mEq per liter	4.2–5.2 mEq per liter	Normal
Serum thyroxine (T_4)	4.6–10.7 ng per ml	6–12.5 ng per ml	Decreased or normal

* Criteria from the Centers for Disease Control: Ten State Nutrition Survey, 1968–1970. DHEW Publication No. (HSM) 72-8134: 72-8133. Washington D.C., U.S. Government Printing Office, 1972

(Aubry RH, Roberts A, Cuenca VG: The assessment of maternal nutrition. Clin Perinatol 2(2):207, 1975)

- Excessive weight gain (more than 2 lb/month)
- Plans to breastfeed (in women with inadequate weight gain, anorexia, or poor health)

Nutritional Risk for the Pregnant Adolescent
The following factors impinge upon the adolescent and place her at nutritional risk:

- Musculoskeletal growth that continues for 1 or 2 years after conception becomes possible
- Nutrient needs for the adolescent's growth and maturation, in addition to those of the fetus, that increase demands for additional protein, calories, and nutrients
- High activity levels
- Abandonment of good eating habits with increased intake of junk food, snacks, and erratic eating habits.
- Influence of commercial advertising targeting products toward teenagers
- Concern with body image and crash diets
- Restriction of food intake during pregnancy to minimize weight or to hide the pregnancy

Assessment of Weight Gain

Adequate weight gain must include repeated measurements of body weight. A satisfactory pattern of weight gain for the average woman is:

- 10 weeks gestation: 650 g (approximately 1.5 lb)
- 20 weeks gestation: 4000 g (approximately 9 lb)
- 30 weeks gestation: 8500 g (approximately 19 lb)
- 40 weeks gestation: 12,500 g (approximately 27.5 lb)

Over the course of the pregnancy, a total weight gain of 25 to 30 pounds is recommended for both nonobese and obese pregnant women. During the second and third trimesters, a gain of about 1 pound per week is considered desirable.

Nursing Interventions

Special Supplemental Feeding Program for Women, Infants, and Children (WIC)

Under the federally funded program known as WIC people considered to be at nutritional risk by health care professionals can receive supplements of high-quality foods. In particular, the program is designed to provide supplemental foods to infants and children under 5 years of age and to pregnant, lactating, and postpartum women. WIC requires that mothers also receive nutritional counseling and routine health care. The eligibility criteria for the WIC program are as follows:

- Recurrent need for medical care
- Conformity with federal income guidelines
- Residence in a local agency's target area
- Determination by a health professional that "nutritional risk" is present

Pregnancy Dietary Counseling

- Counsel mother about changes needed to remedy deficits. Plan prenatal diet with mother to provide adequate nutrition. (Tables 5-8, 5-9, and 5-10)
- Point out value of good nutrition for overall health of mother and family.
- Teach importance of iron and folic acid supplementation during pregnancy. Initiate supplementation to provide 30 to 60 mg/day elemental iron, 400 to 800 mg/day folacin. Encourage intake of foods rich in iron and folic acid.
- Emphasize importance of optimal weight gain. Encourage use of high-quality protein foods to increase protein and caloric intake. Explore concerns about body image.
- Identify foods high in "empty" calories. Encourage use of healthy foods to satisfy hunger.
- Evaluate woman for edema of face and extremities, proteinuria, and glucosuria. Verify that blood pressure is normal.
- Suggest supplemental sources of calcium and vitamin D, such as tofu and foods made with fish/meat bones.
- Explain how the use of alcohol and tobacco adversely affects fetal growth. Provide support for making changes with realistic goal setting.
- For nausea/vomiting, recommend small, frequent meals; hot or cold liquids between meals; and dry crackers or toast before arising from bed in the morning.
- For constipation, encourage increased intake of high-fiber foods, increased daily exercise, regular meals and elimination habits, and adequate fluid intake (6 to 8 glasses of water daily).

FOURTH TRIMESTER

Maternal Nutritional Needs

All new mothers need adequate nutrients to promote healing of tissues traumatized by labor and delivery. The mother's body chemistry and fluid and electrolyte balances are dramatically al-

(*text continues on pg. 138*)

Table 5-8 Pregnancy Food Group Guide

Food Group and Service Size	Servings per Day	Rationale
Protein Foods		
Meat, poultry, fish (2 oz.), eggs (2); beans (1 cup cooked); nut butters (¼ cup) or nuts and seeds (½); tofu (1 cup) or cottage cheese (½ cup)	4	To build tissues in mother and infant. These foods contain iron, protein, zinc, and many other nutrients
Milk/Dairy Foods		
Nonfat, lowfat, or whole milk (1 cup); plain yogurt (1 cup); soymilk or tofu (1 cup); cheese (1.5–2 oz); nonfat milk powder (⅓ cup)	4	To build healthy bones and teeth. These foods are major source of calcium. They provide vitamins A and D, necessary for fetal development.
Grains (Whole grains are best!)		
Bread, rolls (1 slice); macaroni, rice, noodles (½ cup); hot cereal (½ cup); cold cereal (1 oz); wheat germ (1 tbsp).	4+	To provide B vitamins for strong blood and nerves; iron and trace minerals; and fiber for optimal bowel function.

Vitamin C-Rich Foods		
Orange or grapefruit juice (½ cup); 1 orange or ½ grapefruit; bell peppers, greens, tomato, cantalope, broccoli, cabbage, cauliflower (1 cup).	2+	To provide vitamin C (ascorbic acid) for connective tissue and resistence to infection and disease. Daily intake is necessary. Vitamin C intake is especially important for smokers. Whole fruits are preferable to juices; fruit drinks with added sugar should be avoided.
Green Leafy Vegetables		
Broccoli, Brussels sprouts, asparagus, cabbage, greens, red leaf or romaine lettuce, bok choy, watercress (1 cup raw or ¾ cup cooked).	1–2+	To provide folacin and iron and vitamin A for soft skin and good eyesight. These foods also contain vitamin E, C, and K and natural fiber.
Other Fruits and Vegetables		
All fruits and vegetables not listed above, and their juices: apples, carrots, bananas, sweet potatoes, green beans, etc. (about ½ cup).	2+	To promote general health. These foods contain many nutrients and fiber.
Fats and Oils		
Butter, margarine, better-butter, salad dressing, cream cheese, cooking fats, fatty cheeses.	3 tsp.	For energy and healthy skin. These foods, however, should be used in *moderation*.

Table 5-9 Approximate Nutritional Values of Common Foods

Protein

7 g

1 oz lean meat, poultry, fish
1 egg
1 glass of milk
1 oz cheddar or pasteurized, processed cheese
¼ c cottage cheese
½ c dried beans or peas (cooked)
2 tbsp peanut butter

4 g

1 c whole grain cooked cereal
1 c bran flakes
1 c ice cream
½ c milk pudding
2 slices bacon

2 g

1 c ready-to-eat cereal
1 slice bread
1 serving cake, pie or cookies

1 g

½ c fruit or vegetables

Iron

3 mg

1 oz liver
3 oz lean, red meat
4–5 medium oysters
1 c dark greens
1 c green peas
½ c dried beans
1 tbsp blackstrap molasses

1 mg

3 oz fish
2 oz poultry
1 egg
4 prunes or ½ c prune juice
3 tbsp raisins
1 c fruit or vegetable (other than dark green)
2 slices whole grain or enriched bread

Calcium

300 mg

1 c milk
1–1.5 oz cheddar or swiss cheese
1–1½ c ice cream
3 oz sardines
½ c peanuts
1 c collard greens
1–1½ c kale, mustard, turnip greens

150 mg

1 oz pasteurized, processed cheese
3 oz salmon
1–1½ c dried beans
12 medium oysters
1 c broccoli

Vitamin A

10,000 IU

1 oz liver
½ c carrots
⅔ c pumpkin
1 (5 oz) sweet potato, cooked in skin
½ c dark leafy greens
½ cantaloupe (5-in diameter, orange-fleshed)

3,000 IU

3 raw apricots or ½ c canned halves
watermelon, 4 × 8-in wedge

Table 5-9 Approximate Nutritional Values of Common Foods (*continued*)

½ c broccoli
½ c winter squash

1,000 IU

1 raw peach or 1 c canned
1 c fortified dry cereal
1 c green peas
1 raw tomato 2–2.5-in diameter)
½ c canned tomatoes
1 c green leafed lettuce

500 IU

1 c vitamin A-fortified milk
2 oz cheddar cheese
1 c ice cream
2 eggs
1 tbsp butter or fortified margarine
½ c green beans or limas

Ascorbic Acid (vitamin C)

50 mg

½ c orange or orange juice
½ c grapefruit or grapefruit juice
½ c lemon or lime juice
½ c fresh strawberries
¼ c cantaloupe (6.5-in diameter, orange-fleshed)
⅓ c broccoli
1 c fresh raw or lightly cooked cabbage
⅓ c fresh cooked collard greens
½ c cooked dark-green leafy vegetables
½ raw green pepper

25 mg

1 c raw blackberries
watermelon, 4 × 8-in wedge
1 (5 oz) baked potato
1 tomato or 1 c tomato juice
1 baked sweet potato
½ c cauliflower

Thiamine (vitamin B_1)*

0.50 mg

2 oz lean fresh pork

0.25 mg

1 c oysters
3 oz liver
½ c green peas
1 c orange juice
1 c dried beans or peas
½ c peanuts

0.10–0.20 mg

3 oz tuna
3 oz lean beef
1 c milk
1 slice enriched or whole wheat bread
1 c enriched farina

Riboflavin (vitamin B_2)*

1.0–2.0 mg

1 oz liver

0.20–0.30 mg

½ c cottage cheese
8 oz plain yogurt
2 eggs
1 c dark-green vegetables

0.40–0.50 mg

1 c milk or yogurt
1 c oysters
1 c (40%) bran flakes

(*continued*)

Table 5-9 Approximate Nutritional Values of Common Foods (*continued*)

Niacin	2 tbsp peanut butter
	1 c (40%) bran flakes
10 mg	
	2–3 mg
2 oz liver	3 oz ham
2 oz poultry	1 c fresh lima beans or black-eyed peas
3 oz tuna	1 c cooked corn
½ c peanuts	1 med. baked potato or
	1 c cooked potato
5 mg	1 c cooked enriched rice, spaghetti or noodles
3 oz salmon	1 c canned tomatoes or tomato juice
3 oz sardines	
1 c oysters	
3 oz lean beef, pork	

* For levels of B vitamins and iron in fortified cereals, check the labels

tered by labor and delivery and need proper time and nourishment to return to homeostasis. Table 5-11 summarizes the foods and their appropriate amounts for both breastfeeding and nonbreastfeeding women during the fourth trimester. RDAs for adult women are shown in Table 5-12.

---

*Nursing Interventions Self-Care Teaching: Nutritional Recommendations for Optimal Maternal Health**

- Maintain an adequate diet by eating a variety of foods daily. These foods should include:
  - Fruits
  - Vegetables
  - Whole-grain and enriched breads, cereals, and grain products
  - Milk, cheese, and yogurt
  - Meats, poultry, fish, and eggs
- Avoid too much fat, saturated fat, and cholesterol.
  - Choose lean meat, fish, poultry, dry beans, and peas as good protein sources.

(*text continues on pg. 144*)

*(Copyright, B Abrams, Department of OB/GYN and Reproductive Sciences, University of California, San Francisco, Reprinted by permission.)

Table 5-10 Sample Menus from Various Cultures Giving an Adequate Diet

Meals	(X) Mexican	(0) Asian	(—) Black	(√) Lacto-Ovo-Veget.	Pregnancy Guide Number of Servings to Have Each Day: *Protein (4)*	*Milk (4)*	*Grains (4)*	*Vit. C (1–2)*	*Green Veg. (1–2)*	*Other Fruits (2)*	*Fats & Oils (3 tsp)*
Breakfast	2 corn tortillas	1 c steamed rice	½ c grits w/	1 c brown rice	M X	XX	X				X
	1 c beans	½ c tofu	1 c milk	1 tbsp honey	A 0	½	00				0
Time ___	2 oz jack cheese	2 oz fish	2 eggs	1 c milk	B —	—	—				—
	on beans	Tea	1 biscuit	1 c orange juice	L	√	√√	√√			√
	1 c hot chocolate										
	milk										
Snack	1 quesadilla:	2 oz cheese	1 orange *or*	1 piece toast	M	X	X				
	corn tortilla	1 peach or apple	1 c orange	2 tbsp peanut	A	0				0	
Time ___	w/1–2 oz		juice	butter	B			—			
	melted cheese				L √		√				
Lunch	2 corn tortillas	1 c steamed rice	3 oz fried pork	1 c pinto beans	M XX		X	XX	X		X
	1 c beans	2 oz beef strips	w/1 c black-	½ c rice	A 0	0	00		0		0
Time ___	1 c caldo (soup)	w/1 c fried	eyed peas	Salad: ½ c	B —	½	—		—	—	—
	w/2 oz chicken	vegetables:	1 c turnip	spinach	L √	√	√		√		√
	Salad: 1 green	snow peas,	greens	w/tomato,							
	pepper,	broccoli,	1 potato	onion,							
	tomatoes,	chinese cabbage	½ c ice cream	cucumber,							
	lettuce	1 c milk custard	& 1 peach	carrot							
	1 c orange juice			1 c milk							

(continued)

Table 5-10 Sample Menus from Various Cultures Giving an Adequate Diet (*continued*)

Meals	(X) Mexican	(0) Asian	(—) Black	(√) Lacto-Ovo-Veget.	Pregnancy Guide Number of Servings to Have Each Day: *Protein (4)*	*Milk (4)*	*Grains (4)*	*Vit. C (1–2)*	*Green Veg. (1–2)*	*Other Fruits (2)*	*Fats & Oils (3 tsp)*
Snack	Peaches w/1 c	4 rice crackers	1 c buttermilk	Hot sandwich	M X		XX		X		
	cottage cheese	1 oz cheese	4 crackers	w/2 pieces	A ½	0	00				
Time ___		1 c orange juice	1 banana	whole wheat	B —	—			—		
				toast and	L √	√√			√		
				2 oz cheese							
				Peaches							
Dinner	2 oz stewed	2 oz cashew	1 c meat &	1 c rice	M X		XX		X	X	X
or	chicken	chicken	beans	1 c lentils	A 0	0	00		0		0
Supper	2 corn tortillas	1 c fried rice	1 c collard	1 stalk broccoli	B —	½	—		—		—
	1 sweet potato	1 c vegetables:	greens	w/2 oz cheese	L √	√	√√		√	√	√
Time ___	Spinach, raw	bean sprouts,	Cornbread	*or*							
	1 carrot	peppers, green	Pudding made	1 c pineapple							
	Mango juice	onions,	w/½ c milk	juice							
		mushrooms									
		1 c tofu									
		Tea									
Bedtime Snack	1 c flan made	½ c nuts &	1 piece toast	¼ c nuts and	M	½					
	w/½ c milk	seeds	2 oz cheese	seeds on	A 0					0	
Time ___	*or* 1 c hot	Peaches	Strawberries	1 c yogurt	B	—	—	—			
	chocolate			w/fruit	L √	√				√	

Table 5-11 Food Guide for the Fourth Trimester

Food Group	Suggested Servings Per Day			Lower-Calorie Food Choices
	Breastfeeding		*Not Breast-Feeding*	
	Dairy	*No Dairy*		
Protein foods (vegetable or animal) 1 serving = 2 oz cooked meat, poultry, fish 2 eggs 2 tbsp to ¼ cup nutbutter ½ cup nuts or seeds 1 cup cooked beans, peas ½ cup low-fat cottage cheese	4	6–8	4	Trim fat from all meats. Use more fish and poultry (white meat) than red meat. Remove poultry skin. Use water-packed canned fish. Limit luncheon meats (high in fat). Use dry-roasted nuts and old-fashioned style peanut butter.
Dairy products 1 serving = 1 cup milk, yogurt ⅓ cup dry milk powder 1 cup tofu or soymilk 1½ oz hard cheese 1⅓ cup ice cream 1 cup soft frozen yogurt	5	0–1†	2	Nonfat milk or a mixture of nonfat and low-fat. Nonfat or plain yogurt. Limit ice cream. Use yogurt in place of sour cream. Cook with nonfat milk.

(continued)

Table 5-11 Food Guide for the Fourth Trimester (*continued*)

	Suggested Servings Per Day			
	Breastfeeding		*Not Breast-Feeding*	
Food Group	*Dairy*	*No Dairy*		**Lower-Calorie Food Choices**
Grains (whole grains are best) 1 serving = 1 slice bread 1 oz cereal (cold) ½ cup cooked hot cereal ½ cup cooked pasta or rice 1 tbsp wheat germ 1 tortilla	4+	4+	3+	Limit amount of fat (margarine, butter, mayonnaise), sauces, and sweets (jam) you add to grains. Limit sweet rolls, donuts, cookies, croissants, rich crackers (look for fat listed toward the front of the ingredient list). Use cereals without added oil, shortening, sugar, or honey.
Vitamin C-rich vegetables 1 serving = ½ to ¾ cup citrus juice or brocccoli, cabbage, peppers, cantaloupe, tomato, strawberries	2+	2+	1+	Overcooking destroys vitamin C. Use fresh fruits or those canned without added sugar. Drink fruit fizzes (juice and water) in place of full-strength juice.

Leafy green vetegables 1 serving = 1 cup, raw or cooked	1+	1+	1+	Steam or stir-fry or eat raw. Avoid sauces, added fat, etc. Use low-fat salad dressing.
Other fruits and vegetables 1 serving = ½ cup to ¾ cup	2+	2+	2+	Snack on fruits and vegetables often. Limit avocados (high in calories).

* Plus supplemented calcium (1000 mg/day)

† Only for mothers who must avoid milk products because of allergy or lactase deficiency

Table 5-12 Recommended Dietary Allowances for Adult Women

	Woman's Condition		
Nutrients	*Pregnant*	*Lactating*	*Nonlactating*
Calories	2300	2500	2000
Protein (g)	74	64	44
Vitamin A (mcg RE)*	1000	1200	800
Vitamin D (mcg cholecalciferol)	10	10	5
Vitamin E (mg α TE)†	10	11	8
Vitamin C (mg)	80	100	60
Folacin (mg)	800	500	400
Niacin (mg NE)‡	15	18	13
Riboflavin (mg)	1.5	1.7	1.2
Thiamine (mg)	1.4	1.5	1
Vitamin B_6 (mg)	2.6	2.5	2
Vitamin B_{12} (mcg)	4	4	3
Calcium (mg)	1200	1200	800
Phosphorus (mg)	1200	1200	800
Iodine (mcg)	175	200	150
Iron (mg)	18+	18+	18
Magnesium (mg)	450	450	300
Zinc (mg)	20	25	15

* RE = retinol equivalents
† TE = tocopherol equivalents
‡ NE = niacin equivalents
(National Research Council, National Academy of Sciences: Recommended Dietary Allowances, 9th ed. Washington, DC, 1980)

- Use egg yolks and organ meats such as liver in moderation.
- Limit intake of butter, cream, hydrogenated margarines, shortenings, coconut oil, and foods made from such products.
- Trim excess fat from meats.
- Broil, bake, or boil rather than fry.
- Read labels carefully to determine the amounts and types of fat contained in food.
- Eat more meatless or low-meat meals.
- Use nonfat or low-fat dairy products.

- Eat more complex carbohydrates daily.
  - Substitute starches for fats and sugars.
  - Select foods that are good sources of fiber and starch, such as whole-grain breads and cereals, fruits and vegetables, beans, peas and nuts.

- Avoid excessive sugar.
  - Use less of all sugars, including white sugar, brown sugar, raw sugar, honey, and syrups.
  - Eat less food containing these sugars, such as candy, soft drinks, ice cream, cakes, and cookies.
  - Eat fresh fruits or fruits canned without sugar; eat fruits canned in light syrup rather than fruits canned in heavy syrup.
  - Read food labels for clues about sugar content; if an "–ose" word (e.g., sucrose, glucose, maltose, dextrose, lactose, fructose) or the word syrup appears first, the food contains a large amount of sugar.
  - Remember that how often you eat sugar is as important as how much sugar you eat.
- Avoid too much sodium.
  - Learn to enjoy the unsalted flavors of foods.
  - Cook with small amounts of added salt.
  - Add little or no salt to food at the table.
  - Limit your intake of salty foods, such as potato chips, pretzels, salted nuts and popcorn, condiments (soy sauce, steak sauce, garlic salt), cheese, pickled foods, and cured meats.
  - Read food labels carefully to determine the amounts of sodium present in processed foods and snack items.
  - If you crave salt during pregnancy, salt your food to taste and tell your health care provider you are doing so.
- Exercise regularly.
- Assure your baby an adequate diet.
- Breastfeed, unless there are special health problems.
- Delay solid baby foods until the baby is 4 to 6 months old.
- Do not add salt or sugar to the baby's food.

Self-Care Teaching: Keeping Physically and Mentally Fit

- Walk for exercise; it is an excellent way to avoid excessive fatigue and may help to even out mood swings.
- Spend time with other parents of small children, and talk about what you like and don't like about parenthood with each other.
- Take a little more time with your appearance than you ordinarily would early in pregnancy; this may keep your self-confidence up and prevent you from getting discouraged about physical changes.
- Seek out experienced parents and talk about concerns you may have.

- Take time to have fun alone with your partner early in pregnancy; this will help you talk things out and support each other better.

Infant Nutritional Needs in the First Year of Life

- Breast milk is sufficient to meet the nutritional needs of the infant for the first 4 to 6 months of life, although some supplementation for particular nutrients is necessary after 6 months of age.
- Commercially prepared infant formulas are also sufficient to meet the infant's nutritional needs for the first 4 to 6 months of life; after 6 months the diet should be supplemented with solid foods.

Forms for Commercial Formulas

- Concentrated (liquid): Requires dilution with equal amounts of water
- Powdered form: Requires mixing with water according to directions
- Ready-to-use: Requires measuring into individual bottles for feeding
- Ready-to-use, prepackaged: Ready to feed in disposable bottles

See Table 5-13.

Recommended Dietary Allowance for Infants

See Table 5-14.

General Characteristics of a Well-Nourished Infant

- Steady increase in weight and height
- Regular sleeping and elimination patterns
- Vigorous activity and generally happy disposition
- Firm muscles and moderate amount of subcutaneous fat
- Teething at 5 to 6 months

(*text continues on pg. 151*)

Table 5-13 Nutritional Information for Commonly Used Commercial Infant Formulas

	Enfamil	Similac	SMA	Soy Isolates*
Components				
Protein	Nonfat milk	Nonfat milk	Whey and nonfat milk	Soy isolate
Fat	Vegetable oils	Vegetable oils	Vegetable and oleo oils	Vegetable oils
Carbohydrate	Lactose	Lactose	Lactose	Corn syrup and/or sucrose
Major Constituents				
Protein	1.5	1.55	1	1.8–2.5
Fat	3.7	3.6	3.6	3–3.6
Carbohydrates	7.0	7.1	7.2	6.4–6.8
Ash (minerals)	0.36	0.37	0.3	0.4–0.5
Cal per oz†	20	20	20	20
Percent of Calories				
Protein	9	9	9	12–15
Fat	50	48	48	45–48
Carbohydrate	41	43	43	39–40

(*continued*)

Table 5-13 Nutritional Information for Commonly Used Commercial Infant Formulas (*continued*)

	Enfamil	Similac	SMA	Soy Isolates*
Minerals per Liter				
Sodium (mEq)	11	11	6.5	9–24
Potassium (mEq)	19	19	14.3	15–28
Chloride (mEq)	12	17	10	7–15
Calcium (mg)	536	600	445	700–950
Phosphorus (mg)	454	440	300	500–690
Magnesium (mg)	46	40	53	50–80
Copper (mg)	0.6	0.4	0.4	0.4–0.6
Zinc (mg)	4.1	5	3.2	2–5.3
Iodine (mcg)	67	40	69	70–160
Iron (mg)‡	1.5	Trace	12.7	8.5–12.7
Vitamins per Liter				
A (IU)	1650	2500	2650	2100–2500
D (IU)	413	400	423	400–423
E (IU)	12.4	15	9.5	9–11
K (mg)	—§	—§	—§	0.09–0.15
C (mg)	52	55	58	50–55

Thiamine (mcg)	510	650	710	400–700
Riboflavin (mcg)	620	1000	1060	600–1060
Niacin (mg)	8.25	7	7	5–8.4
Pyridoxine (mcg)	410	400	423	400–530
Folacin (mcg)	100	50	32	50–100
B_{12} (mcg)	2	1.5	1.1	2–3
Pantothenate (mg)	3.1	3	2.1	2.6–5

* Prosobee, Isomil, Nursoy, Neo-mulsoy, i-soyalac (contains tapioca starch).
† Diluted per manufacturer's specifications.
‡ Enfamil with iron contains 12.7 mg; Similac with iron, 12 mg per liter.
§ Vitamin K not added because milk base supplies ample amounts.
(Renia D: Infant nutrition. Clin Perinatol 2:384, 1975)

Table 5-14 Recommended Dietary Allowances for Infants

Nutrient	Recommended Dietary Allowance: *Birth to 6 Months*	Recommended Dietary Allowance: *6 Months to 1 Year*
Calories	kg × 115	kg × 105
* Protein (g)	kg × 2.2	kg × 2
Vitamin A (mcg RE)†	420	400
* Vitamin D (mcg, cholecalciferol)	10	10
Vitamin E (mg, α TE)‡	3	4
* Vitamin C (mg)	35	35
Folacin (mcg)	30	45
Niacin (mg, NE)§	6	8
Riboflavin (mg)	0.4	0.6
Thiamin (mg)	0.3	0.5
* Vitamin B_6 (mg)	0.3	0.6
Vitamin B_{12} (mcg)	0.5	1.5
* Calcium (mg)	360	540
* Phosphorus (mg)	240	360
Iodine (mcg)	40	50
Magnesium (mg)	50	70
Zinc (mg)	3	5
* Iron (mg)	10	15

* Only these nutrients have been discussed in this chapter.
† RE = retinol equivalents
‡ TE = tocopherol equivalents
§ NE = niacin equivalents
(National Academy of Sciences, National Research Council: Recommended Dietary Allowances, 9th ed. Washington, DC, Government Printing Office, 1980)

Table 5-15 Typical Pattern of Infant Feedings

Age of Baby	Number of Feedings	Volume per Feeding	Total
Birth–2 weeks	6–10	2–3 oz	12–30 oz
2 weeks to 1 month	6–8	3–4 oz	18–32 oz
1–3 months	5–6	5–6 oz	25–36 oz
3–7 months	4–5	6–7	25–36 oz
7–12 months	3–4	7–8 oz	25–36 oz

Nursing Interventions

Typical patterns of infant feeding are shown in Table 5-15.

---

*Self-Care Teaching: Feeding Your Baby**

- Breast milk or formula is sufficient for the first 4 to 6 months of life for most babies.
- Many babies show signs of readiness for solid food by the age of 6 months. When you are certain your baby is ready for baby food:
  - Introduce the simplest foods first.
  - Add only one new food at a time (no mixtures), and wait 5 to 7 days to see how your baby adjusts to that food. If your baby shows an allergic reaction, discontinue that food and discuss the reaction with your baby's health care provider.
  - Allergy symptoms are vomiting, diarrhea, colic, skin rash, eczema, wheezing, and runny nose. Usually symptoms occur 2 to 3 days after you introduce the food.
  - Foods most likely to cause allergies are cow's milk, egg white, wheat, peanuts, corn, soybeans, citrus, strawberries, tomatoes, chocolate, and fish.
  - At first, offer small amounts (1 tbsp or less) of food from a spoon. Make the food thin and smooth by mixing it with a little breast milk or formula.
  - As your baby grows older, remember to vary the textures of the foods you provide. A 6-month old needs strained (very thin) food; by 8 months most babies do well with mashed, lumpy foods; by 10 months give the baby bits of tender, well-cooked foods to feed himself or herself.
- Store-bought or homemade baby food?
  - It is easy and fun to make food for your baby at home. Ask your nurse or nutritionist for information on making baby food. Your kitchen must be clean, and you will need some inexpensive kitchen equipment.
  - Store-bought baby food is nutritious if you follow these suggestions:

    (1) Buy only single foods (there is as much protein in one jar of strained chicken as in 4.3 jars of chicken and noodles).
    (2) Read labels to avoid sugars, salt, and starches.
    (3) Check the date on the top of the jar for freshness, and make sure the vacuum poptop has not been broken.

*(Copyright, B Abrams, Department of OB/GYN and Reproductive Sciences, University of California. San Francisco. Reprinted by permission)

(4) Do not feed your baby directly from the jar unless she or he can eat the entire portion in one sitting; refrigerated leftovers eaten later can cause food poisoning.

- Better bottle feeding: Bottles are for water, formula, or breast milk only.
  (1) No solids (cereals, etc) should be put in bottles; feed solids with a spoon.
  (2) Koolaid, sodas, and even juices can give a baby cavities when fed from a bottle. Juices should be fed from a cup. Koolaid and sodas should be avoided; they provide only empty calories.
  (3) Always hold your baby when giving a bottle. Your love is as important as the food. "Propping" the bottle can cause problems such as choking, cavities, and ear infections.
- Never force your baby to finish food or milk she or he doesn't want. Overfeeding can lead to weight problems.
- Do not give your baby the following foods during the first year or two of life; nuts, raw carrots, popcorn, seeds and other foods that might cause choking, honey in any form (honey can cause food poisoning).

NOTES

6
Nursing Assessment of the Pregnant Woman

PRENATAL CARE

Maternity care is changing. Women are recognizing their special needs for support and are acquiring knowledge about their bodies, about the bodily changes that occur during pregnancy, and about what might happen during pregnancy and birth. Nurses are health professionals whose ideals seem to best fit the special needs of pregnant women. Consequently, more than ever nurses must prepare themselves to assume responsibility for teaching, informing, and providing care to the pregnant woman and her family.

Nursing Objectives in Prenatal Care

- To ensure that pregnancy will culminate with the delivery of a healthy baby without impairing the mother's health
- To make the family's experience one of positive growth

Possible Nursing Diagnoses Related to Prenatal Care

- Alteration in comfort related to nausea/vomiting from increased estrogen levels, decreased blood sugar, or decreased gastric motility
- Alteration in comfort related to heartburn due to pressure on the cardiac sphincter from enlarged uterus
- Activity intolerance related to fatigue and dyspnea secondary to pressure from the enlarging uterus on the diaphragm and increased blood volume
- Alteration in bowel elimination related to constipation from decreased gastric motility and pressure from the uterus on the lower colon

- Potential disturbance in self-concept related to the effects of pregnancy on biologic and psychosocial patterns
- Potential knowledge deficit of the effects of pregnancy on the body systems, fetal growth and development, nutritional requirements, psychosocial domain, and changes in the family unit

---

Trimesters of Pregnancy

Pregnancy is divided into three trimesters, each approximately 13 weeks:

- Weeks 1 to 13
- Weeks 14 to 27
- Weeks 28 to 40

A fourth trimester is sometimes used to denote the postpartum weeks of recovery.

THE FIRST PRENATAL VISIT

Nursing Objectives in the First Prenatal Visit

- To determine factors in the patient's, partner's, and family's past history that may affect the pregnant woman's prenatal course, pregnancy outcome, and long-term health
- To assess the patient's past and present physical and emotional health
- To inform the patient and her partner about her pregnancy and prenatal needs
- To establish early rapport that will grow as the nurse and the pregnant woman together set priorities for prenatal care and related problems

---

Nursing Assessment

The first prenatal visit is usually extended and may last 1 to 2 hours. The events of this visit generally progress in the following order:

1. Orienting the patient to the setting. Welcome the patient and provide her with a brief description of the setting, its hours of operation, telephone numbers for contacting care providers, and an explanation of what happens during the first prenatal visit.
2. Collecting a health history. The health history is a brief biography and should elicit the following information:
   - Demographic data
   - Menstrual history
   - Present pregnancy: problems, medications, smoking, street drugs, alcohol use, occupational hazards (See Appendix C-1, reported effects of drug exposure on the fetus)
   - Previous pregnancies: abortions (spontaneous, therapeutic); full term; preterm; birthplace; type of delivery, hours of labor, condition of infant; complications of labor and delivery; postpartum complications
   - Past medical history
   - Family history
   - Review of systems (ROS)
3. Pregnancy diagnosis. See Chapter 4.

Calculation of Last Menstrual Period and Expected Date of Confinement

The average length of pregnancy as calculated from the first day of the last menstrual period (LMP) is 280 days: 40 weeks, 10 lunar months, or 9 calendar months. The expected date of confinement (EDC), or the date of delivery, can be estimated by using Nägele's rule.

According to Nägele's rule, the EDC is calculated by adding 7 days to the date of the first day of the last menstrual period and then counting back 3 months: the first day of the LMP plus 7 days minus 3 months equals the EDC. For example, if a women's last normal menstrual period began on February 4, her expected date of delivery would be November 11:

February 4 + 7 = February 11
February 11 − 3 months = November 11 (EDC)

As shown in Table 6–1, the obstetric calendar can be used to determine the EDC. Gestational calculators in the form of wheels can be used not only to determine the EDC but also the weeks of gestation and the estimated length and weight of the fetus for each week of gestation.

(*text continues on pg. 158*)

Table 6-1 Obstetric Calendar

January	1	2	3	4	5	6	7	8	9	10	11	12	13	14	15	16	17	18	19	20	21	22	23	24	25	26	27	28	29	30	31	January
October	8	9	10	11	12	13	14	15	16	17	18	19	20	21	22	23	24	25	26	27	28	29	30	31	1	2	3	4	5	6	7	November
February	1	2	3	4	5	6	7	8	9	10	11	12	13	14	15	16	17	18	19	20	21	22	23	24	25	26	27	28				February
November	8	9	10	11	12	13	14	15	16	17	18	19	20	21	22	23	24	25	26	27	28	29	30	1	2	3	4	5				December
March	1	2	3	4	5	6	7	8	9	10	11	12	13	14	15	16	17	18	19	20	21	22	23	24	25	26	27	28	29	30	31	March
December	6	7	8	9	10	11	12	13	14	15	16	17	18	19	20	21	22	23	24	25	26	27	28	29	30	31	1	2	3	4	5	January
April	1	2	3	4	5	6	7	8	9	10	11	12	13	14	15	16	17	18	19	20	21	22	23	24	25	26	27	28	29	30		April
January	6	7	8	9	10	11	12	13	14	15	16	17	18	19	20	21	22	23	24	25	26	27	28	29	30	31	1	2	3	4		February
May	1	2	3	4	5	6	7	8	9	10	11	12	13	14	15	16	17	18	19	20	21	22	23	24	25	26	27	28	29	30	31	May
February	5	6	7	8	9	10	11	12	13	14	15	16	17	18	19	20	21	22	23	24	25	26	27	28	1	2	3	4	5	6	7	March
June	1	2	3	4	5	6	7	8	9	10	11	12	13	14	15	16	17	18	19	20	21	22	23	24	25	26	27	28	29	30		June
March	8	9	10	11	12	13	14	15	16	17	18	19	20	21	22	23	24	25	26	27	28	29	30	31	1	2	3	4	5	6		April

July	1	2	3	4	5	6	7	8	9	10	11	12	13	14	15	16	17	18	19	20	21	22	23	24	25	26	27	28	29	30	31	July
April	7	8	9	10	11	12	13	14	15	16	17	18	19	20	21	22	23	24	25	26	27	28	29	30	1	2	3	4	5	6	7	May
August	1	2	3	4	5	6	7	8	9	10	11	12	13	14	15	16	17	18	19	20	21	22	23	24	25	26	27	28	29	30	31	Auust
May	8	9	10	11	12	13	14	15	16	17	18	19	20	21	22	23	24	25	26	27	28	29	30	31	1	2	3	4	5	6	7	June
September	1	2	3	4	5	6	7	8	9	10	11	12	13	14	15	16	17	18	19	20	21	22	23	24	25	26	27	28	29	30		September
June	8	9	10	11	12	13	14	15	16	17	18	19	20	21	22	23	24	25	26	27	28	29	30	1	2	3	4	5	6	7		July
October	1	2	3	4	5	6	7	8	9	10	11	12	13	14	15	16	17	18	19	20	21	22	23	24	25	26	27	28	29	30	31	October
July	8	9	10	11	12	13	14	15	16	17	18	19	20	21	22	23	24	25	26	27	28	29	30	31	1	2	3	4	5	6	7	August
November	1	2	3	4	5	6	7	8	9	10	11	12	13	14	15	16	17	18	19	20	21	22	23	24	25	26	27	28	29	30		November
August	8	9	10	11	12	13	14	15	16	17	18	19	20	21	22	23	24	25	26	27	28	29	30	31	1	2	3	4	5	6		September
December	1	2	3	4	5	6	7	8	9	10	11	12	13	14	15	16	17	18	19	20	21	22	23	24	25	26	27	28	29	30	31	December
September	7	8	9	10	11	12	13	14	15	16	17	18	19	20	21	22	23	24	25	26	27	28	29	30	1	2	3	4	5	6	7	October

Locate the date of the first day of the last menstrual period in the top line of any of the above pairs of lines. The date directly below is the expected date of confinement.

SUBSEQUENT PRENATAL VISITS

Schedule for Return Prenatal Visits

- Every 4 weeks until 28 weeks of pregnancy
- Every 2 weeks until 36 weeks of pregnancy
- Every week until delivery

Activities at these visits include:

- Status of pregnancy between visits
- Nutritional assessment of current eating practices
- Physical examination including:
  - Blood pressure
    Blood pressure taken early in pregnancy provides a baseline for evaluation and comparison of readings that may become elevated later in gestation. A systolic increase of 30 mm Hg or a diastolic increase of 15 mm Hg above baseline blood pressure is significant.
  - Weight
    Prepregnant weight is used to assess sequential total pregnancy weight gain. Early loss of weight below prepregnant levels may mean that the woman has experienced nausea and vomiting. Immediate referral for nutritional counseling is needed to avoid dehydration or ketosis. Weight gain that is greater than average in late pregnancy (5 lb or more in 1 week) may indicate overeating, high salt intake, water retention, or, possibly, preeclampsia.

NURSING ASSESSMENT

Complete Physical Examination

A complete physical examination should be performed on every pregnant woman. Physical findings will be different from normal ones in those women in whom pregnancy changes are most dramatic. The physical assessment of these areas includes:

- Palpation of the thyroid
- Auscultation of maternal heart tones
- Inspection and palpation of the breasts
- Inspection and palpation of the abdomen
- Measurement of fundal height
- Auscultation of fetal heart tones
- Pelvic examination

Table 6-2 describes body changes that can be assessed on physical examination.

Abdominal Palpation

Before 12 to 13 weeks gestation the pregnant uterus remains a pelvic organ and cannot be palpated abdominally. From the time it rises into the abdomen at 12 weeks until it reaches the umbilicus at 20 weeks gestation, the uterus is measured in fingerbreadths. After this time it can be measured in either fingerbreadths or centimeters, as shown in Figure 6-1. McDonald's measurements in centimeters can be used instead of fingerbreadths after 20 weeks when uterine height measurement by week approximates centimeters of height. When there is a discrepancy between uterine size and pregnancy dating, the following parameters may be used:

- Size of the uterus at the first prenatal visit
- Presence of the uterus in the pelvis (<12 weeks gestation)
- Presence of the uterus in the abdomen (>12 weeks gestation)
- Date of the first positive pregnancy test
- Weeks of pregnancy as correlated with last menses
- Size of the uterus in relation to estimated fetal gestational age
- Fetal heart sounds heard just above the symphysis with a fetoscope at 20 weeks gestation
- Fetal movement (quickening) felt by 20 weeks gestation—occurs earlier in multigravid women
- Sonography report at 13 to 16 weeks—the optimum time for accurate reporting of fetal age (gestation)

Leopold's Maneuvers

Leopold's maneuvers are used to palpate the fetus to determine its position and presenting part and to determine its attitude, as shown in the accompanying display.

Auscultation of Fetal Heart Tones

Detected as early as 8 weeks with a Doppler ultrasound or at 18 to 20 weeks with a fetoscope, the normal fetal heart rate (FHR) is 120 to 160 beats per minute. Points of maximum intensity for auscultation of fetal heart tones are shown in Figure 6-2.

(*text continues on pg. 166*)

Table 6-2 Body Changes in Pregnancy That Can Be Assessed on Physical Examination

Normal Changes	Discomforts	Problems
Head and Neck		
Increased nasal vascularity	Epistaxis (nosebleeds)	
Chloasma (mask of pregnancy)	Cosmetic concern; may persist	
Epulis (gingival growth)	Bleeding gums, difficulty eating and keeping teeth clean	
Ptyalism (excessive secretion of saliva)	Nausea	Malnutrition
Enlarged, thyroid gland; increased basal metabolic rate	Palpitations, tachycardia, fatigue	
Chest		
Increased circumference of chest wall	Hyperventilation, dyspnea	
Lateral movement of apex of heart		
Exaggerated splitting of first heart sound, loud third sound		
Systolic murmur in 90% of pregnant women; brachial blood pressure—highest when patient is sitting		High blood pressure
Spider angiomas		

Breasts		
Enlargement of breasts, erection of nipples, darkening of areola, secretion of colostrum	Tenderness, tingling	Enlargement of supernumerary breast tissue in axilla
Abdomen/Gastrointestinal Tract		
Increase in uterine size; rising of uterus from pelvis at 12 to 13 weeks gestation	Nausea, vomiting	Weight loss; hyperemesis gravidarum
Sensation of fetal movement at 18 to 20 weeks gestation		Absence of fetal movement; lower abdominal pain
Striae gravidarum		
Linea nigra		
Back		
Increased lumbar curvature		Backache
Pelvis		
Increased white vaginal discharge		Increased risk for vaginal infection due to low *p*H
Increased risk of urinary tract infection; decreased bladder tone	Increased frequency and urgency of urination	Nocturia; dysuria; costovertebral angle tenderness; protein, glucose, ketones in urine

(*continued*)

Table 6-2 Body Changes in Pregnancy That Can Be Assessed on Physical Examination (*continued*)

Normal Changes	Discomforts	Problems
Extremities		
Palmar erythema		Itching hands
Pressure on venous circulation of legs		Varicosities
Dependent edema of feet and legs		Pitting edema

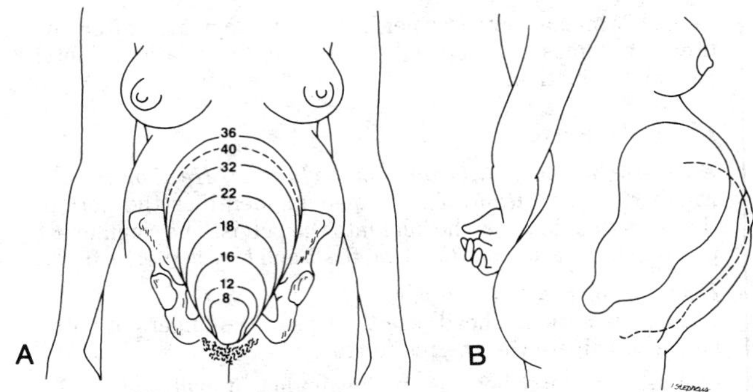

Figure 6-1 *(A)* Fundal height at various weeks of gestation. *(B)* Lightening has occurred and the presenting part has settled into the pelvis. Fundal height decreases and the uterus rests anteriorly against the abdominal wall. (In lay terms, "the baby has dropped.") (Childbirth Graphics)

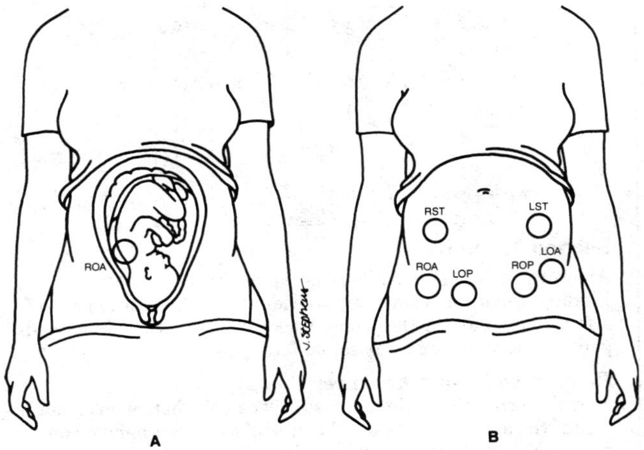

Figure 6-2 Points of maximum intensity for auscultation of fetal heart tones in specific fetal positions. *(A)* Heart tones are best heard through the fetus's back. *(B)* ROA = Right occipital anterior, LOA = Left occipital anterior, LOP = Left occipital posterior, ROP = Right occipital posterior, RST = Right sacrotransverse, LST = Left sacrotransverse (Childbirth Graphics)

LEOPOLD'S MANEUVERS

Leopold's maneuvers are performed in pregnancy after the uterus becomes large enough to allow differentiation of fetal parts by palpation.

First Maneuver

Answers the question: *What is in the fundus? Head or breech?* Finding: *Presentation.* This maneuver identifies the part of the fetus that lies over the inlet into the pelvis. The commonest presentations are *cephalic* (head first) and *breech* (pelvis first).

Performing First Maneuver
Facing the patient's head, use the tips of the fingers of both hands to palpate the uterine fundus.

- When the fetal head is in the fundus, it will feel hard, smooth, globular, mobile, and ballotable.
- When the breech is in the fundus, it will feel soft, irregular, round, and less mobile.

The *lie* of the fetus—the relationship between the long axis of the fetus and the long axis of the mother—can also be determined during the first maneuver. The lie is commonly longitudinal or transverse, but may occasionally be oblique.

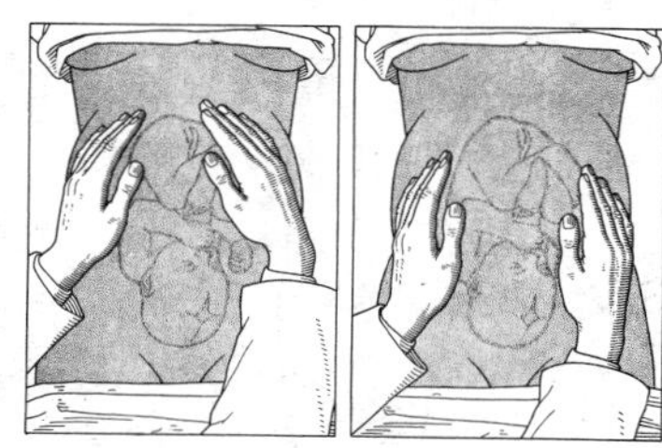

Second Maneuver

Answers the question: *Where is the back?*
Finding: *Position.* This maneuver identifies the relationship of a fetal body part to the front, back, or sides of the maternal pelvis. There are many possible fetal positions.

Performing Second Maneuver
Remain facing the patient's head. Place your hands on either side of the abdomen. Steady the uterus with your hand on one side, and palpate the opposite side to determine the location of the fetal back.

- The back will feel firm, smooth, convex, resistant.
- The small parts (arms and legs) will feel small, irregularly placed, and knobby and may be actively or passively mobile.

Third Maneuver

Answers the question: *What is the presenting part?*
Finding: *Presenting Part.* This maneuver identifies the most dependent part of the fetus—that is, the part that lies nearest the cervix. It is the part of the fetus that first contacts the finger in the vaginal examination, most commonly the head or breech.

Performing Third Maneuver
Turn and face the patient's feet. Place the tips of the first three fingers and thumb of one hand on either side of the patient's abdomen just above the symphysis, and ask the patient to take a deep breath and let it out. As she exhales, sink your fingers down slowly and deeply around the presenting part. Note the contour, size, and consistency of the part.

- The head will feel hard, smooth, and mobile if not engaged, immobile if engaged.
- The breech will feel soft and irregular.

Fourth Maneuver

Answers the question: *Where is the cephalic prominence?*
Finding: *Cephalic Prominence.* This maneuver identifies the greatest prominence of the fetal head palpated over the brim

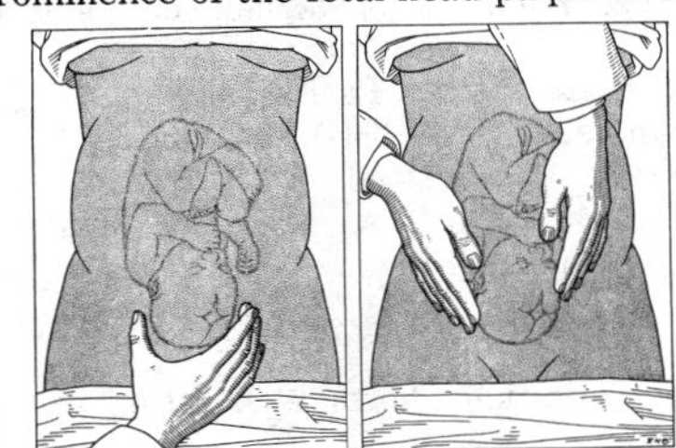

of the pelvis. When the head is flexed (flexion attitude), the forehead forms the cephalic prominence. When the head is extended (extension attitude), the occiput becomes the cephalic prominence.

Performing Fourth Maneuver
Face the patient's feet. Gently move your fingers down the sides of the abdomen toward the pelvis until the fingers of one hand encounter a bony prominence. This is the cephalic prominence. If the prominence is on the opposite side from the back, it is the baby's brow, and the head is flexed. If the head is extended, the cephalic prominence will be located on the same side as the back and will be the occiput.

(Illustrations from Pritchard J, MacDonald P: Williams' Obstetrics, 16th ed. Norwalk, Conn., Appleton-Century-Crofts, 1980. Reprinted by permission)

Pelvic Examination

The pelvic examination includes inspection and palpation of the external genitalia (Table 6-3); speculum examination (Table 6-4); and bimanual and rectovaginal examinations (Table 6-5).

Prenatal Laboratory Studies

Initial Visit

- Complete blood cell count (CBC)
- Rh and blood type
- Antibody screen
- Rubella titer
- VDRL
- Urinalysis and/or urine culture
- Pap smear
- Gonorrhea smear
- Hemoglobin electrophoresis (sickle cell screening for black patients)
- Hepatitis screen (Asians and Pacific Islanders)
- Purified protein derivative (PPD), as indicated
- Chlamydia culture, as indicated
- Alpha-fetoprotein at 16 to 18 weeks of pregnancy
- Wet mount of vaginal secretions, as indicated

See Table 6-6. For additional normal laboratory values and reference tables see Appendix A 1-3.

Repeat Laboratory Studies (as appropriate)

- Urine dipstick for glucose, protein, ketones: each visit
- CBC or Hbg to assess anemia: each trimester
- In Rh−, unsensitized patients, repeat antibody screen at 24, 28, 32, and 36 weeks.
- Cervical smear for gonorrhea early in third trimester
- Wet mount to detect possible vaginal infections
- Other studies as appropriate for individual patients

(*text continues on pg. 194*)

Table 6-3 Inspection and Palpation of the External Genitalia

Organ or Structure	Action	Normal Findings	Pregnancy Changes	Abnormal Findings
Inspection				
Mons Pubis	Adjust the light and sit on a stool at the foot of the table facing the patient's perineum. Inspect the external genitals.	Mature secondary sexual characteristics	None	
		Skin covered by inverse triangle of curly hair (female escutcheon)	None	Pediculosis pubis (crab lice) or nits (eggs on hair shafts). Pruritus (itching), excoriation from scratching, folliculitis (infected hair follicle)

(continued)

Table 6-3 Inspection and Palpation of the External Genitalia (*continued*)

Organ or Structure	Action	Normal Findings	Pregnancy Changes	Abnormal Findings
Inspection				
Labia Majora		Lie in close opposition in nulliparous women, may gap widely in multiparous ones; feel soft; have moist inner surface	Inner surface drier and skinlike	Pruritus, excoriation from scratching, lesions, vesicles, varicosities, discharge between folds from vaginal infection, Bartholin's gland tenderness, edema, redness
Inspection and Palpation				
	Tell the patient she will be touched. With gloved fingers, separate the labia majora, exposing the labia minora.			

Labia Minora		Hidden under labia majora in nulliparous women, project beyond labia majora in multiparous women; vary greatly in size and shape; feel soft	None in multiparas	Redness caused by vaginal infection or allergic reaction to douches, perfumed soap; wartlike growths, lesions
Clitoris	Observe the clitoris and retract its prepuce.	Small, erectile, highly vascular body, rarely exceeds 2 cm in length; covered by retractable prepuce	None	Clitoral hypertrophy, fixed prepuce that cannot be retracted (may interfere with sexual stimulation), lesions, chancres of sexually transmitted diseases
Urethral Meatus	Spread the labia with the index and second fingers of the gloved hand, inspect the urethra.	Vertical slit with pinkish, puckered appearance	None observable; dilatation of urethral canal due to increased progesterone	Polyps, growths, discharge, caruncle, erythema

(continued)

Table 6-3 Inspection and Palpation of the External Genitalia (*continued*)

Organ or Structure	Action	Normal Findings	Pregnancy Changes	Abnormal Findings
Skene's Ducts (on either side of urethra at 4 and 8 o'clock)	Insert the index finger of the right hand 1 inch into the introitus, and gently press upward on the urethra. This is called "milking."	Duct may or may not be observable; no discharge	None	Yellowish-white discharge oozing from Skene's duct (gonorrhea culture needed)
Vaginal Musculature	As the fingers are withdrawn from the vagina, gently spread the vaginal orifice. Holding your fingers steady, ask the patient to cough.	Firm or relaxed muscle tone	More relaxed muscle tone, particularly in multigravidas	Cystocele (prolapse of bladder that protrudes in anterior vagina); rectocele (prolapse of rectum into posterior vagina)
Pubococcygeal Musculature	Insert the fingers further into the vagina and ask the patient to tighten her muscles around your finger.	Tight muscle control	More relaxed muscle tone, particularly in multiparous women	Loss of bladder tone as a result of pregnancy; leaking of urine, especially in older women,

	(These are the muscles used to stop the stream during urination.)			when perineal muscle tone is not maintained
Bartholin's Glands	With the fingers in the vagina, sweep them laterally on either side of the posterior fourchette to palpate the Bartholin's glands at 4 and 8 o'clock.	Glands not felt	None	Gland enlargement from infection, usually unilateral; exudate from duct; reddening of skin; may be extremely painful, with patient unable to walk
Perineum (area between the vagina and anus)	Remove the gloved hand from the vagina and use both hands to spread the buttocks apart to observe the perineum and anus.	No lesions; possibly episiotomy scar from previous delivery	None	Lesions, cysts, infection
Anus		Darker skin	None	Hemorrhoids, inflammation, lesions, fissures

Table 6-4 Procedures in the Speculum Examination

Procedure	Pregnancy Changes	Abnormal Findings
With the light placed for optimum visualization:		
1. Inspect the cervix.	Nulliparous cervical os appears small and round; parous os is slitlike and may have scars from tears during previous delivery. Bluish, friable cervix (bleeds easily); ectopy, white discharge	Dilated os; yellowish, greenish, or foul-smelling discharge at cervical os; inflammation
2. Collect specimens:		
Cervical: Pap smear; gonorrhea or other cervical smears if infection suspected	Increased amount of white, normal discharge	Blood from os, lesions, irregular configuration of ectropion
Vaginal: Wet mount of saline and KOH to diagnose suspected vaginal infections	Bluish vagina, rugae present	Abnormal-appearing discharge, lesions, cysts

3. Remove the speculum in the following manner. Loosen the thumbscrew. Maintaining a downward pressure, rotate the speculum as you slowly withdraw it. Hold the thumb lightly on the thumbscrew to allow you to see the vaginal walls between the blades. As the speculum is withdrawn, it gradually closes and it will be fully closed as it is withdrawn at an oblique angle.	Pinkish blue color, rugae	Structural abnormalities, inflammation, lesions, white plaques, contact bleeding

Table 6-5 Bimanual and Rectovaginal Examination

Procedures	Pregnancy Changes	Abnormal Findings
1. Remove the glove from the left hand and lubricate the first two fingers of the right hand. Insert the lubricated fingers into the vagina, maintaining *downward pressure*. With the fingers well into the vagina rotate the hand until the palm is up. The thumb is kept vertical in the midline, while the other two fingers curve out of the way.		
Cervix		
2. Place the left hand on the abdomen halfway between the symphysis and the umbilicus. Push the vaginal hand forward and backward until each of the fingers is in a lateral fornix with the cervix in between. Palpate the cervix; it should be freely movable.	Os closed until late in pregnancy; feels soft as an earlobe. At term, feels soft as pudding.	Roughened areas, edema, bleeding, dilatation before at term, tenderness with movement.

Uterus		
3. Determine uterine position by passing the fingers along the front and back of the cervix. With the first two fingers over the cervix, push it upward, lifting the uterus into the abdomen. Palpate the uterus between the vaginal and abdominal hands by moving the uterus from side to side with one finger in the lateral fornices so that the surface of the uterus can be felt.	Shape changes from globular to ovoid. Uterine size depends on age of gestation. Feels softer than nonpregnant uterus. Irregular, painless Braxton Hicks contractions may be felt. Becomes an abdominal organ at 12 weeks.	Tenderness with movement, myomas (fibroids) felt as firm irregularities on its surface. Deviations to either side may be due to pelvic masses or adhesions
4. To palpate the adnexa, place the vaginal fingers palm upward in the right lateral fornix and the abdominal hand in the area of the right iliac crest. The hands are brought together and moved together toward the midline. The vaginal fingers will feel the ovaries slip between the fingers while the abdominal hand is pushing them downward. Repeat on the left side. In some women the ovaries are not palpable even in the nonpregnant state.)	When the uterus becomes an abdominal organ, the ovaries cannot be palpated.	Tenderness, cystic masses, firm masses, enlargement (normal size 4×6 cm)

(continued)

Table 6-5 Bimanual and Rectovaginal Examination (*continued*)

Procedures	Pregnancy Changes	Abnormal Findings
Rectovaginal Examination		
1. Wash the secretions from the vaginal examination from the gloves and apply lubricating jelly.	None	Rectal or pelvic masses, fistulas, rectocele, hemorrhoids, polyps
2. Ask the patient to bear down to relax the anal sphincter. Insert the distal half of the middle finger into the anus and the index finger into the vagina. With both fingers reach as high as possible into the pelvis, while pushing the pelvic organs toward the rectal finger with the other hand, which is placed on the abdomen. Assess the rectal tone and rectovaginal septum. The body and fundus of a retroverted uterus can be palpated in the posterior fornix, and the sacral shape, ischial spines, and length of the sacrospinous ligaments can be felt. These findings can be correlated with the pelvimetry for more definitive measurements.		

Table 6-6 Laboratory Data and Procedures to Assess the Prenatal Patient

Laboratory Test	Normal Nonpregnant Value	Normal Pregnant Value	Comments
Blood Tests			
Complete Blood Cell Count (CBC)			
White blood cell count (WBC)	4,500 to 10,000/mm^3	15,000 to 18,000/mm^3 (during pregnancy); 18,000 to 25,000/mm^3 (during delivery and immediate postpartum period)	WBCs are elevated during an infectious process, eclampsia, following hemorrhage, and in response in physiologic stress. Additional tests to detect infection should be performed to avoid unnecessary antibiotic therapy.
Red blood cell count (ml/mm^3)	4,000,000 to 5,000,000 ml/mm^3	Increased 25% to 30%	By 6 to 8 weeks of gestation there is progressive increase in blood plasma and red blood cell volume. It peaks at 28 to 32 weeks and remains constant until delivery. Plasma volume increases 40% to 50% whereas red cell mass

(continued)

Table 6-6 Laboratory Data and Procedures to Assess the Prenatal Patient (*continued*)

Laboratory Test	Normal Nonpregnant Value	Normal Pregnant Value	Comments
Blood Tests			increases only 25% to 30%, resulting in dilutional (physiologic) anemia of pregnancy.
Hemoglobin	12 to 16 g/100 ml	11.5 g/100 ml mean in midpregnancy; 12.3 g/100 ml mean in late pregnancy	Hemoglobin value measures the body's capacity to transport oxygen. Anemia is diagnosed when the value is 10.5 g/100 ml or under. The commonest form is iron deficiency anemia
Hematocrit	36% to 46%	32% to 46%	The percentage expresses the portion of the total blood volume occupied by the red blood cells. This test is also used in the detection of anemia; a value of under 32% indicates anemia.

Red Cell Indices			
Mean corpuscular volume	80 to 95 μm^3	Same	This index describes the size of the cell. A value under 80 is *microcytic*, or smaller than normal, as found in iron deficiency anemia, parasite infestation, or thalassemia. A value over 95 is *macrocytic*, or larger than normal.
Mean corpuscular hemoglobin concentration	32 to 36 g/dl	Same	This test measures the portion of each cell occupied by hemoglobin. A reading of over 39 g/dl occurs in only one condition, hereditary spherocytosis, a congenital abnormality of the cell wall. A decreased reading may indicate anemia.
Red cell morphology			This test measures variability in cell size and shape; the amount of blueness in the cells (amount of retained RNA); the presence of central pallor in the cells; other cells such as sickle cells, spherocytes, cells seen in thalassemia

(*continued*)

Table 6-6 Laboratory Data and Procedures to Assess the Prenatal Patient (*continued*)

Laboratory Test	Normal Nonpregnant Value	Normal Pregnant Value	Comments
Blood Tests			
Platelets	140,000 to 450,000/mm^3	same	
Coagulation Factors			
Fibrinogen Factor (I)	300 mg/dl	450 mg/dl	Platelet counts are unchanged, but certain coagulation factors are altered as shown. Also called thrombocytes, the platelets contribute to hemostasis by forming platelet plugs at bleeding sites and promoting thrombin formation. They are formed in the bone marrow. A decrease in their production is never benign. Low levels are found in leukemia, disseminated intravascular coagulation (DIC), uremia, severe systemic infection, and bone marrow hypofunction.
Factors II, VII, VIII, IX, and X		Increased	
Factors XI and XIII		Decreased	

Prothrombin time	11 to 12 sec	Same	Despite alterations in blood Factors II, VII, VIII, IX, X, XI, and XIII prothrombin and bleeding times remain within the normal nonpregnant range.
Bleeding time	1 to 5 min	Same	
Reticulocytes	0.5% to 1.5%	Increased	Reticulocytes are immature red blood cells that are released from the bone marrow in response to hemolysis, hemorrhage, or iron therapy for anemia. Reticulocytosis (increased production) may reach 3% in response to iron therapy in anemic pregnant women.
Erythrocyte sedimentation rate (ESR)	0 to 15 mm/hr	Not valid in pregnancy	ESR is elevated during infection and helps to document chronic inflammatory processes in patients with vague symptoms. Higher levels of fibrinogen and plasma globulins in pregnancy make this test invalid.

(*continued*)

Table 6-6 Laboratory Data and Procedures to Assess the Prenatal Patient (*continued*)

Laboratory Test	Normal Nonpregnant Value	Normal Pregnant Value	Comments
Blood Tests			
Iron			
Serum iron	50 to 150 mcg/dl	Same	Low serum values usually result from insufficient intake of iron (iron deficiency anemia). Causes include repeated pregnancies, low iron diet (especially in adolescents), heavy menses, pregnancy (600 to 900 mg iron are drained from the mother by the fetus), and IUD use
Total iron-binding capacity (TIBC)	280 to 400 mcg/dl	300 to 450 mcg/dl	The ability of the red blood cells to bind iron is increased in pregnancy because of maternal and fetal needs for iron. A simple formula to rule out iron deficiency anemia is:

			Serum iron ÷ TIBC = % saturation A result of 16% or less is diagnostic of iron deficiency anemia; such a result, in conjunction with mean corpuscular volume less than 80, requires further study.
Serum Folate	1.9 to 14.0 ng/ml		Folate is essential for production of RNA and DNA. The fetus parasitizes large quantities from the mother. Combined iron and folate deficiency is common in pregnancy. Most prenatal vitamins now supply a folate supplemental dose of 1 mg.
Electrolytes			
Sodium	135 to 148 mEq/liter	Increase in retention of 500 to 900 mEq/liter over the norm	Aldosterone is the sodium-conserving hormone of the adrenal cortex. Its excretion is increased throughout pregnancy, causing cumulative total sodium retention.

(*continued*)

Table 6-6 Laboratory Data and Procedures to Assess the Prenatal Patient (*continued*)

Laboratory Test	Normal Nonpregnant Value	Normal Pregnant Value	Comments
Blood Tests			
			Urinary loss of sodium in late pregnancy is normal.
Potassium	3.5 to 5.3 mEq/dl	Same	Aldosterone is also potassium-depleting. However, the increase in its production during pregnancy does not cause potassium wastage.
Chloride	102.7 to 107.0 mEq/liter	98 to 108 mEq/liter	There is no significant change.
Calcium	3.5 to 5.0 mg/dl	Increased	Increased intake is necessary to meet fetal requirements along with increased vitamin D to promote intestinal calcium absorption.
Phosphorus	2.5 to 4.5 mg/dl	Same	

Blood Chemistry			
Albumin	3.5 to 5.0 g/dl	3.0 to 4.2 g/dl	Albumin concentration falls quickly in the first 3 months and more slowly until late pregnancy. Decline in serum albumin below normal pregnancy levels is associated with preeclampsia.
Human chorionic gonadotropin (HCG)	None (placental hormone of pregnancy)	50,000 to 100,000 mIU/ml (early); 10,000 to 20,000 mIU/ml (late)	Concentration peaks at 10 weeks of gestation, then declines and remains at this lower level until delivery. HCG sustains progesterone secretion in early pregnancy and is necessary for growth and preparation of endometrium for implantation. Levels that far exceed normal in conjunction with exaggerated pregnancy symptoms, large-for-dates uterus, bleeding, and absent fetal heart tones may indicate trophoblastic disease.

(*continued*)

Table 6-6 Laboratory Data and Procedures to Assess the Prenatal Patient (*continued*)

Laboratory Test	Normal Nonpregnant Value	Normal Pregnant Value	Comments
Blood Tests			
Serum creatinine	0.8 to 1.4 mg/dl	0.9 to 2.0 mg/dl	Elevated levels may indicate kidney disease or pre-eclampsia.
Thyroid hormone T_3	100 to 200 ng/dl	25% to 35% decrease	T_3 is in lower concentrations than T_4 but is biologically more active and has a shorter serum halflife.
Thyroid hormone T_4	5.0 to 12.0 mcg/dl	5% to 10% increase	T_4 levels directly measure the thyroxine in serum. Increased T_3 levels and decreased T_4 levels may indicate hyper- or hypoactivity of the thyroid gland.
Hemoglobin electrophoresis (% of total hemoglobin)	Hgb A 95% to 97% Hgb A_2 2.0% to 3.5% Hgb F less than 2%	Same	This test identifies hemoglobinopathies, such as sickle cell trait or disease, hemoglobin C disease, and thalassemia, by the changed

			ratios of the three types of normal hemoglobin. (*E.g.*, Hgb A_2 level over 3.5% is diagnostic of thalassemia.)
Glucose-6-phosphate oxidative dehydrogenase (G6PD) (IU/g)	None	None	G6PD is an enzyme that protects hemoglobin from denaturation. When activity of this enzyme is less than 25% of normal, hemolysis occurs. Drugs that can precipitate anemia are acetaminophen, aspirin, sulfa drugs, vitamin K, thiazides, Furadantin, and Macrodantin, and patients should be warned against their use. In pregnancy when serum iron is normal but the patient is anemic, G6PD disease must be ruled out. Pregnancy complications include urinary tract infections, neonatal jaundice, hydrops fetalis, anemia.

(*continued*)

Table 6-6 Laboratory Data and Procedures to Assess the Prenatal Patient (*continued*)

Laboratory Test	Normal Nonpregnant Value	Normal Pregnant Value	Comments
Blood Tests			
Blood Sugar Levels			
Fasting	75 mg/100 ml	65 mg/100 ml	Screening for diabetes mellitus is done in pregnancy when there is consistent spilling of glucose in the urine (glucosuria) or there is a family history of the disease or some other indicator of diabetes.
2-hour postprandial	120 mg/100 ml (upper limit)	145 mg/100 ml (upper limit)	

The normal values for this test are as follows:

Oral glucose tolerance test	*Hour*	*Whole Blood* (mg/dl)	*Plasma* (mg/dl)	*Serum* (mg/dl)	Values that are abnormal in any two specimens constitute a positive test.
	0	90	103	100	
	1	165	188	200	
	2	145	165	150	
	3	125	143	130	

Blood Group and Rh Factor	O, A, B, AB Rh+ Rh−	Same Same Same	If the mother has type O blood and her partner has type A, B, or AB, an ABO incompatibility may exist in the infant. The incidence of clinically significant incompatibility resulting in hemolytic disease in the infant is small. To prevent Rh immunization, screening will identify that 15% of the population that is Rh−. The presence of anti-D serum identifies the Rh-immunized woman. All Rh-negative women are given anti-D globulin after abortion, amniocentesis, or delivery of an Rh+ infant.
Rubella Titer	Depends on sensitization	Same	A result of less than 1.8 indicates that the patient is *not* immune to rubella. Such a patient should be advised to avoid exposure to the disease. If she is exposed, a titer should be obtained in 3 to 4 weeks.

(continued)

Table 6-6 Laboratory Data and Procedures to Assess the Prenatal Patient (*continued*)

Laboratory Test	Normal Nonpregnant Value	Normal Pregnant Value	Comments
Blood Tests			
Serology or VDRL Test	Negative	Negative	A serology test is done to detect syphilis in the pregnant woman at the first prenatal visit. When positive, the VDRL screen is confirmed by an FTA-ABS test specific for syphilis.
Urine Tests			
Urinalysis			
*p*H Color Specific gravity	4.5 to 7.5 Yellow 1.010 to 1.020	Same Same Same	The *p*H test measures acidity or alkalinity of the urine. Levels below the norm indicate high fluid intake; levels above the norm indicate inadequate fluids and dehydration.

Protein	Negative	Negative	Small amounts may occur from vaginal contamination and dehydration. Amounts of 2+ to 4+ may indicate urinary tract or kidney infection or preeclampsia.
Glucose	Negative	Negative or 1+	Urine that registers 1+ may result from decreased renal threshold and increased glomerular filtration rate in pregnancy. High levels of glucose may indicate high levels of blood sugar, gestational diabetes, or diabetes mellitus.
Ketones	Negative	Negative	Ketone bodies are products of fatty acids and fat metabolism. Fasting causes breakdown of fat when carbohydrates and protein are not available. Ketones may be deleterious to the fetus and should be avoided in pregnancy by regular eating habits.

(*continued*)

Table 6-6 Laboratory Data and Procedures to Assess the Prenatal Patient (*continued*)

Laboratory Test	Normal Nonpregnant Value	Normal Pregnant Value	Comments
Blood Tests			
Bilirubin	Negative	Negative	Bilirubin is a product of red blood cell destruction. Its presence in urine suggests liver or gallbladder disease.
Blood	Negative	Negative	Blood in urine suggests urinary tract infection, kidney disease, or vaginal contamination.
White Blood Cells	Negative	Negative	Greater than 5 to 10 per high power field (HPF) may indicate urinary tract or vaginal infection.
Bacteria	Negative	Negative	Trace = rare; 1+ = 1 to 10/HPF; 2+ = 10 to 12/HPF; 3+ = innumerable; and 4+ = closely packed. Result greater than 4/HPF indicates urinary tract infection.

Casts	Negative	Negative	Casts are molds of the kidney tubules and may indicate kidney disease or excessive exercise.
Crystals	Few	Few	These compounds of various chemicals are found in most specimens.
Epithelial Cells	None	None	These are found when the specimen is contaminated by vaginal discharge. A clean-catch specimen should be obtained.
Urine Culture and Sensitivity	Negative	Negative	Specimens for urine cultures should be obtained by clean catch only. The test cannot be accurately read and reported when contaminated with vaginal secretions. A colony count over 100,000 (10^5) represents a positive culture and indicates urinary tract infection. The sensitivity of the infecting organism to various antibiotics is also reported.

NURSING INTERVENTIONS

Self-Care Teaching: Breast Self-Examination

Counseling About Problems in Pregnancy

Danger Signs During Pregnancy

The patient should contact her health care provider if the following symptoms occur:

- Vaginal bleeding
- Edema of the face and hands
- Continuous and severe headache
- Blurring or dimness of vision
- Abdominal pain
- Persistent vomiting
- Cessation of fetal movement
- Chills or fever
- Painful urination
- Fluid escaping from the vagina
- Dizziness when not supine

Vaginal Infections Commonly Found in Pregnant Women

See Table 6-7.

Self-Care Teaching: Vaginal Infections

The pregnant woman can diminish or avoid discomfort caused by vaginal infections and help prevent recurrent infection in the following ways:

- Practice good personal hygiene with frequent bathing and hand washing. Cleanse the perineal area from front to back after a bowel movement to prevent vaginal contamination.
- Sit in a warm sitz bath to relieve vulvar irritation.
- Avoid use of feminine hygiene sprays, bath oils, and strong soaps that may cause irritation or allergy on the vulva or in the vagina.
- Refrain from wearing clothing that fits tightly in the crotch.

(*text continues on pg. 227*)

BREAST SELF-EXAMINATION

Inspection in a Mirror

A. With arms at sides, look in mirror for

- Changes in size and shape of breasts
- Changes in skin: dimpling, puckering, scaling, redness swelling
- Changes in nipples: inversion, scaling, discharge, erosion, nipples pointing in different directions

B. Holding arms over the head, inspect closely in the mirror for masses, breast symmetry, puckering.

C. Press hands firmly on hips, bow slightly forward. Inspect in mirror for lumps or pulling of the skin.

Palpation

D. Lying flat on your back, with your right hand under your head and a pillow or towel under your right shoulder, use your left hand to gently feel your right breast, using concentric circles to cover the entire breast and nipple. Squeeze the nipple for signs of discharge or bleeding. Repeat on your left breast.

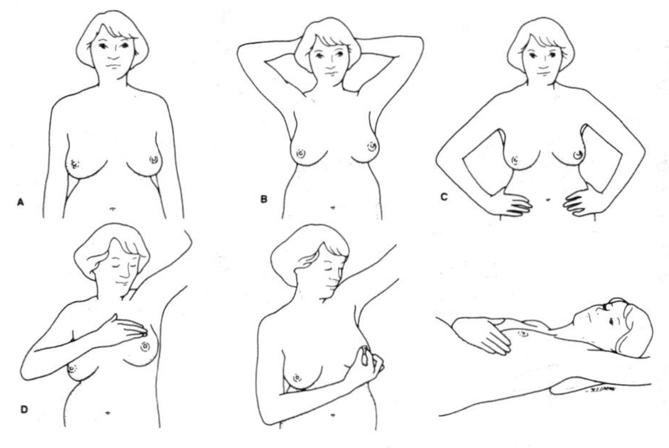

Table 6-7 Vaginal Infections Commonly Found in Pregnant Women

Findings	**Infection**			
	Candidiasis	*Trichomoniasis*	*Gardnerella*	*Herpes Vaginitis*
Causative Organism	*Candida albicans* *Monilia albicans* (Common names: monilia and yeast)	*Trichomonas*—a motile, flagellated protozoa	*Gardnerella* vaginitis Hemophilus vaginitis Nonspecific vaginitis	Herpes hominis type 2 (HVH-2); occasionally HVH-1
Vaginal pH	4.0 to 4.7	5.0 to 5.5	5.0 to 5.5	4.0 to 5.0
Leukorrhea	Profuse, thick, white, curdlike	Profuse, thin, greenish gray, frothy, bubbly	Profuse, grayish green, pasty	Moderate to heavy, thin, whitish
Pruritus	Moderate to severe	Moderate to severe	None or relatively little	Itching and burning at infection site
Odor	None	Malodorous	Malodorous	None
Urinary Symptoms	Burning, frequency	Frequency, urgency, dysuria	Usually none	Burning of lesions with urination

Pain	Dyspareunia	Dyspareunia	Usually none, occasional dyspareunia	Painful lesions
Vaginal/Vulvar Symptoms	White plaques, inflammation, edematous excoriations	Diffuse edema, strawberry patches on cervix	Possible inflammation of introitus and vagina	Vesicles, papules, ulceration, edema
Leukocytes on Wet Mount	Increased—saline Not seen—KOH	Present	Present, absence of lactobacillus after 1 week	Present
Diagnosis	KOH 10% wet mount Pseudomycelia and yeast buds seen; Nickerson's culture media; gram stain	Warm saline wet mount Characteristic movement (when organism is cold it resembles white blood cell)	Saline wet mount Clue cells	Pap smear Tzank test Serologic antibodies

Table 6-8 Discomforts of Pregnancy

Common Complaints and Etiology	Assessment	Intervention and Counseling
Nausa and Vomiting		
Progesterone (decreases gastric emptying time)	Evaluate diet for adequacy of food intake and quality of nutrients.	Reassure the patient that nausea and vomiting usually resolve spontaneously after the first trimester.
Increased levels of human chorionic gonadotropin Decreased gastric secretion of hydrochloric acid and pepsin Inadequate nutrient and liquid intake (empty stomach and dehydration) Altered carbohydrate metabolism Inadequate iron and vitamin intake Decreased maternal blood sugar Ambivalence about pregnancy Acute infection or other illness Fatigue Ptyalism	Assess and document the extent of nausea and vomiting. Observe for weight loss, dehydration, decreased skin turgor, ketonuria. Assess emotional response to pregnancy. Assess possibility of other diagnostic problems—stomach or gastric ulcers, cholecystitis, pancreatitis, hepatitis, gastroenteritis, appendicitis, or intestinal flu.	Advise the patient to: Avoid greasy, spicy foods. Avoid odors that predispose to nausea (use fan while cooking). Eat six small meals a day instead of three large ones. Increase protein snacks (cheese, nuts, eggs). Eat foods high in carbohydrates (better tolerated). Eat dry, unsalted crackers before arising in morning. Drink fluids between meals (decreases dehydration). Avoid liquids with meals.

		Sip carbonated water (not sweet sodas) to prevent onset of nausea. Try spearmint, peppermint, or raspberry tea. Take iron tablets and vitamins after meals. Try 50 to 100 mg/day vitamin B_6 (after a meal) to reduce nausea. Have yogurt, cottage cheese, juice, or milk when awakened by nocturia to decrease nausea in morning. Take frequent fresh air walks. Maintain good posture (to relieve pressure on stomach). Avoid sudden movements.
		Caution the patient to avoid over-the-counter antinausea medications or any medicines without consultation with health care provider.
Fatigue		
Increased hormonal production; possible role of ovarian hormone relaxin Progesterone in first trimester	Assess nutrition for anemia or inadequate caloric intake. Assess hemoglobin (Hgb) and hematocrit (Hct).	Reassure the patient that fatigue is a normal and temporary aspect of pregnancy. Advise the patient to:

(*continued*)

Table 6-8 Discomforts of Pregnancy (*continued*)

Common Complaints and Etiology	Assessment	Intervention and Counseling
Fatigue		
Increased demands on cardiopulmonary systems in last trimester 25% increase in basal metabolic rate Inadequate nutrition Anemia Lack of exercise Excessive activity Excessive weight gain Psychogenic causes Infection Incorrect posture	Assess psychosocial status for anxiety and depression. Assess exercise regimen. Assess activity level and amount of rest. Assess whether fatigue is appropriate for trimester of pregnancy.	Take frequent rest periods (lie down during coffee breaks, etc). Get adequate exercise. Increase social stimulation (when appropriate) with family, friends, or groups. Decrease activities that may cause overexertion. Explore opportunities to participate in activities she enjoys. Get assistance with childcare if possible. Practice deep breathing and relaxation exercises.
Urinary Frequency		
Stretching of the base of the bladder by the enlarging uterus in the first trimester, producing a sensation of fullness; reduction in	Assess for urinary tract infections (urethritis, cystitis, pyelonephritis): Urinalysis Urine culture	Advise the patient to: Maintain hydration during daytime but decrease fluid intake in the evening to reduce nocturia.

bladder capacity through pressure of enlarging uterus on bladder; compression of bladder by presenting part in third trimester Excessive fluid intake Promotion of urine output by kidneys when woman is in supine position, (nocturia) Urinary tract infection	Fever or chills Costovertebral or suprapubic tenderness Assess diet for excessive coffee, tea, or cola intake. Assess for diabetes: excessive thirst, abnormal blood glucose levels.	Void when the urge occurs to avoid bladder distention and urinary stasis. Limit intake of caffeinated beverages (tea, coffee, cola). Do Kegel exercises to strengthen pelvic floor muscles and decrease urinary leakage. Teach the patient the signs of urinary tract infection (urgency or burning) and the importance of prompt medical attention should the signs occur.
Breast Fullness and Tingling		
Fat deposition, caused by estrogen, and development of stromal tissue and ductile system Development of lobules, alveoli proliferation and secretion, and breast swelling, caused by progesterone Increased vascular supply to breasts	Assess whether discomfort is generalized or local. Assess for injury. Assess for supernumerary breast and axillary tissue involvement. Assess for leaking of colostrum, which may cause cracked nipples.	Reassure the patient that breast changes and discomforts are natural; fullness will continue throughout pregnancy, but tenderness usually resolves after first trimester Teach the patient: Anatomy and physiology of breast changes Breast self-examination Breastfeeding preparations at onset of third trimester

(*continued*)

Table 6-8 Discomforts of Pregnancy (*continued*)

Common Complaints and Etiology	Assessment	Intervention and Counseling
Breast Fullness and Tingling		
		Advise the patient to: Wear support bra with wide adjustable straps and smooth interior to decrease irritation. Avoid pressure on breasts. Avoid use of soap on nipples. Apply skin cream to soften crusts formed by colostrum.
Leukorrhea (Vaginal Discharge)		
Increased production of cervical mucus, recognized as a profuse, thin, white or yellowish vaginal discharge, caused by estrogen Increased cervical vascularity and desquamation	Assess type, color, amount, and odor of discharge. Assess whether patient suffers from pruritus. Assess for partner's complaints of symptoms or new or multiple partners. Evaluate for *Candida albicans* or sexually transmitted infection.	Reassure the patient that increased discharge is a normal process of pregnancy. Advise the patient to: Use good perineal hygiene. Keep vulva dry by using hairdryer after washing and dusting with cornstarch. Use external vinegar and water rinse.

		Wear loose cotton undergarments. Avoid pantyhose and tight clothing. Use perineal pads and change them frequently. Report pruritus and foul odor. Caution the patient to avoid: Douching Tampons
Changes in Libido Complicated interplay between physiologic discomforts and hormonal and emotional changes In the first trimester, decreased libido may be due to fatigue, nausea and vomiting, breast tenderness, and ambivalence toward the pregnancy. The second trimester is usually characterized by an increase in libido. There is often a decrease in libido at the end of the third trimester, usually related to physical discomforts, fatigue, and anxiety.	Assess reasons for changes in libido: physical discomforts or emotional origins. Assess couple's psychological response to pregnancy. Assess couple's communication skills and ability to cope with and resolve the perceived difficulties.	Reassure the patient and her partner that variations in sexual interest occur in pregnancy, and that they can enjoy their usual sexual activities unless their health care provider *specifically* contraindicates sexual activity for them. Advise the patient and her partner that: Good communication between partners is essential. Cuddling, kissing, and stroking will often provide emotional satisfaction ad fulfill some physical needs also.

(*continued*)

Table 6-8 Discomforts of Pregnancy (*continued*)

Common Complaints and Etiology	Assessment	Intervention and Counseling
Changes in Libido		
Problems in the couple relationship Fear that intercourse will harm the embryo/fetus Progress through psychosocial tasks of pregnancy Changed body image Discomfort from relaxation of pelvic joints and ligaments Painful contractions from orgasm (third trimester)		Massage is another alternative or adjunct form of sexual expression. Variations in position during intercourse may become necessary for comfort as pregnancy progresses (*e.g.*, intercourse with the woman on top or with the man's entering from behind). Mutual masturbation and oral sex are other adjuncts or alternatives to sexual activity if intercourse becomes too uncomfortable. Refer couple for sexual or couple counseling.
Mood Changes		
Depressant effect of progesterone on the central nervous system	Assess woman's emotional stability and coping mechanisms and	Reassure the patient and her partner that mood swings are a normal

Prominence of physical and emotional changes of pregnancy to the pregnant woman Marked introversion, often secondary to developmental tasks of pregnancy Lack of support system for woman and partner Physical discomforts of pregnancy, fatigue Anxiety Changed body image	compare with prepregnant emotional stability, if known. Assess couple's communication skills, attitude toward pregnancy, and progression through developmental tasks of pregnancy. Assess the support system available to the woman or couple in family, friends, church, community, and workplace. Assess woman's nutritional status with regard to fatigue, anemia, and caloric intake. Assess for dependence on drugs, alcohol, and other substances.	component of pregnancy. Encourage the patient or couple to: Discuss their feelings with a trusted person. Continue activities that bring enjoyment. Take time for good grooming, rest, sleep, and exercise. Refer the patient or couple for counseling if appropriate.
Pyrosis (Heartburn)		
Relaxation of smooth gastrointestinal muscles and cardiac sphincter of stomach by progesterone, allowing gastric reflux of stomach contents to lower esophagus Displacement of stomach and duodenum by enlarging uterus Decreased hydrochloric acid and	Assess nutritional status and habits. Assess psychosocial status for tension or depression. Assess previous medical history for gastrointestinal illness, cholecystitis, or hiatal hernia.	Reassure the patient that normal pregnancy changes are causing the heartburn. Advise the patient to: Eliminate greasy, spicy foods from diet. Eat small bland meals. Eat six small meals a day, not three large ones.

(*continued*)

Table 6-8 Discomforts of Pregnancy (*continued*)

Common Complaints and Etiology	Assessment	Intervention and Counseling
Pyrosis (Heartburn)		
pepsin secretion in the stomach, caused by estrogen Emotional factors		Eat slowly and chew thoroughly. Chew gum (sometimes helpful). Avoid coffee and cigarettes because they irritate the stomach. Drink eight glasses of fluids a day. Drink hot tea. Avoid sodium bicarbonate. Avoid lying down, bending, or stooping after eating. Wear clothes that fit loosely around the waistline. When heartburn occurs, sip water, milk, or carbonated water, or eat 1 tablespoonful of yogurt, heavy cream, or half-and-half. Do flying exercise to decrease heartburn. Try antacids (without phosphorus) if necessary—aluminum hydroxide;

		Gelusil, Amphojel; calcium carbonate; Tums; magnesium hydroxide; Maalox, Mylanta, Riopan. Caution patient to avoid: heartburn medicines containing aspirin (Alka Seltzer, Fizrin) heartburn medicines containing sodium (baking soda, soda mint, Eno, Fizrin, Rolaids, Alka Seltzer).
Ptyalism (Excessive Salivation)		
Possible salivary gland stimulation by starch intake Possible increased acidity of saliva, leading to gland production of saliva Difficulty in swallowing caused by nausea, contributing to the sensation of increased saliva Unusual food cravings or pica Oral infections or lesions	Assess nutrition for iron deficiency or excessive starch intake. Observe for specific oral lesions (salivary calculus, syphilis). Assess emotional status (hysteria). Assess for tonsillitis and stomatitis. Assess previous medical history or current status for gastric, pancreatic, or hepatic disorder.	Reassure the patient that this is a pregnancy-related situation that will resolve. Advise the patient to: Suck hard candy Avoid excessive starch intake Practice good oral hygiene Maintain good nutrition

(continued)

Table 6-8 Discomforts of Pregnancy (*continued*)

Common Complaints and Etiology	Assessment	Intervention and Counseling
Flatulence		
Ingestion of gas-forming food Aerophagia (air-swallowing), ptyalism, or nausea Decreased motility of gut Decreased exercise Uterine compression of gut Constipation Fecal impaction	Assess nutrition status with regard to intake of gas-forming foods. Assess bowel habits. Assess exercise and activity levels. Assess for abdominal pain, eructation, bloating, distention, or passing excessive flatus. Assess antacid use (baking soda will cause flatulence).	Reassure the patient that flatulence is a pregnancy-related phenomenon and will not harm her or the fetus. Advise the patient to: Avoid gas-forming foods (cabbage, beans, fried foods) and large meals. Chew food thoroughly. Decrease salivation by not chewing gum or smoking. Change position frequently. Have regular bowel habits. Exercise regularly.
Headache		
Increased circulating volume and heart rate (contribute to dilation and distention of cerebral arteries)	Assess symptoms to determine whether headache is a normal phenomenon of pregnancy or a	Explain the blood mechanisms that may be responsible for headache. Reassure the patient that symptoms

Vascular congestion of nasal turbinates from tissue edema
Emotional tension, causing spasm of sternocleidomastoid muscles of the neck and shoulders
Fatigue
Second-trimester decrease in blood pressure

warning sign of pregnancy complications:

- Type of headache (front, side, back of head, difference from usual headaches, visual disturbances, frequency of occurrence)
- Causative factors (fatigue, bad lighting, eye strain, stuffy office, emotional stress, poor nutrition, dehydration)
- Assess for other toxemia or preeclampsia symptoms: proteinuria, weight gain, elevated blood pressure, edema, exaggerated reflexes (hyperreflexia), and so on
- Assess for sinusitis, upper respiratory infection, and allergies.
- Assess previous attempts at relief and their effectiveness.
- Assess previous medical history and family history for renal, cardiac, or vascular disease.

are temporary and will respond to treatment.
Advise the patient to:

- Increase rest and relaxation.
- Engage in activities that are relaxing and rewarding.
- Perform relaxation exercises.
- Make dietary changes if causative foods or food allergies are isolated (cheeses, red wines, and shellfish can cause headaches).
- Adjust salts and sugars in diet for relief of symptoms.
- Avoid long periods without eating.
- Maintain hydration.
- Apply cool wet cloth to forehead and back of neck.
- Massage neck, shoulders, face, and scalp.
- Take slow walks in fresh air.
- Arrange for childcare help if appropriate.
- Take acetaminophen (Tylenol; two 325-mg tablets every 4 to 6 hours) after the first trimester if headache is severe.

(*continued*)

Table 6-8 Discomforts of Pregnancy (*continued*)

Common Complaints and Etiology	Assessment	Intervention and Counseling
Headache		
		Caution the patient *not* to use drugs without the health care provider's knowledge. Teach the patient to report signs of toxemia and preeclampsia: Severe, frequent, or long-lasting headaches Blurry vision or spots or bright lights before eyes Edema of face, hands, or legs in the morning Scanty, concentrated urine
Dyspnea (Shortness of Breath)		
Compression of vena cava by gravid uterus, decreasing venous return to the heart and causing arterial	Assess frequency of occurrence of dyspnea, its associations (exercise, sleep, supine position, etc.), and its	Reassure the patient by explaining the physiologic reasons for dyspnea in pregnancy.

hypotension; further compromise of circulatory status by lying in supine position (supine hypotensive syndrome) Prevention of maximum lung expansion by enlarging uterus Increased awareness of breathing	manifestations (dizziness, fainting, etc.). Assess nutrition and Hgb/Hct for anemia. Assess whether client hyperventilates. Assess for thoracic deformities and previous medical history of asthma or pulmonary disease.	Advise the patient to: Sit and stand up straight. Rest after exercise. Avoid overexertion. Sleep and rest in left lateral position or semi-Fowler's position with head elevated.
Backache		
Increased weight of growing uterus, which pulls spine forward and changes center of gravity which leads to compensatory lordosis and muscle strain Lack of support from lax abdominal muscles, which may contribute to compensatory lordosis Relaxation of pelvic ligaments and body joints, caused by estrogen and relaxin Fatigue and muscle tension High-heeled shoes, which cause postural changes and low back strain	Assess posture, lifting techniques, type of footwear worn, and so on. Assess activity level and rest periods. Assess for acute back muscle strain and anatomic musculoskeletal defects.	Advise the patient to: Avoid overexertion and fatigue. Rest frequently in recumbent position. Wear comfortable, low-heeled shoes. Apply local heat to backaches. Get regular daily exercise. Have friend give back massage. Elevate one leg on stool or box while standing. Perform total body relaxation exercises. Avoid lifting small children: have toddlers climb onto lap.

(*continued*)

Table 6-8 Discomforts of Pregnancy (*continued*)

Common Complaints and Etiology	Assessment	Intervention and Counseling
Backache		
Excessive weight gain, which increases strain on back muscles Exaggerated lordosis, which may cause aching and numbness of the upper extremities Increased intercostal respiration and expansion of thoracic cage, which may contribute to upper back pain		Teach the patient to: Exercise. Maintain good posture, especially pelvic cradle posture. Do pelvic tilts several times daily. Sit in tailor position. Use proper lifting techniques.
Round Ligament Pain		
Stretching of round ligaments caused by uterine growth, (round ligaments extend bilaterally from anterior and inferior to the oviducts through the inguinal canal to insert in the superior portion of the labia majora)	Assess cause of onset (exercise, sudden movement, etc.) and site of pain (unilateral or bilateral). Assess uterine activity to distinguish round ligament pain from preterm labor: rhythmic uterine tightening and relaxing and	See all interventions under Backache. Reassure the patient and explain the cause of round ligament pain. Advise the patient to: Avoid sudden jerking or twisting movements.

Sudden jerking or twisting of the torso pulls on these ligaments, causing unilateral or bilateral pain in the lateral lower abdominal wall	sensation of pelvic pressure are symptomatic of preterm labor. Assess for other possible causes of pain: corpus luteal cyst rupture, ectopic pregnancy, Braxton Hicks contractions, constipation, appendicitis, inguinal hernia.	Rise slowly from recumbent position. Apply local heat to the area of discomfort. Do total body relaxation exercises. Avoid excessive exercise, standing, and walking.
Constipation		
Relaxation of muscle tone and decreased peristalsis, caused by progesterone, which allow increased water resorption from the bowel Pressure from the uterus on the colon and rectum Decreased physical exercise Decreased fluid intake Inadequate roughage in diet Changes in eating habits, especially increases in calcium and iron intake Stress Fecal impaction	Assess diet for fiber, fluid, and iron intake. Assess exercise. Assess prepregnant and current bowel habits (irregularity, impaction). Assess psychological status (depression, anxiety). Assess for other possible causes of bowel changes (irritable colon, atonic colon).	Reassure the patient that constipation is pregnancy-related and will resolve. Advise the patient to: Increase fluid intake (6 to 8 glasses/day) and drink warm liquids on arising in the morning. Increase exercise. Increase fiber intake by eating whole-grain breads and cereals (bran); raw, unpeeled or dry fruits; and vegetables. Establish regular bowel habits. Take time for bowel movements, neither forcing them nor resisting the urge.

(continued)

Table 6-8 Discomforts of Pregnancy (*continued*)

Common Complaints and Etiology	Assessment	Intervention and Counseling
Constipation		
		Use extra bulk such as Metamucil, 1 tsp/day as needed. Use a stool-softener such as Colace, 150 to 200 mg/day for 5 to 10 days, or a mild laxative such as milk of magnesia. Raise feet on stool or box during bowel movement to decrease straining.
		Caution the patient to avoid mineral oil as a laxative because it prevents absorption of fat-soluble vitamins from the gut.
Varicosities		
Increased blood volume, putting additional pressure on venous circulation	Assess whether varicosities are associated with mild discomfort or severe pain	Reassure the patient by explaining the cause of varicosities. Explain that varicosities will not resolve during

Increased pressure from enlarging uterus, which restricts venous return from legs and perineum, causing vulvar and leg varicosities and hemorrhoids Congenital predisposition to weakness in the vascular walls Inactivity and poor muscle tone Prolonged standing, which causes venous pooling in lower limbs and pelvis Obesity	Assess previous history and family history of varicosities. Assess levels of activity, exercise, and rest. Assess and document extent of varicosities. With patient supine, observe for signs of venous stasis (pitting, stasis pigmentation, or ulceration). With patient standing, observe for dilated veins in legs.	pregnancy, but steps can be taken to control symptoms (throbbing) and progress of condition. Advise the patient to: Rest in the recumbent position with legs elevated *above* the level of the body twice a day or more. Wear support hose. To put on properly, the patient should lie flat and raise legs to drain the veins, rolling stockings on while legs are still elevated. Hose should be put on *before* arising in the morning. Wear loose clothing and avoid round garters and tight knee-highs. Refrain from crossing legs at the knee. Get up and move around every hour if sedentary. Get regular exercise or walk each day. Wear comfortable shoes to decrease the strain on legs when walking or standing. Wear a pelvic pad supported by a T binder for support of vulvar varicosities.

(*continued*)

Table 6-8 Discomforts of Pregnancy (*continued*)

Common Complaints and Etiology	Assessment	Intervention and Counseling
Hemorrhoids		
See all causes under varicosities. Relaxation of the smooth muscle of the bowel, contributing to constipation and straining at stool, the latter of which predisposes the patient to hemorrhoid formation	Assess nutrition for fiber, fluid, and iron intake. Assess exercise activity. Assess prepregnant and current bowel habits.	Reassure the patient by explaining the causes and ways of preventing hemorrhoids. Advise client to: Avoid constipation (see interventions under Constipation). Take warm or cool sitz baths (whichever is most soothing), and if possible use a finger to gently replace the hemorrhoid into the anal canal. Cleanse the anus carefully after defecation. Place petroleum jelly in the rectum after defecation. Apply cool witch hazel compresses for comfort as necessary. Refrain from straining during bowel movements, since this exacerbates the problem.

		Teach clients to: Lie in knee-chest position for up to 15 min/day. Do Kegel exercises to strengthen perineum and help prevent and control hemorrhoids. Caution the patient to consult her health care provider before using any hemorrhoid medications.
Leg Cramps		
Disturbance in the body's calcium-phosphorus ratio (increased phosphorus predisposes to leg cramps): excessive intake of dairy products, which increases both calcium and phosphorus levels; inadequate intake of dairy products, which decreases calcium levels; high soft drink intake, which increases phosphorus levels Fatigue or muscle strain in the extremities Blood vessel occlusion in the legs Sudden stretching of the leg and foot (pointing the toes)	Assess diet for excessive or inadequate dairy product intake or excessive soft drink intake. Assess for other possible cause of leg pain, such as phlebitis or thrombophlebitis (skin warm to touch, palpable thrombus, positive Homans' sign).	Reassure the patient that leg cramps are a normal occurrence in pregnancy. Advise the patient to: Limit intake of dairy products to four servings/day or take calcium supplements if intake is inadequate (chewable calcium carbonate tablets, 1 g three times/day); decrease the amount of phosphorous in the diet (*e.g.*, by decreasing intake of soft drinks); and take antacids containing aluminum hydroxide (*e.g.*, Amphojel) to bind the phosphorus.

(*continued*)

Table 6-8 Discomforts of Pregnancy (*continued*)

Common Complaints and Etiology	Assessment	Intervention and Counseling
Leg Cramps		
		Dorsiflex foot (point toes toward head) when cramping occurs. Avoid toe-pointing stretch of legs. Apply local heat to sore leg muscles. Keep legs warm. Stretch calf muscles before bedtime. Take a warm bath before bedtime. Loosen heavy covers at end of bed. Elevate and support legs on pillow at night. Stand on affected leg to straighten muscle. Get regular exercise, particularly walking. Caution the patient *not* to massage the calf because of the risk of undetected thrombus.

Skin Changes		
Linea nigra of abdomen, a single thin dark line from pubis to umbilicus: hormone-related *Chloasma* of face (mask of pregnancy), darker pigment, predominantly on forehead and cheeks *Straiae gravidarum* (stretch marks) over abdomen, buttocks, or breasts due to inelasticity of skin: Probable genetic component *Acne:* probably due to increased progesterone and increased activity of sweat and sebaceous glands as a result of increased circulation	Observe for pigment changes of face, abdomen, and breasts (areola will darken).	Reassure the patient that although pigment changes cannot be prevented, the pigmentation will gradually fade after birth. Stretch marks will fade from red or purple to faint silvery lines. Advise the patient to: Maintain good hygiene. Apply moisturizing lotions or oils to abdomen, breasts, and buttocks, although these measures alone will not prevent striae if a woman is genetically predisposed to them. Stay out of the sun or wear a strong sunscreen to prevent further darkening of chloasma. Reassure the patient experiencing acne that it may decrease after the first trimester. Advise the patient experiencing acne to: Thoroughly cleanse the skin with soap and water. Apply topical astringents.

(*continued*)

Table 6-8 Discomforts of Pregnancy (*continued*)

Common Complaints and Etiology	Assessment	Intervention and Counseling
Braxton Hicks Contractions		
Probably increased estrogen levels and distention of the uterus	Assess frequency, strength, regularity, and associated symptoms of Braxton Hicks contractions to distinguish from preterm labor or true labor (see Table 6-9).	Reassure the patient that these contractions are a normal part of pregnancy and a preparation for labor. Advise the patient to: Rest in the left lateral recumbent position. Try walking or exercising, which may make the contractions cease. Teach client to distinguish Braxton Hicks contractions from preterm labor (See Table 6-9) and to call health care provider if signs of preterm or true labor occur.
Food Cravings		
Increased calorie intake required by physiologic changes of pregnancy;	Assess nutritional status for weight gain and anemia. Observe for bizarre eating habits.	Advise the patient to: Eat well-balanced meals. Gain appropriate amounts of weight.

women's choice of foods that most appeal to them Etiology unknown in the case of pica, a craving for substances such as clay, laundry starch, plaster, soap, toothpaste, or ice scraped from freezer	Assess for cultural or socioeconomic factors that might predispose a woman to indulge in pica. Assess for emotional and psychological factors that might contribute to pica.	Take iron and vitamin supplements. Counsel the patient experiencing pica. If nutritional status is adequate and the substance eaten is not harmful, counseling alone is necessary. If pica is interfering with nutrition, then condition counseling is necessary and iron and vitamin supplements must be given. Refer to patient to: Nutritionist for counseling Social worker for financial aid if necessary Counseling for emotional needs if necessary
Epulis (Bleeding Gums)		
Hypertrophy and hyperemia of the gingiva, probably related to estrogen levels	Assess oral hygiene and observe for swollen, reddened gingiva that bleed when touched.	Reassure the patient that this is a normal phenomenon of pregnancy and will resolve spontaneously after delivery.

(continued)

Table 6-8 Discomforts of Pregnancy (*continued*)

Common Complaints and Etiology	Assessment	Intervention and Counseling
Epulis (Bleeding Gums)		Advise the patient to: Maintain good oral hygiene. Use a soft toothbrush; brush from gums toward teeth. Floss gently. Use warm saline mouthwashes to relieve discomfort. Get regular dental checkups and hygienist treatments. Maintain a well-balanced diet, including fresh fruits and vegetables. Cut hard food (apples, carrots) into small pieces before chewing. Refer to a dentist for serious conditions.
Nosebleeds		
Probably high estrogen levels	Assess blood pressure to rule out hypertension as a cause of the nosebleed.	Reassure the patient that this is a common phenomenon of pregnancy.

Dizziness and Fainting		
Increased total blood volume, beginning at 10 to 14 weeks of gestation and peaking at 34 to 36 weeks Anemia, which decreases the oxygen-carrying capacity of red blood cells, causing less oxygen to be supplied to the brain Compression of the vena cava by the uterus in the supine position, causing decreased blood return to the heart and brain (supine hypotension) Lower blood pressure in second trimester Pooling of blood in lower extremities, causing dizziness on sudden change from supine or sitting position to standing Hyperventilation (increased levels of CO_2 in the blood) Hypoglycemia Emotional factors Fatigue Infections	Assess causes of dizziness and associated factors. In first trimester, dizziness can be due to nausea and vomiting, hypoglycemia, lower blood pressure in second trimester or ectopic pregnancy. In last trimester, dizziness can be due to position changes, hypoglycemia, or preeclampsia. Also consider ocular or neurologic causes. Assess nutritional status for anemia, hypoglycemia, and excessive nausea and vomiting. Check Hgb/Hct. Assess emotional status (anxiety). Assess for infection (fever, chills, pain).	Reassure the patient by explaining the possible causes of dizziness. Advise the patient to: Rise slowly from sitting or lying positions. Lie on either side rather than on the back when recumbent. Eat smaller, more frequent meals to prevent hypoglycemia. Avoid crowds and crowded areas. Avoid hyperventilation. Get sufficient rest. Assess factors in her life that may be distressing to her. Take iron and vitamin supplements. Teach the patient to sit down or lie in the left lateral position when she feels slightly dizzy to avoid falling if she faints. Refer to nutritionist or counselor if appropriate.

(*continued*)

Table 6-8 Discomforts of Pregnancy (*continued*)

Common Complaints and Etiology	Assessment	Intervention and Counseling
Insomnia		
Inability to find a comfortable position because of the enlarged abdomen Excessive anxiety about the pregnancy or other concerns Nocturia and subsequent inability to resume sleep Fetal activity A large meal prior to bedtime, indigestion, heartburn Leg cramps Dyspnea	Assess usual sleep habits (somnolence during the day). Observe for fatigue and irritability. Assess emotional status (anxiety or depression). Assess nutritional habits (late meals, stimulants, evening fluid intake, calcium-phosphorus intake).	Reassure the patient that insomnia is not unusual in late pregnancy. Advise the patient to: Avoid late, large meals. Avoid stimulants such as caffeine, tea, and cola drinks before bedtime. Decrease fluid intake in the evening, but maintain adequate intake (6–8 glasses) during the day. Get daily exercise. Take measures to prevent leg cramps (see interventions under Leg Cramps). Sleep with pillows propped to elevate head and chest to avoid heartburn and dyspnea.

		Place a pillow between the legs to support them when in the lateral recumbent position. Take an evening stroll in fresh air. Sleep with the window open. Caution the patient *not* to use sleeping medicine without consulting health care provider first.
Edema		
Increased sodium and water retention and increased capillary permeability, probably related to hormones Increased venous pressure Decreased venous return from dependent structures Varicose veins with congestion Dietary protein deficiency Increased dietary intake of sodium	Assess and document amount and location of edema. Assess nutrition for salt, protein, and fluid intake. Assess rest and activity levels. Assess for other symptoms of preeclampsia (proteinuria, hypertension, weight gain, hyperreflexia, scanty urine output). Also consider other renal or cardiac impairment.	Reassure the patient that physiologic edema is a normal phenomenon of pregnancy. Advise the patient to: Increase rest periods lying on the left side. Elevate legs when sitting. Wear support hose (see interventions under Varicosities). Restrict intake of salty foods (potato chips, pickles, canned soups, etc.), but *not* to adopt a salt-free diet; salt may be used in cooking.

(*continued*)

Table 6-8 Discomforts of Pregnancy (*continued*)

Common Complaints and Etiology	Assessment	Intervention and Counseling
Edema		Increase intake of protein foods (decreased protein contributes to fluid retention in tissues). Decrease intake of carbohydrates (especially simple sugars) and fats, since they also cause fluid retention in tissues. Drink 6 to 8 glasses fluid/day to aid in natural diuresis. Teach the patient to report signs of toxemia and preeclampsia: generalized edema, weight gain, headaches, flashing lights, decreased urine output.

Table 6-9 Distinguishing Between True and False Labor

True Labor	False Labor
Uterine Contractions	
Show regular pattern	Show irregular pattern
Usually become closer together, stronger and longer	Usually vary
Increase in intensity with walking	May stop with walking or position change
Are usually felt in lower back, radiating to lower abdomen	Are usually felt in back, upper fundus
Are not stopped by relaxation techniques such as hot bath, heating pad, alcoholic drink, or sedation	Will eventually stop with relaxation techniques
Cervix	
Softens, effaces, and dilates	May soften; no significant change in dilatation or effacement
Fetus	
Starts descent into pelvis	No noticeable change in position

- Wear loose-fitting, porous cotton underwear that will retain less moisture and heat than those made from polyester.
- Keep the vulva and perineum dry and cool.
- Abstain from intercourse during treatment or have your partner use a condom.
- Continue to use the medication even though symptoms have resolved.

Urinary Tract Infections

Self-Care Teaching: Urinary Tract Infections

- Empty the bladder as soon as you feel the urge to urinate—do not put it off.
- Empty the bladder as frequently as every 3 hours.

- Drink large quantities of liquids (except those with a high sugar content, since sugar provides a growth medium for any bacteria present).
- Observe good perineal hygiene by wiping the perineal area from front to back after urination or defecation.
- Cleanse the perineal area daily, avoiding perfumed sprays or soaps that might cause allergic reactions.
- Avoid wearing underwear while sleeping or tight underwear at any time. The perineal area needs ventilation to help keep it dry and clean.
- Drink a quantity of fluid before sexual intercourse and urinate immediately afterward to wash bacteria from the urethra.
- Wear cotton pants and practice good hygiene.
- Avoid carbohydrate and sugar binges to reduce the incidence of glucosuria.
- Seek immediate treatment for any recurrence of symptoms.

Discomforts of Pregnancy

See Table 6-8.

7
Complications of Pregnancy

The purpose of good prenatal care is to identify the at-risk woman and to initiate early intervention to prevent or alleviate problems.

Nursing Objectives in Pregnancy Complications

- To recognize signs and symptoms indicative of potential maternal or fetal problems
- To assess signs and symptoms of early or ongoing problems during pregnancy
- To apprise the patient and partner of findings as appropriate
- To report findings to the physician to whom you are referring the couple
- To provide ongoing support to and teaching and counseling of the couple as indicated.

HYPEREMESIS GRAVIDARUM

Hyperemesis gravidarum is intractable nausea and vomiting during pregnancy that persists beyond the first trimester.

Assessment

Predisposing Factors

- Rapidly rising levels of human chorionic gonadotropin (HCG) in early pregnancy
- Psychological factors related to the woman's feelings regarding pregnancy

Clinical Signs

- Continual nausea accompanied by excessive vomiting, that can be triggered by the sight or smell of food or by other heavy odors (*e.g.*, cigarette smoke)
- Nausea during the first 16 weeks gestation
- Alteration in nutritional status
  - Weight loss
  - Constipation
  - Thirst
  - Low output of concentrated urine
  - Dehydration
  - Acetonuria
  - Ketosis and ketonuria

Possible Nursing Diagnoses Related to Hyperemesis Gravidarum

- Fluid and electrolyte deficit related to hyperemesis
- Alteration in nutrition, less than body requirements, related to prolonged vomiting
- Ineffective individual coping related to personal vulnerability and emotional stress

---

Nursing Interventions

- Restore and maintain fluid and electrolyte balance
  - Hospitalize, restrict oral intake, and administer intravenous (IV) fluids supplemented with electrolytes and vitamins.
  - Resume oral liquids such as tea and ice chips, gradually adding bland foods to patient's diet.
  - Administer antiemetics as prescribed.
  - Provide a quiet, restful atmosphere to promote patient's needed rest and sleep.
- Psychological support
  - Obtain the assistance of a social worker who may need to coordinate care of patient's children and attend to economic needs.
  - Encourage the patient to verbalize her feelings; be supportive and accepting. Professional psychologic intervention may be indicated.
  - Ensure restriction of visitors to relieve stress during early hospitalization.

MULTIPLE GESTATION

The incidence of 1 in 200 births of monozygotic (identical) twins is the same throughout the world. Fraternal twins in the United States number 1 in 80 live births.

Assessment/Clinical Signs

- Prenatal indicators of multiple pregnancy (ultrasound confirms diagnosis.)
  - Excessive nausea and vomiting
  - Larger uterine size than expected, especially after 20 weeks gestation
  - Polyhydramnios (excessive amniotic fluid)
  - A rapid drop in hemoglobin value
  - Signs of developing pregnancy-induced hypertension
  - Palpable fetal parts in all quadrants of the abdomen
  - Fetal movement felt by the mother in all quadrants
  - Different fetal heart beats heard at two different sites (less valid indication)
- The mother carrying twins is at risk for the six Ps:
  - Preeclampsia
  - Primary anemia
  - Pressure
  - Placenta previa
  - Prematurity
  - Postpartum hemorrhage

  A seventh P—psychological concern—is equally important.

Possible Nursing Diagnoses Related to Multiple Gestation

- Alteration in nutrition less than body requirements, related to increased requirement
- Potential alteration in family processes related to unexpected financial and emotional demands
- Fear related to increased perinatal risk

Nursing Interventions

- Special attention to the following aspects of prenatal nursing care is imperative:
  - Determination of maternal weight gain

- Evaluation of blood pressure (BP)
- Prevention of anemia by dietary iron or folacin supplementation and diet counseling
- Frequent evaluation of hemoglobin and hematocrit
- Administration of nonstress testing to assess fetal response beginning at 37 weeks
- Monitoring ultrasound determinations of sizes and positions of fetuses in late pregnancy

Self-care Teaching

- Encourage regular and more frequent prenatal visits.
- Encourage rest several times each day for one-half hour in the left lateral recumbent position to increase blood flow to the uterus and help avoid excessive water retention.
- Stress the importance of adequate diet. Encourage patient to avoid excessive salt intake, increase fluid intake to eight glasses per day, and consume small, frequent meals to aid digestion.
- Discuss self-monitoring of uterine contractions to detect possible preterm labor.
- Suggest avoiding long periods of standing, which causes pooling of blood in the dependent limbs, and elevating the legs when sitting.

ANEMIA IN PREGNANCY

Approximately 56% of all pregnant women have some degree of anemia as defined by a hemoglobin of 10.0 g or less during the second and third trimesters.

Causes of Anemia

- Nutritional deficiency: iron deficiency; megaloblastic anemia (includes folic acid deficiency and vitamin B_{12} deficiency)
- Hemolysis (increased destruction of red blood cells): congenital sickle cell anemia; thalassemia; glucose-6-phosphate dehydrogenase G6PD deficiency, an enzyme deficiency

---

Possible Nursing Diagnoses Related to Anemia in Pregnancy

- Alteration in nutrition, less than body requirements, related to iron and folacin needed to meet prenatal maternal and fetal demands

- Potential for injury (prenatal iron and folacin deficiencies) related to disturbances of red cell reproduction and oxidation

---

Assessment

Clinical Signs

- Fatigue
- Headache
- Pallor
- Increased susceptibility to infection
- Cheilosis
- Tachycardia

Assessment and Interventions

Table 7-1 describes the anemias and their assessment and interventions.

Rh– BLOOD INCOMPATIBILITY

When a fetus inherits a blood group antigen from the father that the mother with Rh– blood does not possess, the mother's blood forms an immune reaction against the blood group factor on the fetus's red blood cells and a hemolytic process begins.

Assessment

- Determine from past obstetric history if the Rh– mother has had previous spontaneous abortion, induced abortion, ectopic pregnancy, amniocentesis, preterm birth, or term delivery; determine if RhoGAM was given.
- Check current laboratory studies to determine if isoimmunization (antibody titer) has occurred.

Possible Nursing Diagnoses Related to Rh– Blood Incompatibility

- Alteration in family processes related to concerns for fetal well-being
- Anticipatory grieving related to effects of blood incompatibility on the fetus
- Potential alteration in parenting related to disruption in antenatal attachment

---

(*text continues on pg. 237*)

Table 7-1 Types of Anemia

Anemia	Description	Assessment/Intervention
Nutritional		
Iron deficiency	Reduced hemoglobin production from depleted iron stores (inadequate dietary iron intake, malabsorption, blood loss, hemolysis)	• Review laboratory data. • Recognize need for iron supplementation (especially in pregnant teens). • Evaluate 24-hr diet history—refer to nutritionist. • Obtain prescription for ferrous sulfate 320 mg, orally, three times daily; and vitamin C 500 mg, orally, daily, to be taken together for increased absorption.
Folic acid (folacin) deficiency	Folacin is a vitamin that is a coenzyme in the synthesis of DNA. Promotes fetal growth and prevents macrocytic, megaloblastic anemia of pregnancy. Its needs double during gestation to 800 mcg/day	• Review dietary intake of food high in folacin; dark green leafy vegetables, organ meats, eggs, milk, oranges, bananas, dry beans, whole grain breads. • Assess symptoms of folacin lack: nausea, vomiting, anorexia. • Provide dietary counseling and obtain prescription for supplementation, 800 μg/d.

Hemoglobinopathies		
Sickle cell	An inherited disorder usually limited to blacks, resulting from alteration of the beta chain of hemoglobin; increases susceptibility to infection	• Review history of sickle cell disease in family. • Review results of hemoglobin electrophoresis. • Encourage frequent prenatal visits for ongoing monitoring. • Obtain monthly urine cultures. • Obtain prescription for folic acid supplement, 1 to 5 mg daily, and stress the importance of compliance in taking the vitamin. • Assist with hospitalization when infection or sickle crisis occurs. • Counsel the postpartum family about contraceptive methods, permanent sterilization, and the need for genetic counseling.
Thalassemia alpha, beta	A genetic hemoglobin disorder in which the production of alpha or beta hemoglobin chains is decreased, resulting in disruption of red cell function	• Carefully assess the prenatal patient for signs of urinary tract infection, chest colds that may progress to pneumonia, pulmonary congestion. • Assure the patient that normal prenatal activities should be continued. • Advise increased rest. • Counsel postpartally regarding contraception and need for genetic counseling.

(*continued*)

Table 7-1 Types of Anemia (*continued*)

Anemia	Description	Assessment/Intervention
Hemoglobinopathies		
Glucose-6-phosphate dehydrogenase deficiency (G6PD)	G6PD results from deficiency of the red cell enzyme G-6-PD. When certain drugs are ingested, the cell wall is destroyed and the cell becomes hemolyzed. Many drugs cause this reaction, the most common being aspirin products, sulfa drugs, probenecid, quinine, vitamins C and K, and Fava beans.	• During history taking assess patient's complaints of unexplained episodes of jaundice. • Provide a careful explanation of the disease when the patient has been unaware of its presence. The partner need not be screened since this is a female-linked disorder. • Provide the patient with a list of the drugs which, if ingested, will cause oxidation of red blood cells. • Assure the patient that her pregnancy will progress normally. • Be attentive to increased sensitivity for infection in the pregnant woman. • Obtain a prescription for supplemental folacin and iron, and explain their use. • Advise the use of a medicalert bracelet or necklace to protect patient from use of an offending drug in an emergency situation.

Nursing Interventions

- Monitor Rh− antibody titer levels at 24, 28, 32, 36, and 40 weeks in an unimmunized woman. Women with positive titers are followed by an obstetrician.
- Administer Rh− immune globulin at 28 weeks gestation to protect against effects of early transplacental hemorrhage (a crossmatch for Rh-immune globulin is necessary).
- Inform the woman and her family of the procedure to assure their full participation.
- Crossmatch the laboring Rh− negative mother for injection of immune globulin at about 72 hours after delivery.
- Alert the neonatal team to the delivery of a mother who is delivering a sensitized infant.

ABORTION

Abortion is the termination of pregnancy before the conceptus reaches 20 weeks gestation, a mass of 500 g, or a crown-rump length of 18 cm.

Types of Abortion/Clinical Signs

- *Threatened Abortion.* The pregnant woman experiences slight bleeding that may persist for several weeks and is accompanied by uterine cramping and pain. No cervical dilation or effacement occurs, and no tissue is passed. If the bleeding persists, little can be done except to advise bed rest for 48 hours.
- *Inevitable Abortion.* When the abortion reaches the inevitable stage, the cervix is soft and its os is dilated. Bleeding may be profuse, and abdominal cramping begins to resemble the pain of labor. Fetal size is consistent with dates, but its loss is certain.
- *Incomplete Abortion.* When the products of conception are only partially evacuated during abortion, the abortion is incomplete. Tissues that remain in the uterus contain portions of the fetal membrane or placenta. Bleeding and cramping continue and become more severe. Prolonged retention of the tissues predisposes the woman to infection, and immediate medical intervention is needed.
- *Complete Abortion.* When the products of conception (fetus and placenta) are completely passed, abortion is considered complete. Following the abortion there is relief from pain and bleeding usually stops. This type of abortion is more likely to occur early in gestation.
- *Missed Abortion.* When the fetus dies in utero but remains, along with the placenta and tissues, in the uterus, a missed abortion has occurred. Pregnancy symptoms abate, but amenorrhea

continues. When the patient is unaware that a missed abortion has occurred and the abortion is not detected within about 2 months by the health care providers, coagulopathy may occur causing life-threatening illness.

Possible Nursing Diagnoses Related to Abortion

- Fear related to increased perinatal risk
- Knowledge deficit of possible complications, risk factors, and preventive measures
- Grieving related to actual/potential pregnancy loss

Nursing Assessment

- Assess history of past pregnancies.
- Assess the length of present bleeding, the amount (number of sanitary napkins and their saturation), and the appearance of the blood or discharge (*e.g.*, does it contain tissue-like material?)
- Determine the pattern of uterine contractions and their intensity.
- Elicit what the woman has done at home to control bleeding or contractions.

Nursing Interventions

- Reassure the couple that the bleeding is not the result of any maternal behavior.
- Advise bedrest, avoidance of intercourse.
- Reinforce the need to seek immediate care if tissue-like material is passed.
- Offer emotional support when a pregnancy is lost and recommend several days of rest.
- Suggest avoidance of intercourse after loss until after the next menses.
- Administer RhoGAM to all Rh− women after abortion.
- Offer contraceptive counseling to delay pregnancy until full recovery is achieved.

ECTOPIC PREGNANCY

Ectopic pregnancy is a gestation that implants outside the uterine cavity. Rare implantation sites include the abdomen, cervix, ovary, and outer wall of the uterus. This life-threatening event is responsible for 12% of maternal mortality, up from 6% a decade ago.

Assessment

Predisposing Factors

- Pelvic inflammatory disease
- Tubal surgery
- IUD use
- Congenital deformities of the reproductive tract

Clinical Signs

- Missed menstrual period
- Spotting
- Pelvic pain
- Pelvic mass located in area of adnexa
- Internal hemorrhage (emergency)
  - Vertigo
  - Shoulder pain (irritation of phrenic nerve)
  - Decreasing blood pressure
  - Increased pulse rate
- Nausea, vomiting, faintness

Possible Nursing Diagnoses Related to Ectopic Pregnancy

- Alteration in comfort (discomfort) related to pelvic mass and/or blood in the pelvis
- Potential for injury (shock) related to internal bleeding with potential volume deficit
- Anxiety related to symptoms and uncertain pregnancy status
- Alteration in family processes related to unexpected maternal hospitalization

---

Nursing Interventions

- Prepare the patient for a serum pregnancy test and sonography.
- Remain with the patient and make sure that she has been counseled regarding the diagnosis and necessity for surgical removal.
- Reassure the patient with a tubal implantation that fertility may be maintained by the opposite fallopian tube when appropriate.

- Monitor vital signs regularly.
- Order blood crossmatch and start an IV with a large bore needle to maintain an open vein if blood replacement is needed.

HYDATIDIFORM MOLE

Hydatidiform mole is a developmental anomaly of the placenta that occurs when trophoblastic cells continue to grow and form an invasive tumor after death of the embryo.

Assessment/Clinical Signs

- Exaggerated pregnancy symptoms experienced by the patient
- Prenatal history that reveals:
  - Severe nausea and vomiting
  - Elevated BP
  - Proteinuria
  - Uterus may be large for dates
  - Red or brownish vaginal discharge
  - Signs and symptoms of preeclampsia before 20 weeks
  - Absence of fetal movements or heart tones
  - Passage of grapelike clusters from the vagina
  - Ultrasound showing snowlike configuration and absence of a fetus
  - Anemia out of proportion to blood loss
  - Adnexal masses from luteal cysts

Possible Nursing Diagnoses Related to Hydatidiform Mole

- Alteration in comfort (discomfort) related to exaggerated pregnancy symptoms
- Anxiety related to severe symptoms of pregnancy and knowledge deficit regarding the problem
- Alteration in nutrition less than body requirements related to symptoms and anxiety
- Fear related to prognosis

Nursing Interventions

- Provide support to the patient and family when the diagnosis is made. Issues surrounding pregnancy loss, recognition of an abnormal pregnancy, and the need to postpone subsequent pregnancies must be addressed by the physician, nurse, or counselor.

- Encourage the woman to discuss her grief, anger, or fear. (Fifteen percent of patients with hydatidiform mole will progress to either an invasive mole or choriocarcinoma.)
- Prepare the patient for surgery. Depending on the invasiveness of the mole, the procedure will be dilation and curettage (D and C), suction curettage, or hysterectomy (after 14 weeks).
- Observe postsurgery for hemorrhage or uterine perforation.
- Counsel or reinforce the need for close follow-up of HCG titers for at least 1 year. (When HCG titers are maintained and/or continue to rise, the mole is still active.) Negative titers after routine serial testing indicate eradication of the molar tissue.
- Advise that pregnancy should not be attempted for at least 1 year. HCG titers must be monitored to assure a cure. An intervening pregnancy with its high HCG titers would disrupt this process and possibly exacerbate existing molar tissue.

PLACENTA PREVIA

In placenta previa the placenta is implanted and develops in the lower uterine segment and encroaches on or covers the internal cervical os, as shown in Figure 7-1. Its incidence is 1 in 300 pregnancies.

Assessment

Classification of placenta previa is based on the proximity of the placenta to the cervical os, which is the direct determinant of the risk of hemorrhage to the pregnant woman.

- *Total.* The placenta completely covers the internal cervical os.
- *Partial.* The placenta partially covers the internal os (central).
- *Marginal.* The edge of the placenta lies at the border of the os.
- *Low-lying.* The placenta is very near the region of the os.

Women at Greatest Risk

- Age greater than 35 and multiparity. The effect of age is the most important and accounts for one-third of the cases of placenta previa. Of women experiencing placenta previa, 80% are multiparous.
- Prior placenta previa. The incidence of placenta previa among women who have already had one is 12 times the general incidence.
- Incidence increases in women who have recently had a D and C.

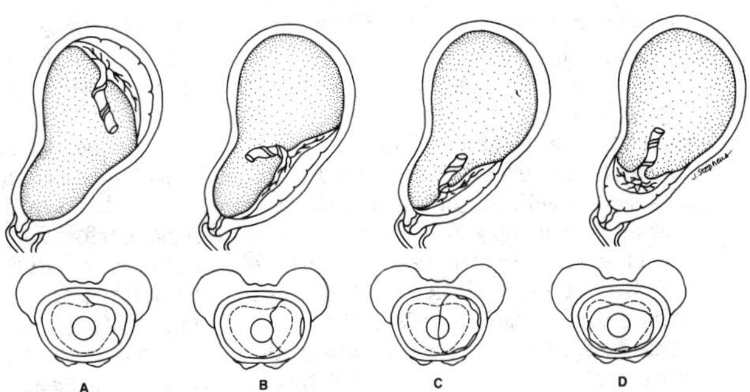

Figure 7-1 Placental positions. *(A)* Normal position. *(B)* Low implantation. *(C)* Partial placenta previa. *(D)* Total placenta previa. (Childbirth Graphics)

Clinical Signs

- The cardinal symptom is painless vaginal bleeding in the latter half of pregnancy. Bleeding occurs during sleep without warning and often without a precipitating factor.
- During subsequent episodes bleeding becomes heavier.
- Bleeding may not occur until labor begins.
- Earlier and more profuse bleeding occurs with total placenta previa.

Possible Nursing Diagnoses Related to Placenta Previa

- Anxiety/fear related to the effects of bleeding on pregnancy and the fetus
- Decreased activity related to increased bleeding in response to activity
- Grieving related to anticipated loss of pregnancy and loss of expected child

---

Nursing Interventions

- Referral to high-risk care is indicated when painless vaginal bleeding occurs at 28 to 30 weeks.
- Assessment of the hospitalized patient

- Monitor hemoglobin, hematocrit, white blood cells (WBCs) to evaluate for anemia and infection.
- Collect history of bleeding, number of episodes, amount of bleeding.
- Routinely monitor vital signs and fetal heart tones.
- Assess fetal movement.
- Enforce bed rest until 3 days after cessation of bleeding.
- Ensure that typed and crossmatched blood is available in the event of sudden hemorrhage.
- Use a fetal monitor if the mother experiences bleeding.
- Be prepared for emergency delivery, possible cesarean section.
- Alert the neonatal team to a possible premature or compromised infant.

ABRUPTIO PLACENTAE

Abruptio placentae is the separation of the normally implanted placenta from the uterine wall prior to the birth of the infant.

Assessment

Predisposing Factors

- High parity
- Previous abruptio placentae
- External trauma
- Short umbilical cord
- Folic acid deficiency
- Woman over 30
- Cigarette smoking
- Poor nutrition
- Previous induced abortion
- Sudden uterine compression
- Vascular disease

Clinical Signs

- Heavy vaginal bleeding
- Boardlike rigidity of the abdomen
- Unremitting, severe uterine pain and extreme tenderness to palpation
- Increased fetal activity due to hypoxia or absent or faint bradycardia
- Moderate to profound maternal shock
- Disseminated intravascular coagulation
- Renal failure

Possible Nursing Diagnoses Related to Abruptio Placentae

- Potential for injury (shock) related to excessive bleeding
- Potential for injury (danger to fetus) related to hypoxia or anoxia
- Anxiety/fear related to effects of bleeding on pregnancy and the fetus

---

Nursing Interventions

- IV infusion of fluids and whole blood as prescribed
- Continuous monitoring of fetal heart tone
- Monitoring of maternal BP, pulse, respirations
- Frequent checks for amount of vaginal bleeding and fundal height (increased with concealed bleeding)
- Collection of blood studies, including complete blood cell count (CBC) and type and crossmatch, and clotting studies, including fibrinogen and platelet studies
- Assistance with placement of CVP line to serve as a guide to the need for blood volume replacement
- Insertion of Foley catheter and hourly monitoring of urine output
- Preparation for immediate delivery, which, depending on the condition of the mother and fetus, will be accomplished vaginally or by cesarean section. Cesarean section is more commonly used because of the immediate delivery of the infant.
- Making sure the couple is informed of what is happening, of the procedures that might be needed, and of the need for a constant vigil of the conditions of mother and infant.

PREGNANCY-INDUCED HYPERTENSION

Pregnancy-induced hypertension (PIH) describes women in the following classes:

- Women who were diagnosed and treated for hypertension prior to pregnancy and had no known underlying disease
- Women who were found to have underlying renal or cardiovascular problems
- Women with no prior history who developed hypertension during pregnancy that resolved in the postpartum period

Assessment

- Screen patients at each prenatal visit for PIH.
  - Blood pressure of 140/90 or greater is considered hypertensive.
  - Dipstick urine for protein. A reading of +1 protein on two or more occasions should be followed by a 24-hour urine specimen to quantify urinary protein.
- Carefully assess total and interval weight gain; retention of fluid may cause as much as a 5-pound weight gain in one week.
- Examine the patient's legs and ankles for degree of edema; facial edema may be an ominous sign of preeclampsia.
- Collect a dietary recall to assess lack of protein intake, excessive salt intake, and to encourage intake of 8 to 10 glasses of fluid per day (without sodium or sugar) to maintain optimum fluid volume.

Clinical Signs and Symptoms

See Table 7-2.

Possible Nursing Diagnoses Related to Pregnancy-Induced Hypertension

- Fluid volume excess (edema) related to retention of water and impaired sodium excretion secondary to impaired renal function
- Knowledge deficit of signs and symptoms of hypertension related to uneventful history
- Fear related to increased perinatal risk
- Potential for injury (seizure) related to hypertension

Nursing Interventions

Preeclampsia, Inpatient

- Request the patient to remain on bed rest in the left lateral recumbent position to optimize kidney function and increase blood flow to the placenta.
- Monitor BP every 4 hours.
- Check deep tendon reflexes twice daily.

(*text continues on pg. 256*)

Table 7-2 Signs and Symptoms of Pregnancy-Induced Hypertension (PIH)

Sign	Early PIH	Mild to Moderate PIH	Severe PIH
Blood Pressure	Rising diastolic pressure, especially in second trimester, but still within normal limits	Increase of 30 mm Hg in systole and 15 mm Hg in diastole over baseline Or, reading between 140/90 and 160/110	Over 160/110
Proteinuria			
Qualitative, dipstick test	Absent	May still be absent +1 or +2 reading may be sporadic or persistent	+3 to +4 reading persistent
Quantitative, 24-hour analysis	Not indicated	0.5 g to 2.5 g total protein lost in 24 hours (variable)	0.5 g or more each 24 hours
Edema	Absent	If present, difficult to differentiate from physiologic edema Present in hands, feet, and ankles	Generalized and noticeable in face; classic facies of coarse features, broad nose, puffy eyes
Reflexes	Unchanged from normal baseline of +1 to +2	May be hyper-reflexion; +3, brisk No clonus	Hyper-reflexion Clonus

Total weight gain	Within normal range, or greater than 2 lb/wk in absence of other signs	2 lb/wk or more Greater than 6 lb/month	2 lb/wk or more Usually total gain over 30 lb in third trimester
Gastric/epigastric function	No problems	Impossible to distinguish from indigestion caused by increasing uterine size	Nausea and vomiting Epigastric pain (classic warning sign of imminent seizure)
Central nervous system function	No signs	No signs	Headache Visual changes: blind spots, photophobia, blurred vision
Renal function	No signs	Proteinuria	Impaired renal function Oliguria (output less than 30 ml/hr)
Placental function	No signs	Decreased blood flow	Decreased blood flow Significant premature calcification found on ultrasound
Fetal wellbeing	No signs	Decreased fetal growth, established by baseline ultrasound	Intrauterine growth retardation Decreased fetal movement

Table 7-3 Drugs That May Be Indicated in Control of PIH

Drug	Dosage	Indications and Adverse Reactions	Nursing Implications
Antihypertensives			
Aldomet (methyldopa)	500 to 1,000 mg orally four times daily	Drug is indicated in essential hypertension and used for outpatient maintenance. It is also an adrenergic blocker with many systemic side effects. Its safety in pregnancy is not established, but no specific fetal effects are known.	Regular interval readings are needed during period of adjustment. Initial sedative effect is beneficial to maintaining bedrest with PIH. Drug may enhance orthostatic hypotension. Observe for symptoms of mental depression. Tolerance may occur in 2 to 3 weeks of therapy, indicated by rise in BP. This must be reported to physician. Compliance tends to be poor because of drug's many side-effects. Encourage patient to keep appointments.

Hydrodiuril (hydrochlorothiazide)	50 to 100 mg orally daily	Drug may be used as first-line therapy for pre-existing hypertension. Usually patient is maintained on previous medications. Because of its diuretic action, drug may be discontinued if moderate or severe PIH develops. There are no known adverse effects to the fetus.	Advise patient to eat potassium-rich foods Check potassium level with periodic serum electrolytes.
Apresoline (hydralazine)	10 to 40 mg IV, every 4 to 6 hours	Drug is reserved for treatment of severe PIH in hospitalized patients. Reduces BP by direct relaxation of vascular smooth muscles. Short-term side-effects are minimal except for cardiovascular changes—palpitation, tachycardia, flushing, hypotension. There are no known adverse effects to the fetus.	Monitor and record BP and pulse every 15 minutes. Observe mental status for signs of mental confusion due to too-rapid fall in BP. Monitor intake and output.

(continued)

Table 7-3 Drugs That May Be Indicated in Control of PIH (*continued*)

Drug	Dosage	Indications and Adverse Reactions	Nursing Implications
Anticonvulsant Sedatives			
Valium (diazepam)	5 to 10 mg orally twice daily	This mild sedative and CNS depressant aids compliance with complete bedrest when patient is being treated at home. It reduces CNS stimulation with progressing PIH. Since it also depresses fetus, it should be discontinued several days before delivery.	If given within 24 hours of delivery, watch for flattened baseline or other changes on the fetal monitor indicating depression. Report such changes to physician.
Magnesium sulfate	*Initial Dose* IV: 2–4 g $MgSO_4$ (USP) as 10% solution injected slowly over 2- to 4-min period IM: 10 g$MgSO_4$ (USP) as 50% solution in H_2O; divided doses, 10 ml in each buttock; 1% procaine may	Drug decreases acetylcholine for neuromuscular transmission. It has a mild hypotensive effect and inhibits uterine contractions. Excessive magnesium in the newborn may cause lethargy and depressed respirations.	If deep tendon reflexes (knee jerk) are depressed, stop drug and call physician. If serum magnesium is above 7 mEq/liter, stop drug. Calcium gluconate is antidote and should be kept at the bedside. Watch for respiratory de-

	be added to reduce pain of injection *Maintenance Dose* IV: 20 g $MgSO_4$ in 1000 ml 5% dextrose in H_2O; usually 1 g/hr, depending on reflexes, respirations, urinary output, etc. IM: 5 g $MgSO_4$ as 50% solution every 4 hr (administered same as initial dose), depending on reflexes, etc.		pression. Rate should be 12 bpm or more. Continue all nursing precautions for the severely preeclamptic patient.
Diuretics			
Lasix (Furosemide)	40 mg IV (slow push)	Drug is reserved for treatment of pulmonary edema resulting from eclamptic seizures. Caution: it may conceal the degree of hypovolemia and oliguria present. It is usually given after delivery.	See section on nursing management of the eclamptic patient. Monitor CVP line. Maintain IV infusion and medications. Monitor hourly urinary output.
Hydrodiuril		Although a diuretic, drug is never used in pregnancy to relieve edema of PIH. It may be used to treat preexisting hypertension	

Table 7-4 TORCH Infections

Infection and Transmission	Maternal Symptoms	Fetal Effects	Nursing Intervention
Toxoplasmosis			
Protozoa transmitted via undercooked meat, cat feces, and transplacentally	Usually asymptomatic or mild and self-limiting symptoms, so most infections are not diagnosed during pregnancy. Swollen cervical lymph nodes in some cases. Difficult to differentiate from mononucleosis. Serologic testing necessary for diagnosis	If disease is acquired during pregnancy, 40% of fetuses will be infected In early pregnancy, increased abortion, stillbirth, intrauterine growth retardation (IUGR), and severe congenital infection In newborns, jaundice, hepatosplenomegaly, encephalitis Sequelae in surviving infected infants: microcephaly, cerebral calcification, chorioretinitis, mental retardation Newborn may be asymptomatic	Instruct pregnant women about the source of disease. Instruct in how to cook meat as recommended. Instruct to avoid cleaning kitty litter box.

Other*			
Syphilis			
Spirochete transmitted via sexual contact and transplacentally	In primary infection, chancre possible in genital area Rash possible on hands and feet Premature labor common Serologic testing required prenatally	Secondary infection with skin rash and purulent nasal discharge. CNS damage Hearing loss Mortality 10% to 30% if untreated.	Include VDRL in laboratory studies on first prenatal visit. Review history for past infections and treatment. Observe preterm newborns for evidence of a palmar rash and "snuffles."
Hepatitis			
Virus A transmitted via contaminated water, fecal-oral route. B transmitted by sexual contact, contaminated needles, and transplacentally.†	Fever, headache, abdominal pain, tea-colored urine, jaundice Virus found in all body fluids, including urine, feces, and semen	Symptomatic chronic hepatitis Jaundice at 3 to 4 months of age Mental retardation possible from high bilirubin levels	Discuss sexual transmission of disease. Make public health referral for evaluation of home environment (many of those affected are drug users). Give HB immune globulin to infants born to women with active hepatitis B. Schedule follow-up pediatric or public health care for repeat of injection monthly for 6 months.

(continued)

Table 7-4 TORCH Infections (*continued*)

Infection and Transmission	Maternal Symptoms	Fetal Effects	Nursing Intervention
Rubella			
Virus transmitted via nasopharynx droplet, transplacentally	Usually mild illness Swollen lymph nodes preceding a rash Rash beginning on face, neck, chest and spreading to abdomen and extremities Joint pain common in adults	In early pregnancy, abortion, stillbirth, gross abnormalities May remain chronically infected for months Classic anomalies: microcephaly, heart defects, cataracts, and deafness	Screen with rubella titer on first prenatal visit. If not immune, schedule immunization in immediate postpartum period. Isolate infected newborns: virus is shed in saliva and urine.
Cytomegalovirus			
Virus transmitted via contact with body fluids, including colostrum, or contact with cervical mucus	Positive antibodies from prior exposure in 50% to 60% of pregnant women Usually asymptomatic Tends to be latent but activated with immunosuppression of pregnancy	May be subclinical to severe, including hyperbilirubinemia, hepatosplenomegaly, pneumonitis, and encephalitis Of those with encephalitis, 5% will die, 85% will have CNS abnormalities	Isolate infected newborns: virus is shed in salvia and urine. No effective treatment known No immunization available

	Serologic testing necessary for diagnosis	If symptomatic at birth: SGA, long-term developmental and learning disabilities Early exposure results in classic tetrad: microcephaly, cerebral calcification, severe mental retardation, and chorioretinitis.	
Herpes Simplex, Type I and II			
Virus transmitted via sexual contact, contact with cervical mucus, or transplacentally	Mostly found in adolescents and young adults Primary infection: painful vesicles on labia, vagina, or cervix, with systemic symptoms of fever, headache, malaise, and anorexia. Recurrent infection: localized painful lesions—systemic symptoms are rare	In early pregnancy, increase in abortions Later in pregnancy, increase in preterm labor Congenital anomalies suspected Infected newborn has 60% risk of mortality Severe neurologic sequelae in 50% of infected survivors	Discuss sexual transmission. Schedule periodic herpes cultures according to protocol (weekly after 34 weeks)—if positive culture is found within 72 hours of delivery, cesarean delivery is indicated. Record and report rupture of membranes during labor. Culture newborn for herpes. Isolate and observe for signs of infection.

* This category includes Group B streptococcal infections, chlamydia, varicella zoster, and AIDS.
† Major effects on fetus relate to Hepatitis B.

- Weigh patient daily.
- Measure daily fluid intake and urinary output.
- Order a high-protein diet (facilitates fluid excretion) and encourage patient to drink 6 to 8 glasses of water daily.
- Monitor fetal activity and heart rate and response to maternal contractions with nonstress testing.
- Order prescribed ultrasound to assess placental function.
- Administer the prescribed antihypertensive drugs and maintain IV infusions.

See Table 7-3.

Eclampsia (at risk for convulsions)

- Provide a darkened, quiet room to reduce central nervous system (CNS) stimuli.
- Provide seizure precautions.
- Monitor hourly urinary output with a Foley catheter.
- Take and record BP and pulse every 15 minutes until stable, then every 30 to 60 minutes.
- Test deep tendon reflexes every 30 to 60 minutes for hyperreflexia and clonus.
- Observe the fetal monitor for signs of fetal distress or spontaneous onset of labor.
- Maintain magnesium sulfate IV infusion and other medications at the rate and dose ordered.
- Transfer patient to ICU if pulmonary edema occurs.

SYSTEMIC INFECTIONS DURING PREGNANCY

A group of systemic infections that occur during pregnancy is known as the TORCH group, so called from the initial letters of the various infections: *t*oxoplasmosis, *o*ther (syphilis and hepatitis), *r*ubella, *c*ytomegalovirus, and *h*erpes. These infections may be sexually transmitted. They share an ability to affect the fetus by crossing the placenta or by way of an ascending infection after rupture of the membranes and cervical dilatation. These conditions receive little attention in maternity nursing because they are thought to be rare. In fact, however, they are increasing in incidence, are often difficult to detect in the adult, and may not be obvious in the newborn until weeks or months after birth. These infections are discussed in Table 7-4.

8
Labor and Delivery

THE PROCESS OF LABOR AND BIRTH

Nursing Objectives in Labor and Birth

- To assess maternal, fetal, and family risk factors that may affect the course of labor and to determine the nursing care required
- To monitor the emotional and physiologic status of family members during the complex process

The Four Ps of Childbirth

Four factors, commonly known as the "four Ps," are of critical importance in the process of childbirth: passage, passenger, powers, and psyche.

- *Passage.* In normal pregnancy the pelvic anatomy, or the passage, must be adequate for the individual fetus.
- *Passenger.* The fetus must be in an advantageous position.
- *Power.* Uterine contractions must be rhythmic, coordinated, and efficient.
- *Psyche.* Maternal efforts must be adequate to accomplish the delivery of the fetus.

Passage: The Pelvis

The passage is determined by maternal pelvic anatomy: the bony pelvis and the muscles of the pelvic floor and perineum. Specific pelvic landmarks and measurements are important when considering the complementary relationship between the bony pelvis and the fetus.

Pelvic Planes and Measurements

For obstetric purposes the pelvis is described as having three planes: the inlet, the midpelvis, and the outlet, as shown in Figure 8-1.

Assessment of Pelvic Capacity

- Pubic arch (subpubic angle) should be wide and rounded at 90 degrees or more to allow pivoting of the descending fetus. A narrow or acute pubic angle will force the fetal head onto the perineum and cause major perineal tears.

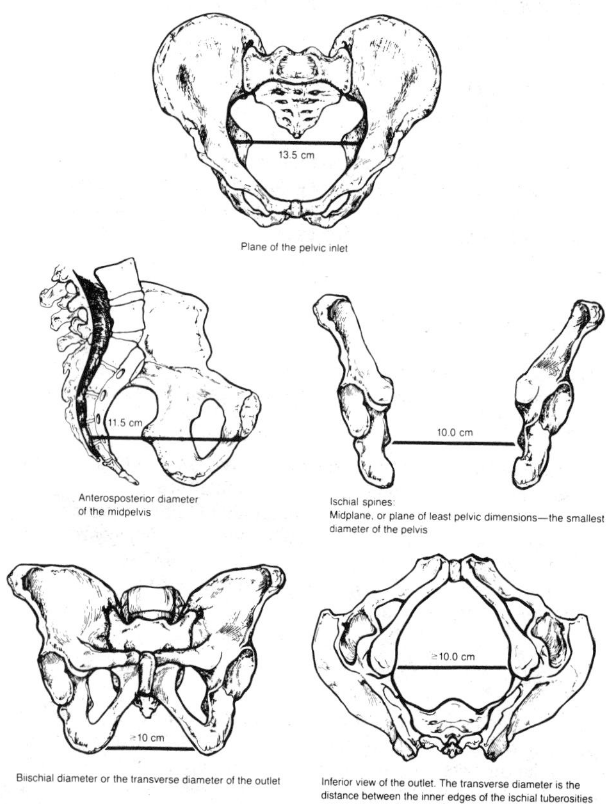

Figure 8-1 Planes of the pelvis. Figures give average measurements. (Childbirth Graphics)

- Ischial spines should be blunt. Sharp encroaching spines decrease the transverse diameter of the midpelvis.
- The sacrum will determine the posterior capacity of the pelvis in all three planes by the configuration of its curvature and length. It may be concave, flat, or convex. A flat or convex configuration will decrease pelvic capacity.

Passenger: The Fetus

The fetus, or passenger, must undergo a series of predictable and synchronized maneuvers to accommodate its descent through the maternal pelvis during normal labor.

Fetal Head

In labor and birth the fetal head is usually the presenting part and is considered the most important part because it:

- Is not compressible, as is the rest of the body
- Represents the largest part of the term infant (along with the shoulders)
- Has the ability to mold by overlapping its cranial bones under pressure—usually without damage to the underlying tissue

Landmarks of the fetal head are shown in Figures 8-2 and 8-3.

Diameters of the Fetal Skull

- Biparietal diameter (average 9.5 cm) is the distance between the parietal bosses. It represents the largest transverse diameter of the fetal head and is considered to be the most obstetrically important consideration.
- Suboccipitobregmatic diameter (average 9.5 cm) extends from the inferior occipital bone to the bregma of the forehead.
- Occipitofrontal diameter (average 11.75 cm) extends from the occipital protuberance to the glabella (elevated area between the orbital ridges).

Fetopelvic Relationships

The following terms are useful in describing the position of the fetus in the pelvis and the level of descent through the pelvis: station, lie, presentation, position, attitude, and synclitism and asynclitism.

Station

Station is the level of fetal presenting part in relation to the ischial spines of the midpelvis. The various levels are defined as:

- 0 station: Presenting part at level of ischial spines (engaged)

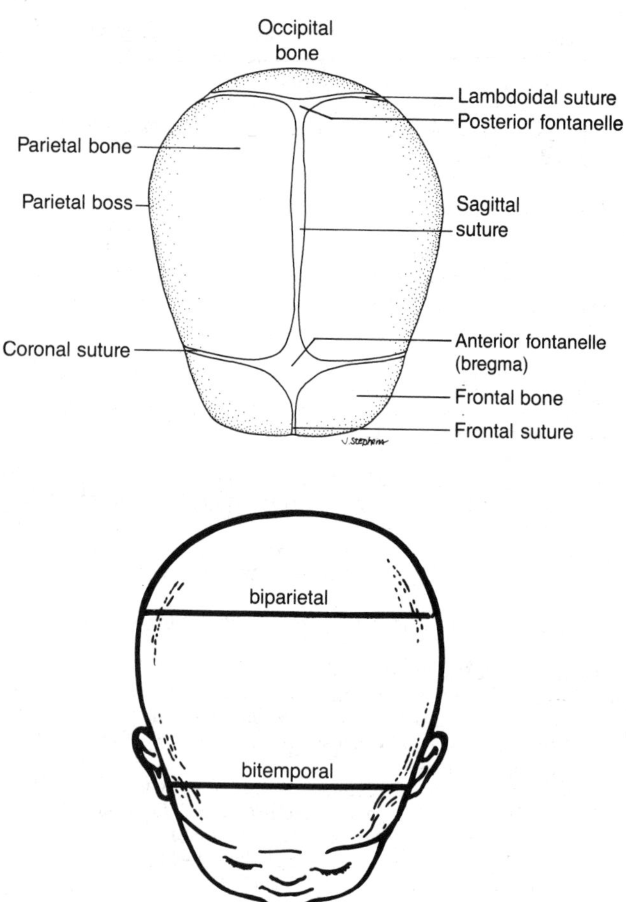

Figure 8-2 Fetal cranium superior. *(A)* Bones. *(B)* Transverse diameters. (Childbirth Graphics)

- −4 to −1 station: Centimeters above the ischial spines (minus stations)
- 1 to 4 station: Centimeters below the ischial spines (plus stations)

See Figure 8-4.

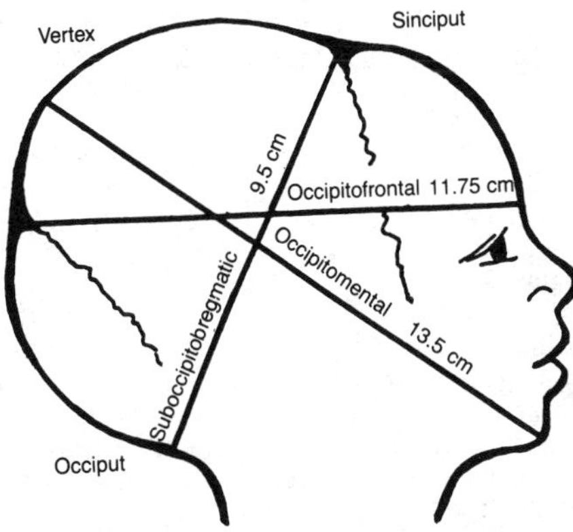

Figure 8-3 Diameters of the fetal skull. (Childbirth Graphics)

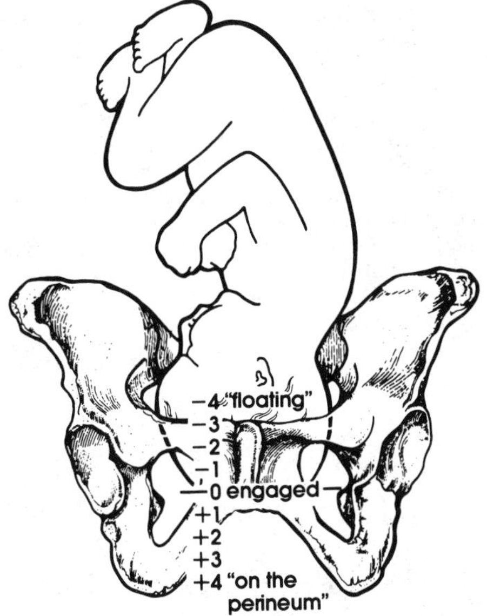

Figure 8-4 Stations of the fetal head.

Fetal Lie

Fetal lie is the relationship of the long axis of the fetus to the long axis of the mother.

- *Longitudinal lie.* Fetal and maternal spines are parallel (most common lie).
- *Oblique lie.* Fetus is at a slight angle off a true transverse lie.

See Figure 8-5.

Presentation

Presentation refers to the part of the fetus that enters, or presents, to the maternal pelvis. The most common is *cephalic* or vertex presentation, which occurs in 95% of labors. *Breech,* or buttock, presentations occur in about 4% of labors and are of three types (Fig. 8-6):

- Frank breech, the most common, is characterized by fetal flexion at the thighs and extension at the knees.
- Complete breech is characterized by fetal flexion at the thighs and knees.
- Footling, or incomplete breech, is characterized by extension at knees and thighs.

Position

Position is the relationship of a particular reference point of the presenting part to the maternal pelvis. Each fetal position is identified by a standard abbreviation with three elements. The elements appear in the following order: the first indicates whether the presenting part is to the left, to the right, or transverse in the maternal pelvis; the second indicates what the presenting part is; and the third indicates whether it is in the anterior or posterior half of the pelvis (Abbreviations are listed in the front of the Manual). See Figure 8-7.

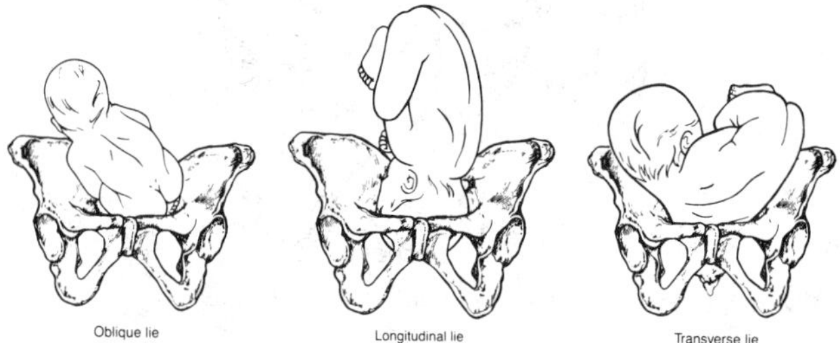

Figure 8-5 Fetal lie. (Childbirth Graphics)

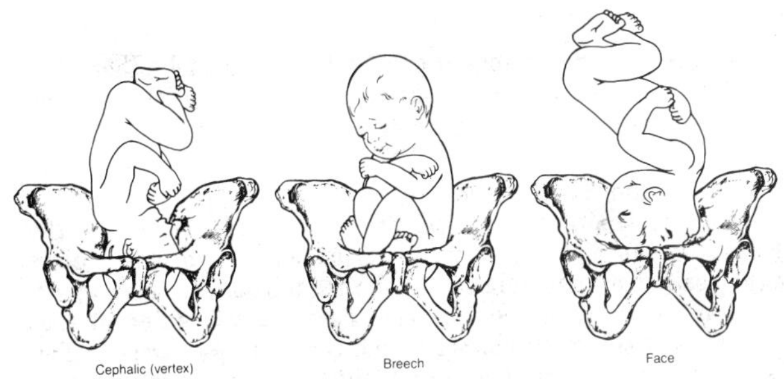

Figure 8-6 Fetal presentations. (Childbirth Graphics)

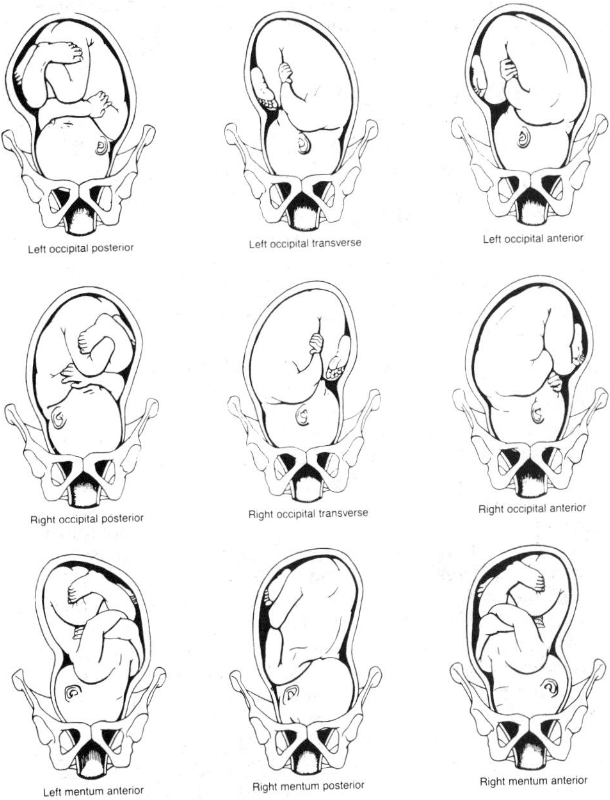

Figure 8-7 Fetal positions. (Childbirth Graphics)

Attitude

Attitude is the relationship of the fetal parts to each other. The attitude of the head determines what part of the skull is the presenting part.

Synclitism and Asynclitism

These terms denote the position of the fetal head in relation to the anteroposterior diameter of the maternal pelvis. Synclitism refers to the position of the fetal head when the sagittal suture is halfway between the sacral promontory and the symphysis pubis, so that the planes of the maternal pelvis and the fetal skull are parallel. Asynclitism refers to the position of the fetal head when the sagittal suture is closer to the sacral promontory or the symphysis pubis. These positions occur normally as the fetal head shifts to accommodate the irregular shape of the pelvic cavity.

Cardinal Movements of Labor

Cardinal movements or mechanisms of labor are a series of passive adjustments of position as the fetus descends through the pelvis during labor. The movements flow smoothly and often overlap as labor progresses. Cardinal movements are:

- *Descent.* The continuous downward movement of the fetus that is brought about by pressure of the uterine contractions. During the second stage of labor maternal bearing-down efforts facilitate descent.
- *Flexion.* A natural attitude conforming to the shape of the uterine cavity and resistance of the pelvic floor during labor. Flexion of the fetal head is important because it causes the smallest diameter of the fetal head to present to the maternal pelvis.
- *Internal Rotation.* The fetal head must rotate to an occiput anterior position when it reaches the midpelvis to accommodate the narrowest transverse diameter of the pelvis. This usually occurs during the second stage of labor or earlier in multiparas.
- *Extension.* Continued downward pressure of uterine contractions and resistance of the pelvic floor causes extension of the fetal head. It remains extended until crowning, so that the smallest diameter of the fetal head presents and distends the perineum. Extension is complete when the head is born.
- *Restitution.* Occurring automatically when the head is born, restitution is the untwisting of the infant's neck to its normal relationship with the shoulders.
- *External Rotation and Expulsion.* May occur in conjunction with restitution. Involves rotation of the infant's shoulders and delivery of the anterior shoulder under the symphysis pubis while the posterior shoulder slides out over the perineum.

Power: The Uterus in Labor

The power of the uterine contractions is a major force in contributing to the process of labor and birth. There are three phases of uterine contractions:

- *Increment.* Period during which the intensity of the contraction increases
- *Acme.* Strongest point of the contraction
- *Decrement.* Period of decreasing intensity

See Figure 8-8.

Interval of Uterine Contractions

During normal labor, contractions occur 2 to 20 minutes apart, last 15 to 19 seconds, and are of varying intensity, depending on the stage of labor.

Purposes of Uterine Contractions

Effacement and dilatation of the cervix
Facilitation of descent and rotation of the fetus
Separation and expulsion of the placenta after birth
Maintenance of hemostasis after expulsion of the placenta by compressing blood vessels
Provision of intervals between contractions that allow the uterine muscle to rest and assure its uninterrupted blood circulation

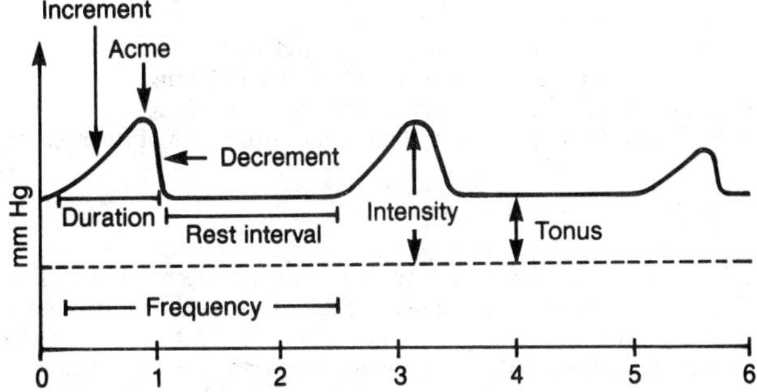

Figure 8-8 Characteristic pattern of uterine contraction. (Childbirth Graphics)

Cervical Effacement and Dilatation

- *Effacement* is the softening, thinning, and shortening of the cervical canal. It is evaluated during labor in terms of percentages: 0% indicates no effacement; 100% indicates complete effacement. In multiparas the cervix may be effaced as much as 50% before labor begins.
- *Dilatation* is the opening and enlargement of the external cervical os from a few millimeters during pregnancy to 10 cm at complete dilatation in labor. It is caused by the retraction of the cervix into the lower uterine segment as a result of labor contractions and pressure of the amniotic sac (Fig. 8-9).

Stages of Labor

- *First stage.* Begins with the onset of regular contractions and ends with complete dilatation of the cervix
- *Second stage.* Begins with complete dilatation of the cervix and ends with birth of the infant
- *Third stage.* Begins with the birth of the infant and ends with delivery of the placenta
- *Fourth stage.* Begins with delivery of the placenta and lasts at least 1 hour or until the mother's condition is stabilized

Duration of Labor
See Table 8-1.

Psyche: Maternal Adaptation of Labor

The woman's psychosocial adaptation is a critical aspect of the process of labor and birth. Her perception is influenced by her:

- Self-confidence
- Pattern of coping with uncertainty and stress
- Attitudes and expectations about labor and birth
- Expectations about her family and care providers
- Response to pain, anxiety, and other alterations of functioning

Pain in Labor and Birth

Most women anticipate and, in fact, do experience some pain in childbirth. Labor pain is sometimes described as the most intense pain a person may experience, and the pain of labor is often the aspect of childbirth most worrisome to expectant parents. There is undoubtedly a physiologic basis for pain in labor, although the intensity of the pain experienced varies a great deal from one

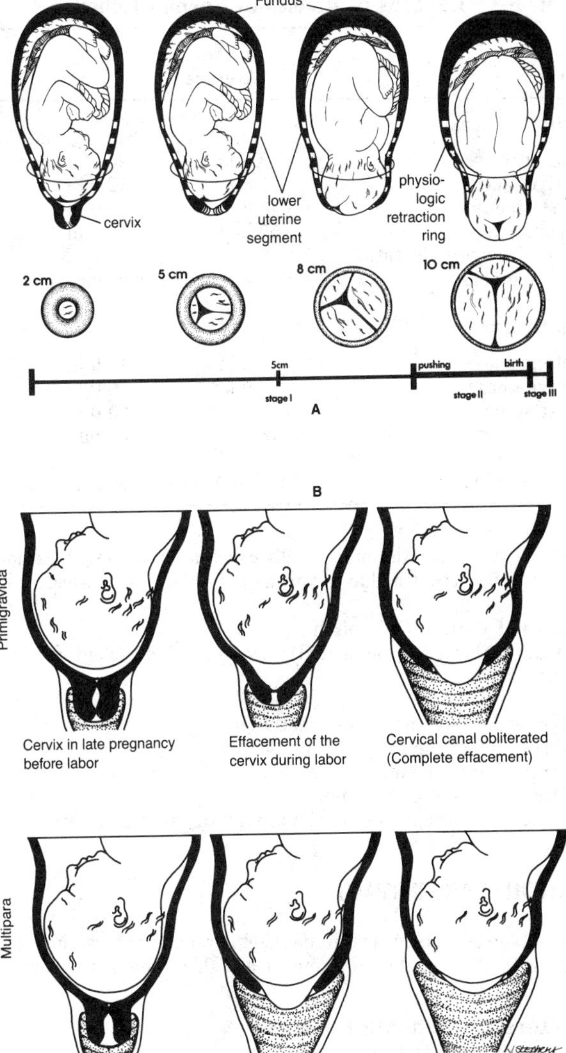

Figure 8-9 Cervical effacement and dilatation. (Childbirth Graphics)

Table 8-1 Lengths of Phases in Normal Labor

Phase	Average	Upper Normal
Primigravidas		
Latent phase	8.6 hr	20.0 hr
Active phase	5.8 hr	12.0 hr
First stage	13.3 hr	28.5 hr
Second stage	57 min	150 min
Rate of cervical dilatation in active phase	Under 1.2 cm/hr is abnormal	
Multiparas		
Latent phase	5.3 hr	14.0 hr
Active phase	2.5 hr	6.0 hr
First stage	7.5 hr	20.0 hr
Second stage	18 min	50 min
Rate of cervical dilatation in active phase	Under 1.5 cm/hr is abnormal	

woman to another. Although usually pain is associated with pathology, in childbirth it is due to normal physiologic processes.

Causes of Pain in Childbirth

Pain during labor may be related to a variety of physiologic factors, including:

- Cervical stretching during dilatation
- Distention of the lower uterine segment
- Stretching of the uterine ligaments
- Traction on the peritoneum
- Pressure on the nerve ganglia around the uterus and vagina

LABOR: FIRST STAGE

First-stage labor begins with the onset of regular contractions and ends with the complete effacement and dilatation of the cervix.

Factors Influencing Progress in Labor and Birth

- *Maternal Age.* The very young woman (under 16 years) may have an immature, small pelvis, increasing the risk of cephalopelvic disproportion, and is at increased risk for preeclampsia.

The older woman (over 35 years) is more likely to have twins, breech, or occiput posterior presentation and a longer second stage of labor.

- *Maternal Weight.* Overweight women are at risk for delays or arrests in latent or active phases of labor and for soft tissue dystocia, the slowing of the second stage.
- *Birth Interval.* When birth intervals are less than 1 year, the woman is at risk for a more rapid labor and a smaller infant.
- *Birth Weight and Gestational Age.* Preterm and small fetuses are usually associated with fast labors, whereas large fetuses are generally associated with longer labors, especially longer second-stage labors. Gestational age of less than 37 weeks is associated with a higher rate of malpresentation, which can affect the progress of labor. Gestational age of more than 42 weeks is associated with macrosomia, or large body size in the fetus, and a higher risk of birth complications.
- *Fetal Position.* Labor progresses most effectively when the fetus is in a well-fixed vertex position.
- *Status of Amniotic Sac.* Early rupture of the amniotic sac may interfere with the progress of labor. There is no evidence that rupture of the amniotic sac shortens labor. Some evidence indicates that the fetus may be at higher risk for acidosis when membranes are ruptured before the second stage of labor.
- *Site of Placental Implantation.* High or fundal implantation of the placenta has been shown to be associated with prolonged labor.
- *Maternal Position During Labor.* Standing or upright positions have been found to be most efficient in dilating the cervix and have been associated with lower incidence of umbilical cord compression and increased maternal comfort. The lateral recumbent position appears to result in less efficient uterine contractions than the upright position. The supine position is associated with more frequent but less efficient contractions. The supine position puts the mother at risk for maternal supine hypotensive syndrome. Maternal symptoms of supine hypotension include dizziness, breathlessness, visual changes, and numbness and tingling in the extremities. Uterine arterial circulation may also be impaired by compression of the abdominal aorta by the uterus.
- *Psychological Factors.* Stress and anxiety stimulate the release of stress hormones called catecholamines, which inhibit uterine activity. Childbirth preparation is helpful in reducing stress and anxiety associated with labor and birth and may contribute to more favorable labor progress and outcome.
- *Medications.* The use of narcotic analgesia has been shown to slow down the active phase of labor. Magnesium sulfate, used in the treatment of preeclampsia, has been shown to diminish the frequency and intensity of uterine contractions as well as reduce the resting tone of the uterus. There is some controversy about

whether regional anesthesia slows the progress of labor and contributes to increased need for oxytocin augmentation and cesarean delivery.

Latent Phase (0 to 4 cm)

Possible Nursing Diagnoses Related to Latent Labor

- Anxiety related to perceived threat of impending labor and expressed feelings of apprehension, nervousness, and frequent requests for reassurance
- Alteration in comfort (pain) related to uncomfortable contractions and restlessness in early labor
- Lack of knowledge of admission procedures and comfort measures related to first pregnancy or inadequate prenatal care

Occasionally women experiencing uterine contractions are not sure that they are actually in labor. The labor nurse is often called on to help in making this determination.

Distinguishing Between True and False Labor

- Signs and symptoms of impending labor are Braxton Hicks' contractions; lightening; cervical changes (softening, effacement, and dilation); increased vaginal discharge, in some cases; persistent backache; weight loss; and nesting behavior.
- Signs of true labor are uterine contractions; spontaneous rupture of membranes; and bloody show.
- Distinguishing characteristics of true and false labor are shown in Table 8-2.

Nursing Assessment: Latent Phase (0 to 4 cm)

Assessing the Pattern of Uterine Contractions

- *Intensity.* Described as mild, moderate, or strong; the contraction will increase and reach a peak, then slowly diminish
- *Duration.* Measures the contraction in seconds from its beginning to end
- *Frequency.* Measured by noting the time in minutes from the beginning of one contraction to the beginning of the next

Table 8-2 Distinguishing Between True and False Labor

True Labor	False Labor
Uterine Contractions	
Show regular pattern	Show irregular pattern
Usually become closer together, stronger, and longer	Usually vary
Increase in intensity with walking	May stop with walking or position change
Are usually felt in lower back, radiating to lower abdomen	Are usually felt in back, upper fundus
Are not stopped by relaxation techniques such as hot bath, heating pad, alcoholic drink, or sedation	Will eventually stop with relaxation techniques
Cervix	
Softens, effaces, and dilates	May soften; no significant change in dilatation or effacement
Fetus	
Starts descent into pelvis	No noticeable change in position

Determining the Status of Amniotic Membranes

- Are membranes intact or ruptured?
  - Mother reports gush of fluid.
  - If ruptured, note time, color, and odor of amniotic fluid. An unpleasant odor, thick consistency, or discoloration suggests possible fetal difficulty.

Tests or Procedures to Assist in Establishing Membrane Status

- *Nitrazine paper test.* Paper will turn bright blue when exposed to the alkalinity of the amniotic fluid.
- *Ferning.* This procedure demonstrates the presence of amniotic fluid, which appears as a frondlike pattern of crystallization when dried on a slide and viewed microscopically.
- Sterile speculum examination. This procedure can detect pooling of fluid in the vagina. If fluid leaks from the cervix when the patient coughs, ruptured membranes are almost assured.

Assessment on Admission to the Labor Unit

When a woman is admitted to the labor unit, the following assessments are routine: complete history, including demographic data, history of present pregnancy, history of past pregnancy, past medical and family history, and present labor history.

Psychosocial and Emotional Status

- Age, educational level, socioeconomic level
- Overall response to pregnancy
- Previous experience with childbearing
- Cultural background
- Family support and partner status
- Nature of contact with care providers (clinic or private patient? consistent prenatal care? preference for particular provider and birth "options"?)
- Extent and type of preparation for birth and parenthood

Physical examination

- General physical assessment
- Abdominal examination to assess fetal size, position, heart tones, movement
- Pelvic examination to assess cervical effacement and dilatation, fetal station, presenting part/position, status of membranes, status of perineum, presence of molding or caput

Laboratory Tests

- Evaluation of prenatal laboratory tests; complete blood cell count (CBC); urinalysis for protein, glucose, ketones; type and cross-match

Monitoring Maternal Vital Signs

In early labor maternal blood pressure (BP), pulse, and respirations show little or no elevation. Pulse and respirations may show slight increases in response to cardiovascular demands of active labor. During labor, vital signs should be monitored as follows:

- Every hour in the latent and active phases
- Every 10 to 15 minutes in the second stage
- Every 5 to 10 minutes in the third stage
- Every 15 minutes for an hour, then every 30 minutes for 2 to 4 hours in the fourth stage

Maternal temperature should be monitored every 4 hours while membranes are intact and temperature is normal. If temperature is over 37.5°C (99.6°F) or membranes have ruptured, temperature should be assessed every 2 hours.

Monitoring Fetal Heart Rate

Fetal heart rate (FHR) should remain between 120 and 160 beats/minute. If the pattern remains within normal limits and no complications arise, it is monitored during labor as follows:

- Every 30 to 60 minutes during the latent phase
- Every 15 minutes during the active phase
- Immediately after rupture of membranes
- Immediately after any change in contraction pattern
- After every contraction during the second stage
- At maternal request

Nurse Alert

Monitoring Maternal and Fetal Wellbeing in Labor

- If maternal BP is greater than 140/90 or shows 10- to 15-mm Hg elevation over pregnant levels, notify the attending physician or nurse midwife: the elevation may signal developing preeclampsia. If pulse rate is over 100 bpm or the respiration rate is over 20 per minute, notify the attending physician or nurse midwife: the elevation may signal maternal dehydration, developing infection, or hemorrhage. Elevation in pulse rate often is the first sign of impending maternal hemorrhage and precedes any drop in BP following rapid blood loss.

Nursing Interventions

Self-Care Teaching: Early Labor

- Rest, relax, and conserve energy.
- Keep your mind occupied with something enjoyable.
- Try comfort measures such as a warm bath, walking, or massage.
- Empty your bladder frequently and eat lightly (unless otherwise directed by your birth attendant).
- Keep taking clear fluids, such as water, juice, or soothing teas.
- Time your contractions, and don't use labor coping techniques (such as breathing techniques) until you really need them to help you stay comfortable.

Active Phase (4 to 7 cm)

Possible Nursing Diagnoses Related to Active Labor

- Alteration in comfort (pain) related to uterine contractions as expressed by grimacing and muscular tension with contractions
- Potential fluid volume deficit related to restriction of oral fluids and increased fluid loss
- Alteration in mobility related to electronic fetal monitoring
- Impaired gas exchange related to hyperventilation with contractions
- Alteration in urinary elimination related to pressure of fetal descent

---

Normally women are admitted to the labor unit in active labor. Characteristics of this phase include increased uterine activity with descent of the fetus into the bony pelvis.

Nursing Assessment: Active Phase (4 to 7 cm)

- Obtain hourly BP.
- Check pulse, respirations, and temperature every 2 to 4 hours (hourly when membranes have ruptured).
- Examine urine with dipstick for protein and ketones at each voiding.
- Palpate the bladder regularly to detect overdistention.
    - Perform a catheterization when bladder distention is a problem; use strict aseptic technique to avoid urinary tract infection.
- Monitor the progress of labor noting:
    - Cervical dilatation and effacement
    - Status of membranes
    - Position and station of presenting part
    - Fetal molding and caput
    - Pattern and intensity of uterine contractions
- Assess the progress of labor before administering pain medication.
- Record progress of labor on a labor graph as noted by periodic vaginal examinations.
- Note behavioral cues of the laboring woman: seriousness, growing apprehension; sense of purpose; introspection; fear of being alone, desire for companionship; change from relaxation to ten-

sion; internal conflict of confidence versus fear; ill-defined doubts and fears.

Nurse Alert

Signs of Inadequate Uterine Relaxation

Placental perfusion is decreased during uterine contraction. Healthy fetuses can tolerate this over the course of labor in the following circumstances:

- If the uterus relaxes well between contractions for long enough (more than 30 seconds) to allow normal perfusion between contractions
- If contractions are not unusually long (*i.e.*, less than 90 seconds)

Abnormally long, strong contractions, termed tetanic contractions, may follow oxytocin administration to stimulate or augment labor. If uterine contractions last more than 90 seconds or occur more often than every 30 seconds:

- Stop oxytocin administration.
- Change mother to left lateral position.
- Administer oxygen by tight face mask at 8 to 12 liter/minute.
- Assess fetal heart rate pattern.
- Notify physician.

Determining Fetal Wellbeing

Additional requirements to auscultate fetal heart tones in the active phase of labor are necessary following:

- Spontaneous or artificial rupture of the fetal membranes
- Sudden change in the labor or contraction pattern:
  - tetanic or prolonged contraction
  - precipitous labor
- An obstetric or medical complication during labor
- An obstetric procedure such as vaginal examination, manual rotation
- Request of the mother

Nursing Intervention

Providing Pain Relief: Analgesia in Labor

In the management of normal labor, the most commonly used types of analgesia are psychoprophylactic techniques and parenteral analgesia. This section focuses on parenteral analgesia, conduction and inhalation analgesia, and anesthesia, which are often the methods of choice in situations where maternal or fetal risk may be increased.

- See Appendix C-2, Drugs Used for Analgesia in Labor
- *Drug Administration.* Administration of these medications and monitoring of their effects during labor are nursing responsibilities. The nurse must be knowledgeable about the patient's condition, the condition of the fetus, and the safe use of each medication in intrapartal care. The following nursing implications relate to the administration of *any* of these medications to the woman in labor:
  - Administration during labor is typically by intramuscular (IM) or intravenous (IV) route. Dosages are kept to the smallest effective dose so that duration of effect can be better predicted and deleterious effects minimized.
  - Intramuscular administration should be done with a needle that is long enough to ensure that the medication is placed in muscle rather than subcutaneous fat, since muscle provides optimal absorption.
  - Intravenous administration should be done slowly at a rate of 1 ml/minute or less to avoid a too rapid physiologic response to the drug. Intravenous medication may also be administered at the beginning of a contraction to decrease the amount of medication transferred to the fetus, since placental circulation is markedly decreased during uterine contraction.
  - Maternal vital signs, FHR, and cervical status should be assessed and recorded prior to administration. Vital signs and FHR should be checked again 10 to 15 minutes after IM administration and 3 to 5 minutes after IV administration to assess possible effects.
  - Effects of any parenteral agent are intensified and potentially more dangerous in the premature or sick fetus or newborn.
  - Routine precautions for administration of these medications should be taken: verify drug and dosage: check for maternal allergies; raise side rails; and closely monitor patient status.
  - Positive suggestion will potentiate the effects of analgesics administered to laboring women.
- Time sequence for nursing support and administration of analgesics/anesthetics during labor: see Table 8-3.

Common Variations in Active Labor

Fetal Heart Rate Variation

Regardless of whether fetal heart tones are assessed with a fetoscope or by electronic fetal monitoring, the nurse may identify FHR patterns during active labor that suggest the need for further, more precise evaluation of fetal status.

Table 8-3 Time Sequence for Nursing Support and Administration of Analgesics/Anesthetics During Labor

Early Labor (1–3 cm dilatation)	Active Labor (4–7 cm dilatation)	Transition (8 cm–complete)	Second Stage (pushing)	Birth
Provide nursing support and promote self-care, using the following: Breathing techniques Back massage Effleurage/stroking Application of heat or cold Position changes, ambulation Praise, encouragement Anticipatory teaching.	Provide nursing support and promote self-care, using the following: Breathing techniques Back massage Effleurage/stroking Application of heat or cold Position changes, ambulation Praise, encouragement Anticipatory teaching.	Provide nursing support and promote self-care, using the following: Breathing techniques Back massage Effleurage/stroking Application of heat or cold Position changes, ambulation Praise, encouragement Anticipatory teaching.	Provide nursing support and promote self-care, using the following: Breathing techniques Back massage Effleurage/stroking Application of heat or cold Position changes, ambulation Praise, encouragement Anticipatory teaching.	

(continued)

Table 8-3 Time Sequence for Nursing Support and Administration of Analgesics/Anesthetics During Labor (*continued*)

Early Labor (1–3 cm dilatation)	Active Labor (4–7 cm dilatation)	Transition (8 cm–complete)	Second Stage (pushing)	Birth
	Caution patient against hyperventilation. Encourage patient to change breathing techniques.	Instruct patient to blow out if she feels urge to push. Do not leave patient alone.	Assist patient with pushing technique, assist with positioning if spinal or epidural anesthetic has been given.	
Sedatives may be provided (Seconal, Nembutal, Restoril, Dalmane).	Analgesics may be provided (Demerol, Nisentil, Stadol, Fentanyl).	Analgesic administration may be repeated if >2 hours before expected delivery.	Local or pudendal anesthesia may be provided.	Narcotic antagonist may be provided.
	Epidural anesthesia may be provided.	Epidural anesthesia may be provided.	Epidural anesthesia may be provided.	Epidural anesthesia may be provided.
		Spinal anesthesia may be provided: Check for bladder distention.		

Nurse Alert

Assessment of FHR Pattern

The following FHR patterns detected by auscultation require further, more precise assessment of FHR pattern:

- Baseline Fetal Heart Rate
  - Tachycardia. FHR of 160 bpm or more for 10 minutes
  - Bradycardia. FHR of 80 to 120 bpm for more than 10 minutes
- Periodic Changes
  - Acceleration. Transitory increase of 15 bpm or more above baseline. Acceleration is not associated with fetal distress, but when it occurs consistently and uniformly with uterine contractions, it may be a forerunner of more serious patterns.
  - Deceleration. Transitory decrease of 15 bpm or more below the baseline. Deceleration that occurs with the onset of contractions and in which FHR returns to baseline rate by the end of the uterine contraction (early deceleration) is not of clinical concern. All other deceleration patterns require further assessment.

If FHR variations are detected:

- Initiate continuous external electronic monitoring of FHR. Place the mother in a side-lying position to eliminate possible maternal supine hypotension or positional cord compression.
- Alert the physician or nurse midwife as to the nature of the FHR variation and response to position change.
- Administer oxygen by tight face mask at 8 to 12 liter/minute to reduce possible fetal hypoxia.
- Explain actions to patient. Explain that more evaluation and possibly treatment may be needed.

Arrest of Labor

Arrest of Labor occurs when cervical dilatation remains the same for 2 hours or more or the rate at which the cervix dilates slows to 1.5 cm/hr in the multigravida or 1.2 cm/hr in the primigravida. The causes of arrest of labor include malposition of the fetus, cephalopelvic disproportion, excessive analgesia, premature administration of regional anesthesia, inadequate uterine contractions, and prior cervical surgery.

When the rate of cervical dilatation is slowed, the labor is sometimes described as dysfunctional. Slow labor without any other abnormality is not harmful to mother or fetus, as long as some progress is being made and there is no fetal distress. Slow labor typically follows one of the following patterns:

- Continuation of slow progress to delivery
- Speeding up of progress to normal rate until delivery
- Slowing to actual arrest pattern

Almost half of all women who experience arrest of labor will resume a normal labor pattern after rest and hydration. Amniotomy and oxytocin administration may also be used to reestablish labor. When cephalopelvic disproportion or malposition is the causative factor, delivery is often by cesarean.

Transition Phase (7 to 10 cm)

The last part of active-phase labor is typically called transition, reflecting the impending shift from first stage of labor to the second stage.

Possible Nursing Diagnoses Related to Transition

- Ineffective individual coping related to exhaustion and sensory overload
- Sensory perceptual alteration related to sensory overload
- Fear related to mate's unexpected behavior changes

Nursing Assessment

During this phase the nursing assessment is geared toward careful monitoring of the maternal and fetal status. Because of the intensity of this phase the woman needs additional support in maintaining control because she may be experiencing any of the following: acute sensitivity and irritability; difficulties in controlling behaviors; uninhibited behavior; fatigue, sleepiness; amnesia; horror of being left alone but little desire for interaction; discouragement and fright; frustration; pronounced introspection; many physical symptoms, including leg cramps, shaking and chills, perspiration, hiccoughing, belching, flatulence, nausea and vomiting, heavy bloody show, pulling and stretching sensations low in the pelvis, and severe backache.

Nursing Intervention

See Table 8-4.

Table 8-4 Nursing Interventions During Transition

Common Physiologic Characteristic	Nursing Support Measures
Shaking, chills	Hold extremities; use warm blankets.
Perspiration, feeling hot	Use fan; wipe with cool cloth; give ice chips.
Restlessness, irritability, increased apprehension	Give encouragement; work on relaxation techniques; avoid behaviors irritating to patient; increase verbal cues for relaxation.
Inability to focus; confusion	Give firm but kind instruction; repeat instruction and show understanding; breathe with patient; use eye contact.
Increased pain, especially sacral	Apply sacral counterpressure; give other comfort measures.
Inability to cope	Give reassurance; maintain physical presence; focus on shortness of phase. Give overwhelming support—"baby is almost here." Take one contraction at a time.
Exhaustion	Facilitate rest and sleep between contractions. Alert patient to beginning of contraction.
Hiccoughing, burping, flatulence	Patient is often embarrassed. Reassure that this is normal.
Nausea and vomiting	Reassure that this is normal and will be over soon; use comfort measure, such as cold cloth to throat; position with head elevated or on left side.
Urge to push	Check for complete dilatation. If not complete, try side-lying position and "blowing contractions away."
Carpopedal spasm	Extend patient's leg and flex foot; check for warmth of extremities; provide blanket as needed.

LABOR: SECOND STAGE

The second stage of labor begins with complete dilatation of the cervix and ends with birth of the infant.

Possible Nursing Diagnoses Related to the Second Stage of Labor

- Alteration in comfort (pain) related to stretching of the cervix, vagina, and perineum
- Potential for perineal injury related to uncontrolled bearing-down efforts
- Anxiety related to an extended second stage
- Fear related to laboring spouse's negative comments, focus, or abandonment of efforts to provide support

---

Nursing Assessment: Maternal and Fetal Monitoring

- Monitor the mother's BP, pulse, and respirations every 5 to 15 minutes throughout the second stage.
- Monitor effects of increased physical activity and fatigue as reflected by flushing, increased perspiration, muscle weakness, and tremors.
- Encourage the mother to void and assess for bladder distention frequently, especially if IV or oral fluids were administered.
- Monitor the fetal heart continuously or after every contraction.
- Observe the mother's bearing-down efforts and assist her in positioning and pushing efforts that will result in labor progress.
- Allow the mother to assume her preferred position and encourage her to use the diaphragm and abdominal muscles to assist in bearing down, while keeping other muscle groups as relaxed as possible to decrease fatigue.
- Observe that the fetal head advances with bearing-down efforts and makes steady progress toward the perineum.
- Determine FHR between and after each contraction to assess changes in baseline FHR and variations in response to contractions and maternal bearing-down efforts. Fetal heart rate will best be heard over the midline in the lower abdomen as fetal descent progresses.

Uterine Activity

- Early second stage uterine activity decreases in intensity and frequency.

- As the stage progresses, uterine contractions increase in frequency from 1 to 3 minutes apart and from 60 to 90 seconds in duration.
- The urge to bear down is initiated by stimulation of sacral and obturator nerves as the fetal head descends into the pelvis.
- The perineum begins to bulge and flatten as the fetal head descends, and bloody show occurs.
- The fetal head advances with each contraction, the labia begin to separate, and the perineum thins.
- As the head appears at the vaginal opening, the introitus expands from a slit to a circular opening.
- Crowning occurs when the largest diameter of the fetal head appears at the vaginal outlet.

Maternal Position

The delivery position used should allow the bearing-down efforts of the mother to be aided by gravity, promote fetal descent and rotation, and avoid supine hypotension. The traditional lithotomy position is not optimum and may cause a more painful and difficult labor; it is the position of choice only when operative procedures are needed to complete delivery.

Varied positions may be used during delivery to promote comfort, enhance or slow down fetal descent, rotate a malpositioned infant, avoid exacerbation of hemorrhoids, increase bearing-down sensations, protect the perineum from lacerations or episiotomy, or intervene when fetal distress occurs due to umbilical cord compression or supine hypotension.

These positions may include: semisitting; supported squat; semilithotomy; hands and knees; sitting on toilet or commode; lying on back, legs pulled back, raising head to push; squatting; and side-lying.

Nursing Interventions

Preparation for Birth

The nurse assumes a key role in preparation for delivery. She must prepare for implementing procedures aimed at:

- Preserving asepsis during delivery
- Gathering necessary equipment, supplies, and personnel
- Assisting the anesthesiologist in preparing the patient for anesthesia when appropriate (See Appendix C-3, Regional and General Anesthesia)
- Monitoring maternal and fetal status on a continuous basis
- Assisting the father in preparations for the birth

Nursing Responsibilities at Delivery

The atmosphere surrounding birth often appears chaotic, since nursing tasks during this time are varied and urgent. The following are common nursing interventions:

- Monitoring maternal vital signs at 5- to 10-minute intervals throughout the second stage
- Monitoring FHR after each contraction
- Assisting the mother and father with position changes and viewing of birth
- Assisting the birth attendant with equipment as needed
- Supporting the mother's bearing-down efforts and instructing her as necessary
- Administering medications, including analgesics and oxytocics as ordered
- Performing the initial assessment of the newborn
- Following identification procedures for newborn

Episiotomy

Episiotomy is an incision made during the second stage of labor to enlarge the opening and accommodate the fetal head. The incision extends from the lower aspect of the vaginal opening into the perineum. Episiotomy is the second most common surgical procedure performed, excluding cutting of the umbilical cord. Over 65% of vaginal deliveries in the United States include episiotomy. Among primigravidas the incidence reaches 80%.

Benefits and Risks of Episiotomy

Benefits of Episiotomy

- The following list reflects general beliefs that are based on observations during clinical practice and are not necessarily documented by clinical research.

- Maternal
  - May maintain pelvic floor integrity
  - May lower incidence of serious lacerations with delivery of a large infant
  - Heals more rapidly than a laceration
- Fetal
  - Shortens second stage, which may be important with compromised fetus

  - May prevent fetal brain damage by reducing pressure on fetal head from pelvic floor; may be important with premature fetus

- Obstetric
  - Facilitates obstetric maneuvers, such as forceps delivery, vacuum extraction
  - Facilitates delivery of malpresenting or large infants
  - Shortens second stage

Risks of Episiotomy

The following risks have been documented in clinical research and practice:

- Severe postepisiotomy pain is estimated to occur in 60% of women.
- Risk of infection is increased.
- Pain and edema may inhibit urination and defecation after delivery.
- Risk of significant blood loss is increased.
- Risk of persistent dyspareunia, which may last 6 months or more, is increased.

Techniques to Avoid Episiotomy

When the client wishes to avoid episiotomy and the birth attendant is cooperative, the following techniques may be used by the nurse to maximize chances for avoiding the procedure.

- Apply hot compresses to the perineum during the second stage of labor to promote relaxation, increased circulation, and increased pliability of the perineal tissues.
- Encourage the patient to avoid bearing-down efforts when crowning occurs.
- Use a lubricant to massage the perineum during the second stage.
- Apply an ice-pack on the clitoral or peri-urethral area during crowning to reduce burning and stinging that accompanies stretching of the vagina and to enhance perineal relaxation.
- Use maternal positions for delivery that avoid overstretching the perineum, such as the side-lying or semisitting positions. When stirrups are used, position patient to avoid hyperextension of the legs and extreme perineal stretching.

Lacerations of the Perineum and Vaginal Tract

Lacerations or spontaneous tears of the perineum, vagina, and occasionally the cervix, may occur during delivery. Factors associated with lacerations of the perineum and vagina include:

- Rapid, precipitous, uncontrolled delivery
- Malpresentations, such as occiput posterior or face presentation
- Use of exaggerated lithotomy position
- Use of perineal anesthesia
- Friable or tense maternal tissue
- Operative delivery

Classification of Lacerations

- *First degree.* Involves the skin or vaginal mucosa but does not extend into the muscular layers
- *Second degree.* Extends from the skin and vaginal mucosa into the muscles of the perineum
- *Third degree.* Extends from the skin, vaginal mucosa, and muscle into the anal sphincter
- *Fourth degree.* Extends through the rectal mucosa into the lumen of the rectum

Immediate Care of the Newborn

As soon as the infant is born, the nurse notes the exact time. When respiration is established, newborn assessment begins. The Apgar scoring system is used to assess fetal response in each of the following:

Heart rate. Indicates the degree of possible asphyxia. A heart rate of less than 100 bpm indicates that resuscitation is needed.

Respiratory effort. Observed along with heart rate. Crying indicates good respiratory effort.

Muscle tone. The degree of flexion and resistance present in the infant's extremities

Reflex irritability. Elicited by initiating the "startle reflex" through sudden contact with cold, noise, or jarring of the supporting surface under the neonate

Color. Immediately after birth the newborn's body is pink while the extremities are often blue (acrocyanosis). Color of the mucous membranes should also be assessed.

See Apgar scoring, Table 8-5

Table 8-5 Apgar Scoring

Sign	Score*		
	0	*1*	*2*
Heart rate	Absent	Slow (below 100)	Over 100
Respiratory rate	Absent	Slow, irregular	Good, crying
Muscle tone	Flaccid	Some flexion of extremities	Active motion
Reflex irritability†	No response	Grimace	Cry
Color	Blue, pale	Body pink, extremities blue	Completely pink

*This method is used for evaluating the immediate postnatal adjustment of the newborn baby. The total score of the five signs is 8 to 10 when the initial adjustment is good. Infants with lower scores require special attention. Scores under 4 indicate that the child is seriously depressed.

†Tested by inserting the tip of a catheter into the nostril.

(Courtesy of Virginia Apgar, MD, and Smith, Kline & French Laboratories, Philadelphia, Pennsylvania)

Support of the Newborn
Positioning of the normal, healthy baby immediately after birth should meet the following criteria:

- Allow for the maintenance of an airway.
- Provide a safe, secure location for the newborn.
- Provide for the thermoregulation of the newborn.
- Allow for frequent assessment by the staff.
- Facilitate the drainage of secretions.
- Facilitate family interaction and bonding.

Maintaining body heat in the normal newborn is accomplished by the following procedures:

- Provide a warm, draft-free environment for delivery.
- Avoid placing the infant in contact with cold objects such as instruments, hands, blankets.
- Dry the baby thoroughly immediately after delivery.
- Use radiant heat or skin-to-skin contact and cover the infant with warm blankets.
- Place a hat on the infant to prevent evaporation heat loss from wet hair.

Resuscitation of the newborn is covered in detail in Chapter 11.

LABOR: THIRD STAGE

The third stage of labor lasts 5 to 30 minutes and involves separation and expulsion of the placenta.

Possible Nursing Diagnoses Related to Third Stage of Labor

- Potential for injury (excessive uterine bleeding) related to uterine atony
- Alteration in comfort related to episiotomy repair and/or massaging of the postpartum uterus
- Family anxiety related to the wellbeing of the newborn.

Placental Separation and Expulsion

Classic signs of placental separation are the following:

- A gush of blood from the vagina
- A change in the size, shape, and consistency of the uterus

- Lengthening of the umbilical cord from the vagina
- Maternal report of a contraction

Nursing Assessment

Nursing assessment centers on monitoring maternal and infant status during placental delivery, assessing famiy responses to the newborn, and examining the placenta and cord for significant abnormalities. (Monitoring maternal status and examining the placenta are discussed here. Assessing family responses is discussed under Fourth Stage.)

Monitoring Maternal Status

- Assess maternal pulse rate and rhythm every 15 minutes for the first hour postpartum.
- Assess maternal BP every 15 minutes until stable.
- Palpate uterine consistency and position every 10 to 15 minutes to assess amount of bleeding.
- Assess maternal affect and response to infant.

Examination of the Placenta, Membranes, and Umbilical Cord

The nurse or birth attendant should examine the placenta and membranes to determine completeness and to check for any abnormality. A technique for examination of the placenta and membranes follows:

- With the placenta maternal side down, grasp the membranes and approximate the edges to determine if they are complete.
- Inspect the fetal side.
  - Check the location of the insertion of the cord (central, marginal, or velamentous).
  - Trace blood vessels to the periphery to detect any torn vessels, which might indicate a succenturiate, or extra, lobe of the placenta.
- Inspect the maternal surface.
  - Check the cotyledons to determine if they are all present.
  - Observe for areas of abruption, infarction, or calcification.
- Inspect the umbilical cord.
  - Check the number of blood vessels (two arteries and one vein).
  - Check the length of the cord (appropriate [54-61 cm], long, or short).
  - Check for the presence of a true knot, varicosities, or other abnormalities.

The nurse should chart the examination of the placenta, noting particularly any abnormalities, since these may have significance for the newborn.

Nursing Interventions

- Immediately after delivery, allow the mother and/or father to see and hold the baby when desired.
- Assure the couple that their baby is normal and well.
- Palpate and massage the uterus every 15 minutes to ensure its contracted state to prevent excessive bleeding.
- Record BP and pulse every 15 minutes for 1 hour.
- Assess amount of bleeding; an estimated loss of 300 ml of blood or more is excessive and medical intervention is needed.
- Institute an IV infusion of Pitocin as ordered.
- Inform the mother that uterine contractions will occur as a result of the Pitocin infusion.
- Encourage frequent voiding to prevent bladder distention.
- Reassure the father if he expresses anxiety.

Nurse Alerts

Signs of Impending Postpartum Hemorrhage

Immediate nursing action is required if any of the following conditions are noted in the first 1 to 2 hours after delivery:

- Two perineal pads are soaked within 30 minutes (excessive bleeding).
- Mother complains of lightheadedness, nausea, or visual disturbances (possible impending hypovolemic shock).
- Mother is anxious, skin color is pale or ashen, skin is clammy and cool (impending hypovolemic shock).
- Pulse and respirations are elevated, BP is unchanged or slightly lowered (impending hypovolemic shock).

If any of the above are noted in the newly delivered woman, the nurse should take the following steps in this order:

1. Summon help immediately by emergency call light; have care provider notified.
2. Check uterine tone, massage fundus gently if not firm, and assess effect on bleeding and presence of clots, if any.
3. Elevate patient's legs, lower head of bed to facilitate blood return.
4. Increase IV infusion, if present, and start O_2 at 7 to 8 liter/minute by mask.

LABOR: FOURTH STAGE

The fourth stage of labor is the first hour following completion of the third stage. Although not technically a part of labor, it has been so labeled because of the great importance of the immediate postpartum period.

Possible Nursing Diagnoses Related to Fourth Stage of Labor

- Alteration in comfort (pain) related to perineal trauma
- Alteration in urinary output related to perineal edema

Nursing Assessment of Family Responses to the Newborn

Interaction between the newborn and its parents increases feelings of attraction and connectedness to the newborn. It may lay the groundwork for and facilitate the longer process of parent–infant attachment. Behaviors that are thought to signify the beginning of positive parent–infant interaction include:

- Progression of touch from tentative touch with fingertips to more confident touch and enfolding of the infant.
- Active reaching for the infant rather than passive receiving
- Active attempts to make and hold eye contact with the infant in the same vertical plane, known as *en face positioning*
- Expressions of approval or satisfaction with infant's sex, weight, condition, appearance, and size

Nursing Intervention

Nursing care for the woman and her family is directed at supporting maternal and neonatal physiologic status, providing for comfort needs, and supporting family interaction.

Supporting Maternal Physiologic Status

- Continue close monitoring of uterine tone and application of fundal massage to prevent excessive bleeding.
- Administer oxytocics as ordered.
- Re-establish normal nutrition and elimination.
  - Offer clear liquids when the mother is stable and alert.
  - Provide a high-residue diet when clear liquids have been tolerated.

- Encourage urination even though no urge to void is felt and monitor intake and output.
- Assist the mother to the bathroom and remain with her until she voids (running tap water, pouring warm water over the vulva, and gentle suprapubic pressure may help to assist voiding).
- If less than 100 ml of urine is voided, be alert that this may be overflow from an overdistended bladder.
- If the bladder is palpable and the women is unable to void, straight catheterization is indicated.

Supporting Neonatal Physiologic Status

(For immediate care of the newborn, please refer to Chapter 11.)

- Using a bulb syringe to keep the infant's upper airway clear of excessive mucus as signaled by bubbling from the mouth, sneezing, or noisy respiration.
- Make sure the neonate is well covered at all times and is wearing a hat to prevent heat loss from the head.

Providing Comfort Needs

- Offer a sponge bath to the mother and assist her into a clean gown.
- Provide gentle perineal hygiene to promote comfort.
- Apply an ice pack to the perineum to ease swelling and promote comfort.
- Instruct the woman in how to do her own fundal massage and its importance, even though it is uncomfortable.
- Reassure the woman experiencing a shaking chill that this is a normal phenomenon.
  - Cover the mother with warmed blankets and offer warm, nonstimulating liquids such as soup or herbal tea.
- Encourage the mother to rest and help her to find a comfortable position for breastfeeding as needed. Also encourage the father to rest or sleep.

Supporting Family Interaction

This stage of labor provides an excellent opportunity for parent–newborn interaction for the following reasons:

- The newborn is likely to be in a quiet, alert state for 1 to 2 hours, will gaze at faces, and will initiate breastfeeding.
- Early contact with the alert newborn provides the parents with

cues about its temperament and its needs that will help them interact with the newborn as the reward for their hard work in labor; fatigue and discomfort may not be significant enough to interfere with this interaction.

- Parents may feel a special closeness with each other and with the newborn during this time, and interaction takes on special significance.

Nursing Support

- Teach the parents about their newborn while performing its routine assessment.
- Assist with early breastfeeding, since the newborn will not nurse long and will be more interested in gazing at faces. Ensure correct positioning of the mother to support the newborn at breast without undue fatigue or strain.
- Assess how much contact the father wants with the newborn and facilitate this interaction as appropriate.
- Provide private time for the family without interruptions.

NOTES

9
Intrapartal Risk Reduction and Complications

Modern maternity care includes a range of treatments and procedures that are designed to reduce intrapartal risk to the mother and fetus/newborn. Each procedure entails specific nursing responsibilities and specialized nursing assessment and intervention. In general, risk reduction procedures in intrapartal care can be grouped into four major categories:

- Close monitoring of fetal status
- Effective management of maternal pain
- Modification of the pattern of labor
- Modification of the mode of delivery

Nursing Objectives in Intrapartal Risk Reduction

- To screen all patients for factors that increase obstetric risk and identify those who are likely to benefit from more active obstetric management in the intrapartal period
- To be sensitive in assessing and meeting the emotional needs of the woman and her family when active obstetric management is required
- To be prepared to answer questions about indications and relative advantages and disadvantages of risk reduction procedures in collaboration with the physician or midwife
- To encourage the couple to ask questions and seek explanations about intrapartal care
- To assess maternal and fetal status systemically during the obstetric procedures and respond appropriately to support maternal and fetal well-being
- To provide appropriate comfort measures and family-centered support when active obstetric management is necessary

---

Possible Nursing Diagnoses Related to Intrapartal Risk Reduction

- Potential disturbance in self-esteem related to intrapartal problems
- Alteration in cardiac output related to blood loss from episiotomy, cesarean delivery, perineal or vaginal lacerations, or other unanticipated events
- Alteration in comfort (pain) related to cesarean birth, perineal or vaginal lacerations, episiotomy, ruptured uterus
- Alteration in comfort (psychological discomfort) related to anxiety or fear
- Ineffective individual coping related to impairment of adaptive behaviors and problem-solving abilities due to personal vulnerability or situational crisis
- Anticipatory grieving related to risk of infant with problems
- Ineffective family coping related to management of adaptive tasks required by health challenge

---

MONITORING FETAL STATUS: FETAL DISTRESS

Fetal distress results from physiologic deprivation that places the fetus at risk when additional demands such as those of labor and delivery are placed on it.

Acute fetal distress may be manifested by the following indicators:

- Presence of heavy meconium in the amniotic fluid
- Presence of nonreassuring patterns on electronic fetal monitoring, such as:
  - Peristent late decelerations
  - Persistent severe variable decelerations
  - Prolonged fetal bradycardia
  - Absent or decreased beat-to-beat variability

Chronic fetal distress occurs when the physiologic exchange of nutrients, oxygen, and metabolites from the mother is disrupted over a period because of maternal systemic problems. These may include:

- Vascular abnormalities associated with maternal hypertension, preeclampsia/eclampsia, diabetes with vascular complications, and pelvic vascular abnormalities

- Inadequate systemic perfusion due to cardiac or pulmonary disease
- Placental abnormalities such as "aging" in prolonged pregnancy

Chronic fetal distress may also result from:

- Multiple gestation in which there is twin-to-twin transfusion (shared fetoplacental circulation)
- Congenital anomalies or infection
- Rh disease (erythroblastosis fetalis)

When the fetus has been chronically stressed by inadequate fetal–maternal exchange, the extent to which repetitive uterine contractions contribute to fetal distress depends upon the extent of previous compromise. When uterine activity is decreased, the distressed infant will benefit.

Electronic Fetal Monitoring

The electronic fetal monitor (EFM) is a device that provides a graphic display of fetal heart rate (FHR) and monitoring of uterine activity by digital readout and tracing. It can be either external, which is noninvasive, or internal, which is invasive and requires attachment of an electrode to the fetal presenting part or introduction of a pressure-sensing catheter into the uterus. The nurse may initiate external EFM, while internal EFM is generally done by a physician, nurse-midwife, or specially trained nurse clinicians.

External (Indirect) Monitoring

Advantages of External EFM Are:

- Most beneficial as an adjunct to repeated nursing assessments of fetal status and labor pattern by auscultation and palpation
- Can be initiated by the nurse
- Is noninvasive and can be used when membranes are intact and cervix is undilated
- Provides useful information about fetal response to labor
- May be reassuring and helpful to the woman as she copes with labor

Disadvantages of External EFM Are:

- Limits maternal ambulation and position change
- Relative lack of accuracy in recording FHR and uterine contraction strength
- May record artifact sounds, such as maternal bowel or cardiac sounds; may be affected by fetal or maternal movement

- Requires frequent repositioning of belts; inaccurate measurements may occur even when belts are properly positioned
- Accuracy further limited by maternal obesity, polyhydramnios, or very active fetus

Indications for External EFM
- Variations in FHR detected by auscultation
- Meconium-stained amniotic fluid
- Induction of labor
- Oxytocin augmentation of labor
- High risk for uteroplacental insufficiency or fetal compromise in patients with hypertension, bleeding, preterm or post-term pregnancies, intrauterine growth retardation (IUGR), abnormal fetal presentation, previous stillbirth, diabetes, sickle cell disease, and hemolytic disease of the fetus.

Internal (Direct) Monitoring

Because of its invasiveness and potential risks, the disadvantages of EFM outweigh its advantages for routine use. But when accurate information about a potentially compromised fetus is essential, internal EFM provides information on fetal status that allows an otherwise impossible margin of safety (Fig. 9-1).

Advantages of Internal EFM
- Provides beat-by-beat assessment of fetal heart rate
- Provides information on uterine contractility when palpation is difficult or when its assessment must be continuous, such as during vaginal delivery after previous cesarean section birth or during oxytocin infusion
- Continuous recording of contractions not affected by maternal or fetal position changes

Disadvantages of Internal EFM Are:
- Membranes must be ruptured before it can be used, the fetus must have descended, and the cervix must be dilated 1 cm.
- Skilled personnel are needed to apply the equipment and maintain its operation.
- Fetal scalp abscess or laceration of the scalp or other body part may result from insertion of the spiral electrode.
- There is risk of infection to the mother.
- There is risk of perforation of the uterus by the intrauterine catheter.
- Maternal movement is restricted.
- The incidence of cesarean birth is increased.
- Maternal stress can be induced by early amniotomy.
- Trauma to the fetal head may occur due to loss of the amniotic fluid cushion to protect it.

A

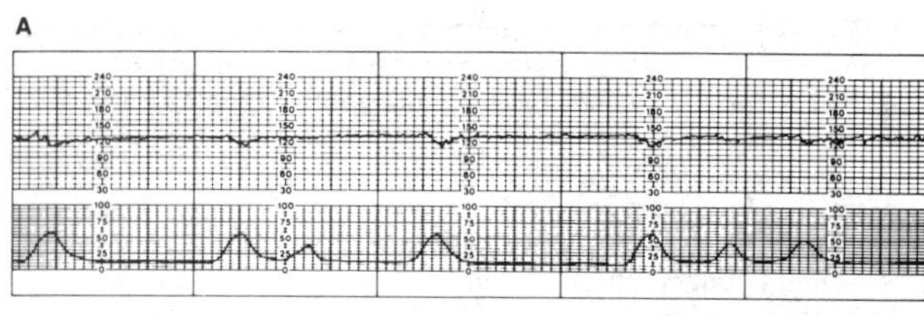

B

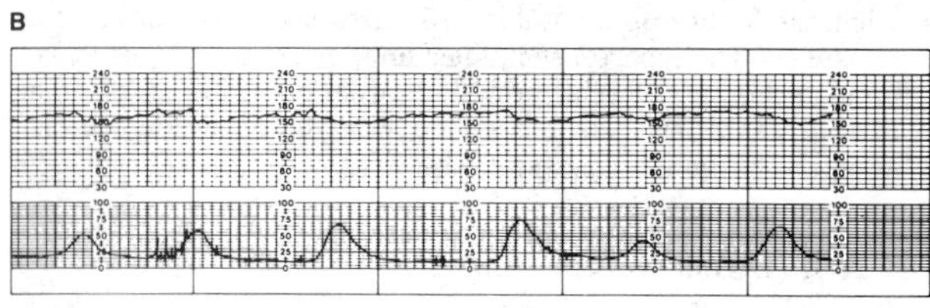

C

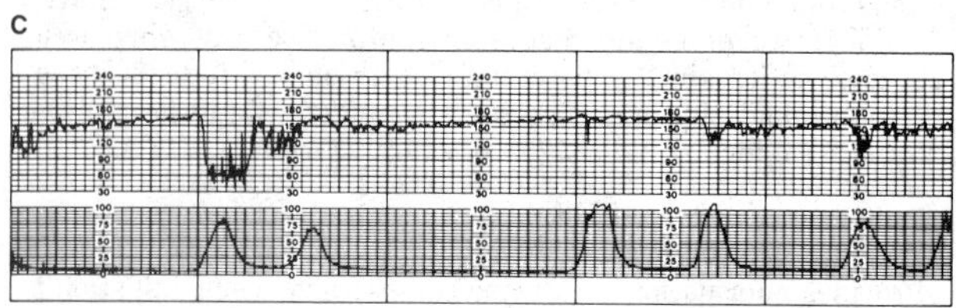

Figure 9-1 Mechanical and physiologic effects of uterine activity on the fetus. *(A)* Early deceleration. Cause: head compression. *(B)* Late deceleration. Cause: uteroplacental insufficiency. *(C)* Variable deceleration. Cause: umbilical cord compression.

- There can be a loss of attention to the laboring mother when the focus of attention is on the monitor.

Fetal Heart Rate

During each uterine contraction, a transient, temporary reduction in maternal blood flow through the placenta occurs. Labor has been described as a stress test for the fetus, who becomes handicapped when certain conditions exist, such as placental abnormality; maternal disease such as diabetes, pregnancy-induced hypertension (PIH), or decreased perfusion; maternal hypotension; fetal disease, such as erythroblastosis fetalis, cord compression; and analgesic drugs or anesthesia.

Assessment and Interpretation

Baseline Fetal Heart Rate

Baseline fetal heart rate (FHR) is determined by the range of the FHR in a 10-minute period in the absence of or between contractions. The normal baseline FHR is 120 to 160 beats per minute. Causes of baseline changes in FHR are given in Table 9-1.

Periodic Changes in Fetal Heart Rate

Periodic FHR changes are fluctuations from the baseline rate that are associated with uterine contractions:

- Acceleration is a transient increase in the baseline.
- Deceleration is a decrease in the baseline.

Variability

Variability is the beat-to-beat difference in the interval between fetal heart beats.

- Short-term: beat-to-beat changes in FHR.
- Long-term: irregular or rhythmic changes or waves of three to five cycles per minute.
    - —Normal long-term variability has an amplitude range greater than 6 beats per minute.
    - —Decreased long-term variability: <6 BPM
    - —Absent: <2 BPM

Fetal Heart Rate Patterns

Reassuring patterns are those with normal baseline FHR and average variability with:

- Mild variable decelerations (less than 30 seconds in duration with rapid return to baseline)
- Early decelerations (concurrent "mirror image" decrease with contraction)
- Accelerations without other changes

Nonreassuring patterns (warning signs) are:

- Moderate tachycardia (160 to 180 bpm)
- Decrease in baseline variability
- Progressive increase or decrease in baseline FHR
- Intermittent late decelerations with good variability

Table 9-1 Causes of Baseline Changes in Fetal Heart Rate

Fetal Bradycardia	Fetal Tachycardia	Reduction in FHR Variability
Fetal hypoxia	Prematurity	Deep fetal sleep (should persist only 20–30 minutes)
Maternal drugs (anesthetics, oxytocics)	Mild hypoxia resulting in increased cardiac rate to compensate for oxygen debt	Prematurity
Maternal hypotension	Tocolytic agents given to mother to treat preterm labor	Congenital anomalies
Prolonged cord compression	Maternal fever, which increases maternal metabolic levels, and increased fetal oxygen needs	Parasympathetic blocking agents (phenothiazines, atropine)
Congenital fetal cardiac lesion	Maternal anemia or hyperthyroidism	Maternal analgesics
	Administration of phenothiazines or other atropine-like drugs, which interrupt vagal response in fetus	Fetal hypoxia
	Fetal activity	
	Fetal infection	

Ominous patterns are:

- Persistent late decelerations, especially with decreasing variability
- Variable decelerations with loss of variability, tachycardia, or late return to baseline
- Absence of variability
- Severe bradycardia

Nursing Interventions with Nonreassuring FHR Patterns

Nursing interventions are directed at maximizing uteroplacental perfusion, providing support and reassurance to the couple, and preparing for additional obstetric intervention as necessary. When nonreassuring patterns reflect decreasing fetal reserve to cope with uterine contractions, the physician or nurse-midwife should be notified and the following actions taken:

- Position the mother on either the left or right side to reduce the possibility of cord compression.
- Discontinue oxytocin infusion to avoid overstimulation of the uterine muscle and decreased perfusion.
- Administer oxygen by face mask or prongs at 8 to 12 liter/minute to increase oxygenation.
- Reassure and support the mother to decrease detrimental effects of fear on uterine blood flow.
- Insert intravenous line for administration of fluids and emergency drugs as ordered. With nonreassuring patterns, this should be done immediately.

Nurse Alerts

Suspected FHR Abnormalities

- Observe EFM recording strip and identify nature of abnormality.
- Check that monitor straps and lines are properly secured and connected.
- Explain actions and provide reassurance to woman and partner.
- Alert physician or nurse-midwife.
- Change mother to lateral position to decrease supine hypotension and correct for possible cord compression.
- If maternal hypotension persists, elevate legs and increase rate of maintenance IV infusion.
- If severe variable decelerations are present, assess for prolapsed compressed cord. If cord is prolapsed, move mother to

knee-chest position to relieve pressure on cord; prepare for emergency cesarean delivery.
- Administer oxygen by face mask at 8 to 12 liter/minute.
- Discontinue oxytocin infusion to decrease uterine activity and promote placental perfusion.

Fetal Blood Sampling

Fetal blood sampling supplies information about fetal blood chemistry. A blood sample is drawn most commonly from the fetal scalp and analyzed to determine *p*H, oxygen, and carbon dioxide levels. This information in conjunction with the FHR data assists in decision making regarding fetal management.

Fetal blood *p*H values are interpreted as follows:

- *Normal pH* (7.2 to 7.35). No intervention needed; continue to monitor.
- *Borderline pH* (7.2 to 7.25). Evaluate second sample in 15 to 30 minutes to check for downward trend. Continue to monitor.
- *Acidotic pH* (7.2 or less on two consecutive measurements): Severely compromised fetus; immediate forceps or cesarean delivery is necessary.

Advantages of Fetal Blood Sampling

- Provides direct information about fetal physiologic status and avoids unnecessary obstetric intervention
- Corroborates and clarifies inconclusive FHR findings

Disadvantages of Fetal Blood Sampling

- Requires considerable skill in its performance
- Immediate, high-quality laboratory support necessary for accurate assessment of blood specimen
- Provides only intermittent data that can be influenced by examiner skill and maternal status
- May not accurately reflect *p*H and blood gas levels when the fetal head is well applied to the cervix and labor is advanced.
- Incision sites make fetus vulnerable to hemorrhage or infection

Nursing Interventions in Fetal Blood Sampling

- Describe the procedure and provide support to the couple.
- Gather the needed equipment and assist with the procedure while also informing the woman of what is happening and how she can help.

- Optimize maternal and fetal status while awaiting the *p*H results by:
  - Providing oxygen
  - Discontinuing an oxytocin infusion (with permission) to decrease intensity and frequency of uterine contractions and increase uterine blood flow
  - Alternating maternal position from left to right to attempt relief of possible compression of the cord and great vessels
- Preparing the patient for delivery when fetal *p*H is less than 7.20. Cesarean birth or forceps delivery may be necessary depending on cervical dilatation.
- Interpreting fetal *p*H results to the couple and keeping them apprised of rapidly changing events

MANAGING MATERNAL PAIN: ANESTHESIA IN INTRAPARTAL CARE

When comfort measures and relaxation techniques do not successfully help the mother to cope with labor pain, pharmacologic pain relief may be suggested to the woman. Both analgesia, the absence or decreased awareness of pain without loss of consciousness, and anesthesia, the partial or complete loss of sensation with or without loss of consciousness, may be used in intrapartal care. See Appendix B.

MODIFYING THE LABOR PATTERN

Maternal–fetal risk in the intrapartal period can be reduced by modifying the pattern of labor, either by induction of labor or by stimulation of labor.

- Induction of labor is typically used when either the maternal or fetal status would be improved by delivery, but there is no need for cesarean delivery.

Induction of Labor

Induction of labor refers to the deliberate initiation of uterine contractions before they begin spontaneously. Its use as a routine for delivery is controversial, but it can be a life-saving measure when medical indications exist. In addition to resolving the medical condition for which induction is indicated, labor induction offers other advantages to the mother at risk, such as:

- Opportunity for physical and emotional preparation for labor and delivery

- Decreased anesthetic risk, since the patient can be kept NPO and well-hydrated
- Adjustment of timing can allow for physician attendance and suitable nursing staff levels

Indications for Induction

- Pregnancy-induced hypertension. This condition may progressively worsen unless relieved by delivery of the fetus.
- Maternal diabetes, classes B to R. Induction and delivery of the fetus 2 to 3 weeks before EDC may be indicated to prevent fetal demise from placental insufficiency, especially if the diabetes is not well controlled during pregnancy.
- Premature rupture of the membranes. Induction may be indicated to prevent uterine infection when membranes have been ruptured 24 hours or more.
- Rh isoimmunization. A rising Rh-antibody titer in late pregnancy may indicate maternal sensitization and the need for prompt delivery to prevent erythroblastosis fetalis.
- Postmaturity (more than 42 weeks gestation). Placental insufficiency and fetal compromise may result from prolonged pregnancy.
- Intrauterine fetal demise. If fetal death has been diagnosed but labor does not ensure, induction may be indicated to reduce maternal risk of disseminated intravascular coagulation and unwarranted emotional distress.
- Previous cesarean section patients may be considered for induction.

Contraindications to Induction

Maternal
- Abnormalities of the uterus, vagina, or pelvis
- Placental abnormalities (previa or suspected abruption)
- Herpesvirus Type II in genital tract
- Grand multiparity
- Overdistention of uterus (from multiple gestation, polyhydramnios)

Fetal
- Abnormal fetal lie (transverse position)
- Low-birth-weight or preterm fetus
- Fetal distress shown by EFM
- Positive (abnormal) contraction stress test

Assessment of Readiness for Induction

The Bishop score is used to predict cervical favorability for successful induction of labor (see Chapter 12).

Amniotomy

One method of labor induction is amniotomy, the artifical rupture of the membranes (AROM). It is performed by inserting a sterile instrument (Amnihook) into the vaginal canal and puncturing the amniotic sac. Its effectiveness is thought to be the promotion of descent of the presenting part on the parous uterus to initiate uterine contractions.

Indications for the use of amniotomy in induction are:

- Contraindications to use of oxytocin infusion
- Desire for direct fetal monitoring

Contraindications to the use of amniotomy in induction are:

- High or unengaged presenting part (−2 station or above)
- Unknown presenting part or abnormal presentation, such as transverse lie or breech
- Uncertain EDC
- Placenta previa
- Herpesvirus Type II present in vaginal tract

Nursing Actions Following Amniotomy

- Assess fetal heart tones.
- Observe the color, amount, and odor of the fluid and record.
- Note the time of amniotomy and cervical status on the EFM graph.
- Explain to the couple the results of the procedure and what to expect:
  - Onset of uterine contractions
  - More intense contractions
  - Leakage of fluid
- Change bed linens for patient comfort.
- Monitor the patient's temperature every 2 hours to assess for possible infection.

Intravenous Oxytocin Infusion

Oxytocin is the most efficient and frequently used drug for induction of labor. It is a powerful drug, and the patient must be carefully assessed prior to and throughout oxytocin administration.

Indications for oxytocin infusion are:

- Pregnancy-induced hypertension
- Maternal diabetes, classes B to R, especially if diabetes is not well controlled during pregnancy
- Premature rupture of the membranes
- Rh isoimmunization
- Postmaturity (more than 42 weeks gestation): placental insufficiency and fetal compromise may result from prolonged pregnancy
- Intrauterine fetal demise

Contraindications to oxytocin infusion are:

- Cephalopelvic disproportion (CPD)
- Abnormal fetal presentation (transverse, breech)
- Placental abnormalities (placenta previa, suspected abruption)
- Documented fetal distress
- Prematurity (unless maternal or fetal condition warrants delivery)
- Predisposition to uterine rupture (multiple gestation; or other overdistention of the uterus such as polyhydramnios, grand multiparity, history of uterine trauma, infection)

The FDA has banned the use of oxytocin for elective inductions and recommends it only for medically indicated inductions.

Modifying the Mode of Delivery

Maternal and fetal risk in the intrapartal period may also be reduced by modifying the mode of delivery. These include *version,* a procedure that may convert malpresentation of the fetus; *forceps* or *vacuum extraction,* procedures that shorten the second stage and facilitate delivery; *cesarean birth,* or operative abdominal delivery; and *trial of labor* and *vaginal birth after previous cesarean.*

Version

Version is the manipulation of the fetus to obtain a more favorable position for delivery.

- *External version* refers to manipulation of the fetus through the maternal abdominal wall, usually to convert a breech presentation to vertex or a persistent transverse lie into a longitudinal presentation. This procedure is usually done around 37 weeks of gestation or may be done in early labor.
- *Internal podalic version,* or direct manual manipulation of the

fetus inside the uterus, was done in the past to convert malpresentation of a second twin. This procedure poses significant risk to the fetus and is now used only in extreme emergencies.

External version may be attempted if a breech or transverse presentation is diagnosed and the following conditions exist:

- Ultrasound evaluation has been done to localize the placenta and rule out multiple gestation.
- The presenting part is not engaged in the pelvis.
- The maternal abdominal wall is thin, permitting accurate palpation of fetal position.
- The uterus is not irritable (prone to contraction with manipulation). Tocolytics may be administered.
- There is enough amniotic fluid to allow easy movement of the fetus.
- Manipulation can be done without anesthesia to avoid application of undue force.

Contraindications to external version are:

- Absence of any of the above conditions
- Previous uterine trauma or surgery
- Any condition that would prohibit a vaginal delivery
- Evidence of third-trimester bleeding or low-lying placenta

Nursing Responsibilities

Nursing responsibilities after version focus on close monitoring of maternal–fetal status for signs of impending hemorrhage or fetal compromise. Maternal BP should be monitored every 5 minutes throughout the procedures, and continuous FHR monitoring should be in place. The procedure should be discontinued if abnormalities in the FHR appear.

Forceps Application

Obstetric forceps are curved metal tongs used to facilitate the birth of the baby's head by providing traction and rotation.

Indications for forceps application include those conditions that require a shortened second-stage labor either because mother or fetus is in jeopardy or because assistance with maternal bearing-down efforts is needed. The following conditions must exist for a safe forceps delivery:

- Fetal head engaged
- Complete dilation of the cervix and ruptured membranes

- Diagnosed vertex, breech, or face (mentum anterior) presentation
- Absence of cephalopelvic disproportion, sacral or pelvic outlet abnormalities
- Adequate regional or general anesthesia

Without these conditions, forceps delivery is unsafe, and cesarean birth is likely indicated.

Advantages of forceps applications include possible avoidance of cesarean delivery when vaginal birth can be safely achieved with mechanical assistance, protection of the preterm fetus's vulnerable head during the second stage, and avoidance of maternal exhaustion from prolonged pushing.

Disadvantages of forceps applications center on trauma to maternal tissue and the fetal head during delivery. These effects may include:

- Lacerations of the vagina and cervix
- Extension of an episiotomy into the rectum
- Rupture of the uterus
- Increased risk of uterine atony and excessive bleeding
- Increased risk of infection
- Fracture of the coccyx and bladder trauma
- Potential trauma and bruising of neonate's head

Vacuum Extraction

Vacuum extraction of the infant is accomplished by use of a specialized vacuum extractor. This device has a caplike suction cup that is applied to the fetal head to facilitate traction and descent of the infant. Once the optimum level of suction is obtained the physician applies traction on the cup during uterine contractions.

Indications for use of vacuum extraction are similar to those for forceps application. In addition, vacuum extraction can be safely used through a partially dilated cervix to shorten first-stage labor in some cases.

Contraindications include profound fetal or maternal distress requiring rapid delivery, evidence of cephalopelvic disproportion, and face or breech presentation.

Vacuum extraction has the following advantages over forceps application:

- Less trauma to bladder and vaginal tissue
- Lower risk of perineal tearing
- Easier application when the presenting part fits snugly in the birth canal
- Less risk of excessive pressure on fetal head
- No routine need for anesthesia

Disadvantages are:

- Cannot assist in an emergency where rapid delivery is needed
- Usually cannot actively achieve rotation of the presenting part (although spontaneous rotation sometimes occurs when traction is applied)
- Risk of fetal scalp bruising, avulsion, and other cerebral trauma from excessive suction or prolonged use (greater than 30 minutes)
- Increased incidence of cephalhematoma

Nursing Responsibilities

- Inform the mother about the procedure.
- Continue to monitor maternal and fetal status.
- Assist the birth attendant with the procedure.
- Auscultate fetal heart rate every 5 minutes if electronic monitoring has not been established.
- Prepare for possible forceps application and neonatal resuscitation when prompt delivery is necessary.
- Postdelivery the infant must be assessed and observed for signs of cerebral trauma secondary to vacuum extraction (a caput succedaneum at the suction cap site is normal and will resolve within 24 hours).

Cesarean Birth

Cesarean birth is a major operative procedure in which the fetus is delivered through a surgical incision in the maternal abdominal wall and uterus.

Types of Cesarean Birth

There are two major types of cesarean deliveries: low-segment and classic. The most commonly used is the low-segment procedure.

Low-segment Delivery
In the low-segment procedure, a horizontal skin incision called *Pfannenstiel's,* incision or more popularly the "bikini cut," is performed by a transverse cut made on the skin at the level of the mons pubis.

Advantages of Pfannenstiel's incision are:

- The low skin incision is hidden by the pubic hair.
- Blood loss is minimal.
- There is less chance of uterine scar rupture with subsequent pregnancies.

- Less postoperative abdominal distention occurs.
- The chance of uterine weakening and scar rupture is decreased because the tissue of the lower uterine segment is less contractile than the body of the uterus.

Disadvantages are:

- The procedure takes longer to perform.
- It is not useful in an emergency because the anatomic features of the area limit stretching of the incision, and there is limited space in which to work.

Classic Cesarean Delivery

Classic cesarean delivery is performed by making a vertical midline incision in the skin and wall of the body of the uterus. This type of cesarean is commonly used in emergency delivery because more rapid access to the fetus is possible.

Advantages of the classic type are:

- Easier access to the fetus in a transverse lie
- Better access when abdominal adhesions from previous surgery are present
- Rapid delivery when maternal wellbeing is threatened
- Used when vaginal delivery presents maternal or fetal risk

Disadvantages are:

- Increased blood loss from severing of large vessels in the myometrium
- Weakened uterine musculature from a midline incision
- Increased risk of uterine rupture in subsequent pregnancies
- Major abdominal surgery
- Higher maternal morbidity and mortality than with vaginal delivery
- Surgical complications such as hemorrhage, anesthetic reactions, injury to pelvic or abdominal organs
- Increased risk of infection

Indications for Cesarean Delivery

- Cephalopelvic disproportion
- Malpresentation of fetus
- Uterine dysfunction
- Previous cesarean delivery
- Soft-tissue dystocia
- Pregnancy-induced hypertension (PIH)
- Herpesvirus infection of genital tract
- Maternal diabetes
- Maternal complications

- Placental insufficiency
- High-risk obstetric factors: placenta previa, placental abruption, umbilical cord prolapse, fetal distress, previous fetal death or damage, prolonged rupture of membranes with intraparatal infection

Nursing Interventions

Pre-operative Care

- Pre-operative teaching of the couple
- Provision of emotional and family-centered care
- Preoperative preparation of the patient
  - Shave the abdominal area beginning just below the breasts and including pubic region.
  - Insert an indwelling urinary catheter to dependent drainage to prevent bladder distention during delivery.
  - Obtain preoperative laboratory tests, including complete blood cell count (CBC), electrolytes, clotting studies, and type and crossmatch (necessary when ordering units of blood replacement).
  - Insert an IV line or assess the patency of an existing line to ensure an open route for administration of medications, fluids, and blood. The bore of the needle must be large enough for the administration of blood replacement (18 gauge or larger). Infusion of antibiotics may be ordered in the event of prolonged rupture of the membranes and possible ensuing infection. The mother should be kept NPO.
  - Help the father or support person with preparations to attend in the delivery room or keep him well informed about preparations and patient status.
  - Ensure that patient identification is correct. It is also helpful to prepare the baby's identification before delivery to affix it to the front of the mother's chart.
  - Administer a nonparticulate antacid 15 minutes before induction of anesthesia. In the event of aspiration during anesthesia induction, the stomach contents will have been neutralized, which helps to prevent aspiration pneumonitis.
  - Attend the anesthetist when anesthesia is administered.
  - Scrub the entire operative field with antiseptic solution.
  - Notify other members of the health care team that the delivery is imminent: pediatrician, intensive care nursery staff, and anesthesia staff. Notify the blood bank when blood replacement is needed.

Postoperative Care

- Check vital signs every 5 minutes until stable, then every 5 minutes for 1 hour; then every 1 to 2 hours for 8 hours.
- Check uterine fundus and its state of contraction every 15 minutes for 1 hour or more often as indicated.

- Massage fundus carefully and gently. Monitor dressing for amount of bleeding.
- Suction mouth and throat.
- Position patient on side to promote mucous drainage.
- Assist patient to cough every 2 hours for 24 hours.
- Splint incision while patient coughs.
- Check hematocrit and hemoglobin 8 hours after delivery and the first postop day.
- Assess laboratory values: Hgb <10.5 gm, Hct <30%. Assess for symptoms of dizziness, lightheadedness, fainting.
- Check patency of indwelling catheter to dependent drainage.
- Monitor adequate intake and output.
- Remove catheter as ordered.
- Check ability of patient to void and adequency of the amount.
- Assist the patient to the bathroom.
- Check for symptoms of burning with urination, frequency, urgency.
- Collect urine culture.
- Maintain IV flow rate as ordered.
- Add medications such as oxytocics and antibiotics as ordered.
- Assess for swelling, redness, pain, heat. If present, remove needle from IV site and place at another site.
- Offer ice chips when ordered. Advance progressively to clear liquids, regular diet.
- Remove IV as ordered, usually within 24 to 48 hours postop.
- Administer pain medication as ordered.
- Provide other comfort measures such as heat, positioning, incision splinting to relieve pain from the incision, gas, or uterine involution.
- Assess vital signs before administering pain medication.
- Confirm that medication is not contraindicated in breastfeeding mothers.
- Administer antiemetic as needed. Check vital signs prior to administration.
- Check incision for swelling, redness, drainage, warmth.
- Outline area of drainage on dressing, marking it with date and time every 4 hours for the first 24 hours postop.
- Notify physician and assist with culture of wound if infection is present. Administer antibiotic as ordered.
- Encourage progressive ambulation starting within 24 hours postop. Offer pain medication prior to ambulation and remain with the patient.
- Explain the rationale and importance of early ambulation to the patient.
- Administer stool softener as ordered, and encourage increased fluid intake.
- Encourage family interaction as soon as possible.
- Provide parents early information about their baby.

- Provide infant and self-care instruction.
- Encourage discussion of feelings about the cesarean birth and the mother's self-image.

Trial of Labor/Vaginal Birth after Cesarean Delivery

In the past, fear of uterine rupture during a subsequent labor prevented physicians from considering a trial of labor and vaginal birth after cesarean (VBAC) as a safe mode of delivery, since the uterine musculature was believed to be significantly weakened. However, more recent research suggests that the risks of VBAC may have been overestimated, and the trend toward trial of labor appears to be increasing.

Maternal and neonatal risks of elective repeat cesarean may be greater than careful management of trial labor and VBAC. Recent studies show that 60% of women permitted a trial of labor go on to deliver vaginally and that the risk of uterine rupture appears to be small, even among women with a previous midline uterine incision.

Requirements for Vaginal Birth After Cesarean

- Only one previous uterine incision, preferably low-segment incision
- No repeating cause for previous cesarean
- Capability for internal monitoring during labor, with available emergency surgical facilities
- Constant physician attendance in labor

Contraindications are:

- Any contraindications for vaginal delivery
- More than one previous uterine incision
- Previous classic (verticle) uterine incision (considered by some to be a relative, not an absolute contraindication)
- Malpresentation or possible cephalopelvic disproportion
- Lack of capability for continuous monitoring and emergency operative delivery if necessary

INTRAPARTAL COMPLICATIONS

Usually labor and birth progress with few problems, and outcomes for mother, newborn, and family are generally positive. However, when complications arise in the intrapartal period they develop rapidly and may have devastating effects on maternal and fetal/ newborn wellbeing. Care providers must identify the nature of the problem and intervene to reduce or limit detrimental effects to mother and fetus/newborn.

When complications develop in the intrapartal period, the nursing care given must be adapted to the particular needs of the high-risk patient and her family. The specific types of nursing assessments and interventions will vary with the nature of the complication. Overall objectives for nursing care of the woman with intrapartal complications include an emphasis on early detection and treatment of intrapartal problems, careful assessment of maternal and fetal status, and efficient implementation of appropriate obstetric care.

Nursing Objective in Intrapartal Complications

- To assess maternal and fetal status carefully to detect problems and to evaluate response to obstetric interventions
- To assess the emotional status of the woman, her partner, and other family members, and to provide needed support
- To explain to the family, in collaboration with the physician or nurse midwife, the nature of the complication and the needed obstetric treatment
- To understand emergency procedures that may be required during intrapartal crises and to be prepared to take necessary nursing action
- To integrate family-centered practices into the care of families with complications within the limits of safety and feasibility
- To coordinate activities with other staff members to provide for maximum effectiveness and continuity of care for families experiencing intrapartal complications

---

Nursing Interventions

Common Problems

Complications occurring in the intrapartal period may place the fetus or mother at risk, but in most cases both are involved and are at some measure of jeopardy. Table 9-2 summarizes many of the most common problems encountered in the intrapartal period and discuss the maternal and fetal implications, treatment, and nursing responsibilities.

See Table 9-3 for medical management of missed abortion/intrauterine fetal demise.

(*text continues on pg. 341*)

Table 9-2 Intrapartal Complications

Disorder	Etiology/ Predisposing Factors	Maternal Implications	Fetal/ Neonatal Implications	Treatment	Nursing Responsibilities
Placental Problems					
Placental Previa	• Largely unknown • Multiparity • Uterine scarring • Advanced maternal age • Multiple gestation • Increased placental size	• Severe hemorrhage • Embolism • Risk of emergency operative delivery • Endometritis • Postpartum hemorrhage	• Prematurity • Intrauterine asphyxia • Hemorrhage • Fetal vessel injury from vaginal examination • Congenital anomaly • Malposition or malpresentation	• Monitor bleeding • Bedrest to extend period of gestation • At 36 wk delivery may be planned • Vaginal delivery with partial previa (30%) • Pitocin-induced labor if presenting part is low (with partial previa) • Amniotomy induction to promote descent of presenting part	• *Never perform a rectal or vaginal examination.* • Monitor vital signs, FHT, contractions. • Monitor Hgb, HCt, WBC, and differential. • Prepare for sonography. • Facilitate bed rest. • Lab tests: CBC, type and crossmatch, coagulation studies. • Prepare for delivery.

(continued)

Table 9-2 Intrapartal Complications (*continued*)

Disorder	Etiology/ Predisposing Factors	Maternal Implications	Fetal/ Neonatal Implications	Treatment	Nursing Responsibilities
Placental Problems					
Abruptio Placentae	• Exact cause unknown • External trauma • High parity • Overdistended uterus • History of previous pregnancy loss • Age over 30 years • Hypertensive disease	• Maternal mortality 0.5 to 5.0% • Concealed hemorrhage • Uterine irritability with poor relaxation • Sudden, extreme pain • Rapid increase in uterine size, rigidity • Hypovolemic shock • Disseminated intravascular coagulation	• Perinatal mortality 50% to 80% • Signs of acute fetal distress • Absense of fetal heart tones • Morbidity from hypoxia, birth trauma, prematurity	• IV fluids, whole blood • Monitor vaginal bleeding • Monitor urinary intake and output • Frequent vital signs • Continuous fetal monitoring • Cesarean section for immediate delivery of infant	• Monitor BP, pulse, respiration, FHT. • Provide oxygen therapy as needed. • Monitor uterine bleeding. • Prepare for delivery. • Support patient and partner. • *Never perform a vaginal or rectal examination.*
Placenta Accreta, Percreta Increta (Estimated incidence 1 in 7000 deliveries)	• Probable cause: failure of the decidua to develop in the placental bed • Uterine scarring from previous cesarean birth • History of uterine curettage	• Mortality may be as high as 10%. • About one-third of emergency postpartum hysterectomies result from abnormal placental attachment.	• Placenta functions normally. • In the absence of current problems such as placenta previa, fetus is generally unaffected.	• For minor degrees of adherence, placental tissue can be removed by curettage. • Zealous attempts to remove the	• Maintain maternal physiologic status. • Prepare the patient for curettage or hysterectomy. • Institute emergency measures for hemorrhagic shock.

	• Previous manual removal of placenta • Previous uterine sepsis • Uterine malformation	• Zealous attempts to remove adherent placenta may cause uterine rupture, hemorrhage, exsanguination.		placenta may cause excessive bleeding and hemorrhagic shock. • Emergency laparotomy and hysterectomy may be life-saving. • Subsequent pregnancy may be at risk for placental abnormality.	• Support the patient and keep her informed when surgery is anticipated.
Placenta Infarction	• Associated with vascular disease of the uteroplacental unit secondary to maternal hypertension. In the presence of preeclampsia nearly 33% will contain infarctions.	• Central placental infarctions may cause underperfusion of the placenta. • Marginal placental infarctions may occur. • Infarctions pose no threat to the mother.	• Reduced fetal circulation • Limited capacity for metabolic exchange • Marginal infarctions pose no fetal threat. • Fetus can survive when as much as 20% to 30% of the placenta is infarcted. • Small areas of infarcts do not affect the fetus.	• Placental infarctions cannot be treated. • Treatment of underlying maternal disease can decrease the severity and incidence of placental infarcts.	• Commonly the nurse is responsible for examination of the placenta after delivery. Otherwise the nurse is not directly involved.

(continued)

Table 9-2 Intrapartal Complications (*continued*)

Disorder	Etiology/ Predisposing Factors	Maternal Implications	Fetal/ Neonatal Implications	Treatment	Nursing Responsibilities
Placental Problems					
Retained Placental Fragments	• Placental fragments may adhere to the uterine wall after placental delivery when: • Overvigorous attempts are made to hasten placental delivery. • The contracted uterus has been kneaded to excess. • The placenta has become fragmented.	• Steady postpartum bleeding for the first 24 hours after birth even though the uterus is well contracted. • Late postpartum hemorrhage—after 24 hours • Bleeding that resumes 1 to 2 weeks after delivery • Failure of uterine involution • Endometritis • Rehospitalization may be necessary.	• None	• Exploration of the uterine cavity • Curettage of the uterine lining • Blood replacement when bleeding has been excessive • Antibiotic therapy when infection (endometritis) occurs • Administration of oxytocics or methergine after removal of placental fragments	• After delivery and examination of the placenta, by the nurse, areas of missing tissue should be brought to the birth attendant's attention. • Monitor the amount and pattern of the patient's postpartum bleeding.

Membrane, Amniotic Fluid, and Cord Problems

Premature Rupture of the Membranes (PROM)	• Cause unknown • Associated with malpresentations, possible weak areas in the amnion and chorion, subclinical infection, and possibly incompetent cervix	• Maternal sepsis subsequent to PROM is usually not serious and can be effectively treated with antibiotics. More active obstetric intervention may be necessary, including induction of labor and cesarean delivery.	• The fetal defense mechanism is lost. The leading cause of fetal death associated with PROM is infection. About 7% of term neonates and 25% of preterm neonates do not survive chorioamnionitis. High risk for premature birth and respiratory distress syndrome	• Active management: induction of labor or cesarean delivery if labor does not commence within 24 hours • Conservative management: careful observation without intervention unless amnionitis or fetal distress occurs	• Instruct pregnant woman to seek immediate care if persistent leaking or a gush of fluid from the vagina occurs. • Counsel pregnant woman not to douche, have intercourse, or take a tub bath when the membranes have possibly ruptured. • When hospitalized, assess for signs of developing infection; temperature; pulse; respiration; uterine tenderness; and color, odor, and amount of amniotic fluid.

Chorioamnionitis	• Premature rupture of the membranes
	• Poor nutritional status
	• Repeated vaginal or rectal examinations
	• Internal fetal monitoring
	• Vaginitis, cervicitis
	• Previous cervical cerclage
		• Cesarean delivery three times more common
		• Increased risk of postpartum complications
		  • Septicemia
		  • Pelvic peritonitis
		  • Abscess formation
		  • Septic thrombophlebitis
			• High risk for sepsis
			• Neonatal pneumonia; changes in color, muscle tone, feeding, activity; impaired thermoregulation, abdominal distention, death
				• Delivery of the infant and antibiotic treatment for mother, and possibly infant
				• Vaginal delivery; cesarean delivery is controversial in the presence of infection
					• Closely observe fetal and maternal status.
					• Take maternal pulse, temperature, respiration hourly.
					• Note and report signs of maternal sepsis.
					• Monitor intake and output.
					• Maintain IV infusion for hydration and administration of antibiotics.

(*continued*)

Table 9-2 Intrapartal Complications (*continued*)

Disorder	Etiology/ Predisposing Factors	Maternal Implications	Fetal/ Neonatal Implications	Treatment	Nursing Responsibilities
Membrane, Amniotic Fluid, and Cord Problems					
		• Infection unresponsive to antibiotic therapy may require hysterectomy.			

Hydramnios	• Etiology unknown
	• Occurs in 1.5% of pregnancies
	• Possible disruption of water transport in and out of the amniotic cavity
		• Enlarged uterus
		• Detected at about 7 mo
		• Difficult to palpate uterus and to detect fetal heart tones
		• Severe hydramnios
		  • Abdominal discomfort
		  • Generalized edema
		  • Dyspnea
		  • Difficult mobility
		• At increased risk for postpartum hemorrhage from uterine atony
			• Increased risk of preterm labor and PROM
			• Cord prolapse
			• Common associated congenital anomalies:
			  • Upper gastrointestinal abnormalities
			  • Anencephaly
			  • Hydrops
			  • Hydrocephalus
			  • Neural tube defects
				• Mild hydramnios requires no treatment.
				• Severely symptomatic:
				  • Hospitalization
				  • Bed rest
				  • Amniocentesis to withdraw fluid in an attempt to alleviate symptoms
					• Promote comfort.
					• Provide emotional support
					• Provide anticipatory guidance
					• Be alert for cord prolapse if membranes rupture.

Oligohydramnios	• Etiology unknown
	• Post-term pregnancy
	• Chronic leakage of amniotic fluid
	• Placental insufficiency
	• Fetal renal anomalies
		• Uterine fundus small for dates
		• Fetal outline easily palpable thorugh the abdominal wall
		• Risk for preterm or dysfunctional labor
		• Severe discomfort during labor and birth
		• Risk of bearing a deformed infant (1 in 4,000 births)
			• May assume a flexed, cramped attitude
			• Chronic cord compression may result in:
			  • Intrauterine growth retardation
			  • Meconium staining
			  • Fetal hypoxia
			  • Skeletal deformities
			  • Wizened appearance at birth
				• No current treatment
				• May require cesarean delivery in advance of labor onset due to in utero fetal distress
					• Provide comfort measures to relieve extreme maternal discomfort during labor.
					• Closely monitor fetus to identify signs of distress.
					• Offer emotional support to families if serious fetal anomalies have been diagnosed.

Umbilical Cord Prolapse	• Occurs in approximately 1 of 200 pregnancies
	• Abnormal fetal position
	• Multiple gestation (6 times greater than with single gestation)
	• Premature rupture of membranes
	• Fetopelvic disproportion
	• Low-lying placenta
	• Abnormally long umbilical cord
		• At increased risk when membranes rupture before descent of fetal head
		• An emergency situation
		• Concern for fetal well-being
		• Immediate delivery attempted by forceps or cesarean delivery
		• Increased risk for trauma to birth canal, excessive blood loss, infection, uterine atony
			• Risk for perinatal morbidity and mortality
			• Prematurity
			• Birth trauma
			• Meconium aspiration
			• Hypoxia
			• Fetal survival:
			  • Delivery within 60 minutes, 70% to 75%
			  • Delivery more than 1 hour, may exceed 50%
				• Deliver infant as soon as possible
				• Vaginal delivery when appropriate or cesarean delivery when labor has not begun
				• Relieve pressure on prolapsed cord
				• With fetal death, surgical intervention is unnecessary and labor is allowed to proceed.
					• Identify and monitor woman at risk for cord prolapse.
					• When membranes rupture, ausculate FHR for 1 minute and with next uterine contraction to identify signs of cord compression.
					• Examine vaginally to determine engagement of the fetal head or prolapsed cord.

(continued)

Table 9-2 Intrapartal Complications (*continued*)

Disorder	Etiology/ Predisposing Factors	Maternal Implications	Fetal/ Neonatal Implications	Treatment	Nursing Responsibilities
Membrane, Amniotic Fluid, and Cord Problems					
Velamentous Insertion	• Etiology unknown • More common with multiple gestations	• Usually asymptomatic and diagnosed after delivery • Unprotected vessels of the umbilical cord may rupture during labor and delivery • Amniotic fluid may become blood-stained	• Increased incidence of fetal anomalies • Majority of deliveries without incident, but if cord vessels tear, risk of fetal exsanguination is 60% to 70%	• No treatment • Evidence of fetal hemorrhage requires emergency cesarean delivery	• Recognize abnormality, such as pulsating vessels at cervical os and blood-stained amniotic fluid. • Alert physician immediately. • Keep patient on bedrest with IV line to facilitate emergency management. • Prepare for cesarean delivery and neonatal support.
Fetal Problems					
Multiple Gestation (Delivery)	• Factors affecting mode of delivery: • Age of fetuses when delivery is imminent	• Small increase in morbidity with twin pregnancy • Increased risk of: • Abnormal fetal	• Preterm delivery and low birth weight • Immature neonate • Complexities of descent and delivery	• Cesarean delivery • Fetuses under 34 weeks and delivery is imminent	• Palpate the fundus and auscultate for two separate heart beats. • Establish external fetal heart monitoring.

• Presence of fetal problems such as: • Hypoxia • Abnormal positions • Premature separation of one placenta • PROM • Number of fetuses	presentations • Premature labor • PROM • Extended labor • Hydramnios • Placenta previa • Postpartum hemorrhage • Febrile complications	• Abnormal positions that disrupt circulation to one fetus • Intrauterine fetal demise • Cord accidents and entanglement	• Compromised maternal condition • Avoid fetal hypoxia and trauma associated with preterm vaginal birth • Fetuses not in vertex position • Monoamniotic twins (single sac): mortality greater than 50% due to cord accidents • Term pregnancy when first twin is in transverse lie or breech • Hyperextension of the first fetal head • Vaginal Delivery • Prepare for immediate cesarean delivery • Continuous EFM	• Alert the delivery and neonatal teams. • Plan for possible emergency cesarean delivery. • Type and crossmatch blood. • After delivery of first twin, rule out cord prolapse by vaginal examination. • Continue to monitor second twin's FHR. • Accurately identify each twin. • Monitor maternal postpartum bleeding.

(continued)

Table 9-2 Intrapartal Complications (*continued*)

Disorder	Etiology/ Predisposing Factors	Maternal Implications	Fetal/ Neonatal Implications	Treatment	Nursing Responsibilities
Fetal Problems					
Macrosomia	• Fetal birth weight that exceeds 4000 g occurs in approximately 5% of births • Disorder associated with: • Poorly controlled maternal diabetes • Genetic predisposition for large babies • Maternal obesity or other metabolic disease	• Shoulder dystocia at delivery • Cephalopelvic disproportion where fetal head is too large to accommodate pelvis • CPD may also cause: • Distention of the myometrium and uterine inertia, requiring cesarean delivery • Increased risk for perineal trauma, uterine rupture, and postpartum hemorrhage	• Fractured clavicle with vaginal delivery	• Cesarean delivery	• Monitor fetal heart tones and activity. • Assess labor progress and notify the physician. • Prepare for cesarean delivery.

Hydrocephalus	• Women with a previous hydrocephalic infant have a 2% to 5% risk of recurrence. • Rapid uterine growth in last trimester • Hydramnios • Failure of fetal head to engage	• Difficult last trimester with dyspnea, back and abdominal pain, nausea and vomiting • Risk for dystocia and uterine rupture	• Possible damage to fetal brain • When not diagnosed risk of traumatic delivery lowers chance of fetal survival	• At present antenatal treatment is not available.	• Provide emotional and physical support to the woman and her partner.
Anencephaly	• The fetal cerebrum and cranium fail to develop, conditions that are incompatible with life. • Commonly accompanied by hydramnios	• Prolonged pregnancy • Presence of hydramnios • Emotional trauma, grief	• Neonatal death	• Once diagnosed induction of labor is difficult. • Slow aspiration of amniotic fluid in combination with serial induction is necessary to initiate labor.	• Provide emotional and physical support to the woman and her partner. (See fetal demise.)
Dystocia (Complications involving fetal descent)	• Dystocia means difficult labor; involving fetal descent are: • Pelvic size and internal shape • Fetal size, presentation, and ability of fetal head to mold in the pelvis • Ability of uterus to contract efficiently	• Uterine and pelvic factors: • Hypotonic labor • Hypertonic labor • Precipitous labor • Prolonged labor • Inlet contracture • Midpelvic contracture • Outlet contracture	• Fetal factors: • Abnormal position • Unusually large • Anomaly that prevents descent into pelvis	• Labor augmentation with pitocin may be attempted if uterine forces are inadequate • Forceps or cesarean delivery may be indicated	• Monitor labor progress closely • Continuous fetal monitoring • Identify signs of delayed fetal engagement and alert birth attendant • Administer and monitor pitocin in conjunction with birth attendant

(continued)

Table 9-2 Intrapartal Complications (*continued*)

Disorder	Etiology/ Predisposing Factors	Maternal Implications	Fetal/ Neonatal Implications	Treatment	Nursing Responsibilities
Fetal Problems					
		• PROM • Pathologic retraction rings • Dysfunctional labor pattern			• Keep the parents informed about labor progress and fetal status

Malpresentations and Malpositions	*Breech Presentation*
	• Commonly found in 2nd trimester
	• A major reason for cesarean delivery in some settings
	• Breech presentation diagnosed prenatally
	  • Frank breech (65%)
	  • Incomplete breech (10%)
	  • Complete breech (10%)
		• Increased risk of cord prolapse or infection
		• Prolonged, inefficient labor
		• Premature rupture of membranes
		• Laceration of lower uterine segment, cervix, vagina, and perineum
		• Possible forceps delivery
			• Entrapment of fetal head resulting in:
			  • Erb's palsy
			  • CNS damage from hypoxia
			  • Separation of the occipital bone and subdural hemorrhage
			  • Vertebral and medullary injuries in infants with hype extended heads
				• Decision about mode of delivery early in labor
				• Vaginal delivery
				  • Frank or complete breech without hyperextension of fetal head
				  • Fetal weight less than 3500 g
				  • Adequate pelvic size
					• Be prepared to answer couple's questions.
					• Be prepared for prompt action when problems occur from aftercoming head.
					• Constantly monitor fetus for evidence of compromise

• Dystocia results from large, less compressible head delivering last	• Possible cesarean delivery	• Muscle damage • Aspiration of amniotic fluid • Meconium aspiration	• Gestational age 36 to 42 weeks • Birth attendant skilled in vaginal breech deliveries • Pediatric support • Cesarean delivery • Absence of labor when fetal status requires delivery • Premature infant • Previous history of perinatal death of child with birth trauma	
Brow Presentation • Fetus in head-down position • Brow and orbital ridges are presenting part • May be caused by conditions that allow fetal body to sag forward	• An adequate maternal pelvis may allow conversion to face or vertex presentation. • Vaginal delivery with persistent brow may result in perineal and vaginal lacerations.	• Increased danger of trauma to head, neck, and larynx • Possible damage to CNS • Possible trauma from forceps delivery	• Intervention not needed when pelvis is adequate and labor is progressing • In presence of arrested labor or fetal distress, cesarean delivery is indicated	• Closely monitor labor progress and fetal status • Explain the problem to the parents and prepare them for a long, difficult delivery. • Prepare for forceps or cesarean delivery.
Face Presentation • Fetus is in a head-down position with	• In mentum (chin) posterior positions the chin may be	• Fetal distress is uncommon when the maternal pelvis is	• Vaginal delivery may occur in up to 80% of face	• Closely monitor labor progress and fetal status.

(continued)

Table 9-2 Intrapartal Complications (*continued*)

Disorder	Etiology/ Predisposing Factors	Maternal Implications	Fetal/ Neonatal Implications	Treatment	Nursing Responsibilities
Fetal Problems					
	head hyperextended so that the face is the presenting part. • Factors that favor extension of the head while preventing flexion may lead to face presentation, including: • Small pelvis • Large infant • Weakness in maternal abdominal wall • Preterm labor	arrested against the maternal sacrum, arresting labor. • Prolonged labor • Fetal descent may be more painful • Increased risk to genital tract	adequate and the fetus is anterior. • The fetal face becomes swollen, misshapen, and bruised. • Molding of the fetal head may be pronounced. • Transient respiratory distress from edema to larynx.	presentations when the maternal pelvis is adequate and the fetal chin is anterior. • Fetal arrest is an indication for cesarean birth.	• Prepare for emergency delivery and resuscitation of the infant. • Discuss with the parents the infant's facial appearance at birth, and assure them of its resolution in 3 to 5 days.
Shoulder Dystocia	• Shoulder dystocia occurs during second-stage labor when the fetal head is born but the shoulders are too broad to deliver be-	• Increased risk of vaginal and perineal trauma	• Asphyxia from cord compression • Trauma from overstretching of the neck and clavicle fractures sustained	• Should be prevented by careful assessment of fetal size • When a fetus is large, arrests in	• Monitor labor progress. • With slow and difficult descent be alert for any arrest of progress of the fetal head or shoulders at the symphysis.

	tween the symphysis and sacrum. • Caused by macrosomia and/or a tight or contracted pelvic outlet		during emergency delivery • Possible cervical nerve damage	the midpelvis with use of vacuum or forceps increases the risk for shoulder dystocia. • Application of suprapubic pressure may help deliver the shoulder under the pubis.	• Assist with suprapubic pressure as requested.
Dysfunctional Labor Patterns					
Hypotonic Labor	• In early labor may exhibit normal pattern • Infrequent contractions with poor intensity and low-resting tone develop. • Pattern characterized by slowing or arrest of dilatation and fetal descent • May result from overstretching of the uterus, administration of sedation in early labor	• Contractions seldom painful • Increased risk of prolonged labor and PROM. • Maternal discouragement from slow labor • At risk for uterine atony with consequent postpartum hemorrhage	• No effects on normal fetus • Fetal distress in late hypotonic labor • Neonatal sepsis	• Rule out cephalopelvic disproportion, malpresentation, obstruction from uterine abnormalities; when these are absent it is uterine dysfunction • IV oxytocin to augment labor	• Closely monitor labor progress and maternal-fetal status. • Document contraction pattern that shows slowing or arrest of fetal descent and report to birth attendant. • Evaluate maternal anxiety, sedation, or dehydration that may slow labor. • Facilitate uterine contractions by change of patient position, ambulation, and rest.

(continued)

Table 9-2 Intrapartal Complications (*continued*)

Disorder	Etiology/ Predisposing Factors	Maternal Implications	Fetal/ Neonatal Implications	Treatment	Nursing Responsibilities
Dysfunctional Labor Patterns					• Monitor intake and output. • If oxytocin is administered, closely monitor its effects.

Hypertonic Labor	• Fundal dominance of contraction pattern is altered.
	• More frequent contractions of moderate intensity
	• Resting tone of the uterus increased
	• Uterus does not relax sufficiently between contractions to allow its optimum perfusion.
		• The patient becomes discouraged and exhausted
		• Little progress is made; painful contractions earlier in labor
		• Depletion of physiologic reserves:
		  • Dehydration
		  • Acute fatigue
		  • Increasing anxiety
			• Decreased placental perfusion to the fetus
			• Increased risk for uteroplacental insufficiency
			• Fetal reserves are taxed and fetal distress may occur
			• Excessive pressure to the fetal head may cause excessive mold ing and cephalohematoma
				• Stop incoordinate labor and promote more effective contractions by encouraging relaxation and sleep through comfort measures.
				• Rest will often result in a more normal labor pattern.
				• Rehydrate with
					• Carefully evaluate fetal heart rate patterns to detect early fetal distress.
					• Monitor uterine tone for tetanic contractions or development of pathologic contraction rings.
					• Keep patient hydrated and monitor intake and output.
					• Support the couple in coping with this unanticipated event.

	• Increased pain with contractions, although of moderate intensity			IV or oral fluids. • Amniotomy or oxytocin administration may be necessary to establish effective uterine contractions.	

Precipitous Labor	• Precipitous labor is labor that lasts less than 3 hours before spontaneous delivery.
	• Occurs when there is low resistance of maternal tissue, allowing easy passage of the fetus through the pelvis
	• Other causes:
	  • Strong, frequent contractions
	  • Multiparity
	  • Previous precipitous labor
	  • Small vertex fetus
		• Rare maternal problems when maternal tissues are pliable and the cervix effaced and dilated
		• Risk of maternal complications exists when:
		  • Cervix is long and firm
		  • Contractions are vigorous
		  • Maternal tissues are firm and resistant to stretching
		• Associated risks:
		  • Uterine rupture
		  • Amniotic fluid embolism
		  • Postpartum hemorrhage
			• If the fetus is chronically stressed, its condition may worsen with an abnormally brisk labor.
			• Perfusion to the fetus is reduced by uterine hypermobility
			• Trauma to the fetal head may occur when maternal tissues are resistant.
			• When delivery is unattended, neonatal aspiration or hypothermia may result.
				• Delivery	• In women who present in advanced active labor, immediately assess the labor pattern, stage of cervical effacement, and fetal station and presentation
					• Auscultate fetal heart tones and monitor for fetal distress.
					• Alert the birth attendant and staff.
					• Prepare an emergency delivery pack and assist with the delivery.

(continued)

Table 9-2 Intrapartal Complications (*continued*)

Disorder	Etiology/ Predisposing Factors	Maternal Implications	Fetal/ Neonatal Implications	Treatment	Nursing Responsibilities
Dysfunctional Labor Patterns					
Prolonged Labor	• Labor that lasts longer than 24 hours without spontaneous delivery is prolonged; occurs in 1% to 7% of labors. • Usually the first stage is prolonged, and either the latent or active may be longer than normal. • A major cause is myometrial dysfunction.	• Increased risk for uterine atony and lacerations • Increased risk for hemorrhage, infection, and maternal exhaustion and stress from a difficult labor that is not progressing	• Risk of fetal morbidity and mortality increases as labor is prolonged • Potential for asphyxia, infection, and cord prolapse when the presenting part is not engaged • Soft tissue damage or cerebral trauma may occur, especially when immediate delivery is necessary	• Management depends on cervical status: • Ripe cervix: nipple stimulation, amniotomy, or oxytocin may be indicated • Unripe cervix: comfort measures such as fluids, sedation, and promotion of rest • When dysfunctional labor continues, amniotomy and oxytocin are used.	• Monitor maternal and fetal status for adverse effects of protracted labor: • Fetal distress • Infection • Risk of uterine rupture • Administer and evaluate effect of medications such as analgesics, sedatives, and oxytocin. • Provide emotional support and comfort measures to the couple.

				• Cesarean delivery is indicated when cephalopelvic disproportion is suspected.	

Complications of Uterine Function

Preterm Labor and Birth	• Labor begins before 37 weeks of pregnancy—the greatest single problem in obstetrics; 75% of perinatal mortality and 85% of neonatal deaths are attributed to complications of preterm delivery
	• Cause of preterm labor is not always known; predisposing factors include:
	  • Spontaneous rupture of membranes
	  • Incompetent cervix
	  • Uterine anomalies
	  • Overdistention of uterus from hydramnios or multiple gestation
		• Significant emotional stress for the mother accompanies preterm labor because of risk to the infant.
		• Parents commonly blame themselves and feel anger and guilt.
		• Maternal depression may occur
		• The mother must monitor uterine activity during the course of therapy, which causes her to focus intensely on her body and its failure to perform normally.
			• Infant mortality is high among those born at less than 32 weeks gestation.
			• Prematurity is responsible for almost two-thirds of neonatal deaths.
			• Risk for long-term disability
			• Respiratory distress syndrome
			• Immature organ systems
			• Lack of fat storage
			• Problems of thermoregulation
			• Increased risk of intracranial trauma and hemorrhage during delivery
				• Suppression of preterm labor includes:
				  • Bedrest
				  • Use of tocolytic agents such as: Beta-sympathomimetics, progestins, antioxytocins, and prostaglandin inhibitor (See Appendix C-1, Drugs Used in Treatment of Preterm Labor)
				• Magnesium sulfate may be used in conjunction with other tocolytic drugs or when there are
					• Restrict patient to bed rest and continue monitoring of:
					  • Uterine activity
					  • Fetal status
					  • Maternal vital signs
					  • Intake and output
					  • Cervical consistency, effacement, and dilatation
					• After the initial sterile vaginal examination, if membranes have ruptured, vaginal examinations should be minimal, and the patient should be instructed to maintain perineal hygiene.
					• Collect a urine specimen for culture.
					• Initiate an IV line and

(continued)

Table 9-2 Intrapartal Complications (*continued*)

Disorder	Etiology/ Predisposing Factors	Maternal Implications	Fetal/ Neonatal Implications	Treatment	Nursing Responsibilities
Complications of Uterine Function					
	• Maternal illness; preeclampsia, cardiac disease, infection • Elective induction of labor or repeat cesarean delivery			contraindications to their use. • When preterm labor is suppressed, the mother may be discharged on a regimen of bedrest and oral tocolytics. • Use of telemetric monitoring of uterine activity is now available in some areas. • When preterm labor is unresponsive to therapy, delivery of a preterm infant may be inevitable.	hydrate the patient as ordered. • Provide diversions such as books, radio, television, crafts. • Prepare the couple for delivery when labor cannot be suppressed.

Table 9-3 Medical Management of Missed Abortion/Intrauterine Fetal Demise

Medical Management	Rationale	Laboratory Studies	Nursing Implications
12 Weeks			
Confirmation of diagnosis	To diagnose fetal death as soon as possible	Ultrasound	Prepare patient for ultrasound.
Dilatation and curettage of uterine contents Prescription analgesic	To evacuate the uterus	Pregnancy test (converts from positive to negative)	Obtain repeat pregnancy test.
Blood studies	To control possible hemorrhage following uterine evacuation and curettage	Tests: • Hemoglobin (Hgb), hematocrit (Hct), white blood count • Fibrinogen • Platelets • Type and crossmatch	Administer oxytocin as ordered Order two units of blood, fresh frozen plasma, and cryoprecipitate before curettage. Routinely monitor postoperative vital signs. Monitor state of uterine contractions every 15 minutes and massage uterus to maintain firmness. Permit the patient's partner to remain to offer support. Prepare the patient for discharge when her condition stabilizes at 10 to 12 hours.

(*continued*)

Table 9-3 Medical Management of Missed Abortion/Intrauterine Fetal Demise (*continued*)

Medical Management	Rationale	Laboratory Studies	Nursing Implications
13–28 Weeks			
Confirmation of diagnosis	Medical intervention is not appropriate until after 3 weeks of fetal death: spontaneous labor begins in 89% of women during this period.	Untrasound Weekly Hgb, Hct, and fibrinogen-level tests (if fibrinogen levels drop to 0.2 g/dL, delivery is indicated)	Prepare patient for ultrasound. Schedule weekly counseling visits. Obtain type and crossmatch for two units of whole blood. Order cryoprecipitate and fresh frozen plasma for emergency use.
After 3 weeks of fetal death, induction of labor with vaginal prostaglandin E_2, suppositories (20 mg)	Drop in fibrinogen causes risk of DIC. (See Appendix B-4, Blood Coagulation Factors and Laboratory Tests for DIC)		Assist patients who experience nausea and vomiting from prostaglandin use. Give medication before prostaglandin use to minimize side-effects.
Prescription of analgesic.	To decrease patient discomfort from uterine contractions.		Offer patient analgesic.

Labor and delivery of products of conception (takes 10 to 12 hours)			
Prescription of Methergine	To enhance postoperative uterine contractions and reduce blood loss.		Give IM Methergine 0.2 mg as ordered.
Uterine curettage	To ensure removal of all tissue		
Cervical inspection for trauma from procedure		Hct and fibrinogen levels, collected 4 hours after uterine evacuation	
Discharge after 24 hours of stable vital signs	The patient will be eager for discharge. No further risk of DIC exists.		Prepare the patient for discharge. Schedule counseling session with a professional counselor for 2 weeks after discharge or sooner if deemed necessary. Refer for genetic counseling regarding possible risk in future pregnancies. Refer to parent support group.

(*continued*)

Table 9-3 Medical Management of Missed Abortion/Intrauterine Fetal Demise (*continued*)

Medical Management	Rationale	Laboratory Studies	Nursing Implications
Greater than 28 Weeks			
Confirmation of diagnosis	Medical intervention is not appropriate until after 3 weeks of fetal death.	Ultrasound	Offer support to grieving couple.
Scheduling of weekly visits	To monitor for early signs of DIC	Weekly Hgb, Hct, and fibrinogen level tests (if fibrinogen levels drop to 0.2 g/dL, delivery is indicated)	Keep patient informed of need for close surveillance of her blood levels and signs of bleeding.
After 3 weeks, collection of blood coagulation studies every 6 hours	Patient is at greater risk for DIC.		Obtain type and crossmatch for two units of whole blood. Order cryoprecipitate and fresh frozen plasma for emergency use.
Induction of labor	Low fibrinogen levels increase DIC risk.		Discuss need for induced labor with couple and answer questions.
Induction options: • Laminaria placed in cervix 12 hours before induction	To speed cervical ripening or dilatation or to initiate labor		Assure couple that a nurse will be with them throughout procedure. Obtain type and crossmatch

• Prostaglandin gel applied to cervix • Prostaglandin E_2 suppository inserted high in posterior vaginal fornix • Prostaglandin or oxytocin infusions			for two units of whole blood. Order cryoprecipitate and fresh frozen plasma for emergency use. Assist with insertion of laminaria or suppository, informing patient about what is happening and why. Establish an IV line with Ringer's lactate or similar solution.
• Amniotomy and insertion of transcervical pressure catheter between amnion and uterine wall	To permit accurate monitoring of uterine pressure and reduce risk of uterine rupture		Collect equipment and assist with placement of pressure catheter. Place an external pressure monitor when amniotomy cannot be performed.
		Coagulation studies, collected every 4 hours	Ensure collection of blood specimen and expedite its transport to the laboratory. Monitor vital signs every 2 to 4 hours.

(*continued*)

Table 9-3 Medical Management of Missed Abortion/Intrauterine Fetal Demise (*continued*)

Medical Management	Rationale	Laboratory Studies	Nursing Implications
Greater than 28 Weeks			
Prescription of antiemetic and antidiarrheal medication	Nausea, vomiting, and diarrhea may occur with prostaglandin use.		Give patient medications before prostaglandin use to minimize side-effects.
Prescription of analgesic	To decrease patient discomfort from uterine contractions		Offer patient-ordered analgesic. Encourage partner to support patient during labor and delivery.
Delivery of infant			Support couple and assist in their grieving process and its resolution. After delivery, fetus should be cleaned, wrapped in a blanket, and given to parents to hold. They may prefer to be left alone at this time. Refer the couple to a parent support group if they desire.

Self-Care Teaching: Risk Reduction Strategies for Preterm Labor

- Recognize the signs and symptoms of preterm labor and seek obstetric care immediately when they occur.
- Maintain a schedule of regular weekly prenatal check-ups to allow ongoing assessment of cervical status and uterine activity.
- Curtail work activities and maintain bedrest as prescribed.
- Refrain from sexual intercourse and orgasm (sexual stimulation and uterine contractions associated with orgasm may trigger labor).
- Restrict travel outside your immediate community in case labor ensues.
- Optimize health by maintaining an adequate diet, taking prenatal vitamins or iron, practicing good hygiene, and avoiding people with infectious diseases.

Care of Patients with Pre-existing Maternal Diseases

Hypertensive Cardiovascular Disease

Intrapartal management is similar to that for PIH. If placental function is compromised, early delivery may be necessary. Close monitoring of maternal BP is needed throughout labor to detect possible PIH superimposed on already elevated BP. Spinal anesthesia may be avoided because of the risk of abrupt hypotension and fetal compromise.

Cardiac Disease

About 1% of all pregnant women suffer from pre-existing cardiac disease. Patients are usually hospitalized before delivery, with earlier hospitalization in more severe cases. Vaginal delivery is preferable to cesarean delivery if no other complications arise. It is important, however, to minimize maternal anxiety and pain because of their detrimental effects on maternal cardiorespiratory status. Systemic analgesia and pudendal block are customary for vaginal birth. Continuous epidural block may be used, but constant vigilance regarding maternal BP is required to avoid maternal hypotension, which can be fatal to some cardiac patients.

Pulse, respirations, and BP should be monitored every 15 minutes through first-stage labor, and every 5 to 10 minutes through second-stage labor. Increasing pulse (over 100 bpm) and respiratory rate (over 24 per minute) may signal developing cardiac embarrassment. The patient should be maintained on bedrest in the early postpartum period until cardiac function is fully recovered; cardiac decompensation may occur up to 7 days after delivery because of mobilization of extravascular fluid and resulting cardiac overload. Stress and energy expenditure during this time must be minimized.

Hyperthyroidism

There is an increased incidence of preterm labor and birth with hyperthyroidism. Intrapartal management is not unusual, except for closer monitoring of blood and electrolyte values. A cord blood sample should be tested for free T_4 to determine the thyroid status of the neonate.

Acquired Immune Deficiency Syndrome

Acquired immune deficiency syndrome (AIDS) has been reported among pregnant women whose partners had the disease or were in high-risk groups and among women who have received artificial insemination with donor sperm. Intrapartal management requires vigilance to decrease the risk of infection, since the mother's immune system is compromised. To avoid spreading AIDS, health care providers should take the following precautions: scrupulous handwashing, avoidance of accidental needle sticks, gown-glove, eye goggle precautions when in contact with bodily fluids and excretions, and the use of masks if the patient is coughing or has pneumocystosis. The patient's cytomegalovirus titer may be elevated. The probability of transmission to the fetus/newborn is as yet unknown, but potentially high.

Care of Grieving Parents

Acknowledge Shock and Grief

- Express your feelings about the baby's death with consoling words.
- Touch parents in a caring fashion; words are not always necessary.

Sharpen the Reality of the Baby's Death

- Provide as much factual information about the baby's death as is available.
- Describe the baby's appearance in factual and tender terms before bringing the baby to the parents.
- Encourage the parents to see and hold the baby. Stay with them as they examine the baby for the first time.
- Acknowledge the baby's death at first contact with the parents and daily thereafter; do not act as if the death has not occurred.
- Provide parents with physical tokens of the baby: wisp of hair, instant photograph, blanket, identification bracelet.

Assist Parents in Grieving

- Encourage the parents to grieve openly.
- Spend extra time with the parents to review events surrounding the baby's death.
- Encourage the parents to make arrangement for a spiritual or religious ritual to mark the baby's death (baptism, funeral, memorial service).

Help Parents to Prepare for Homegoing

- Suggest a "dry run" of discharge to help the parents work through their feeling about going home without a baby.
- Help parents prepare themselves for telling family and friends and responding to others who do not know of the baby's death.
- Involve other family members or support people in preparations for homegoing.
- Discuss possible difficult times: dismantling the nursery, renewing their sexual relationship, seeing other newborns.
- Provide referral to support services, such as parent support groups or counseling.
- Maintain postdischarge contact with parents through the first year.

Adapted from Estok P, Lehman A: Perinatal death: Grief support for families. Birth 10: 17, 1983

NOTES

10
Normal and Complicated Postpartum Period

Nursing Objectives in the Normal Postpartum

- To monitor maternal physiologic and psychological adaptation in the early postpartum period
- To promote the restoration of maternal bodily functions
- To promote maternal rest and comfort
- To promote parent–infant acquaintance
- To facilitate parental caretaking
- To teach effective self-care and infant care

Possible Nursing Diagnoses Related to Normal Postpartum

- Anxiety related to breastfeeding
- Potential alterations in bowel elimination (constipation) related to decreased bowel motility and perineal/rectal pain
- Alteration in comfort (pain) related to uterine contractions and alterations of the perineum or rectum
- Fluid volume deficit related to abnormal fluid loss and dehydration
- Alteration in patterns of urinary elimination related to bladder trauma and postdelivery diuresis
- Alteration in family processes related to new family member

PHYSIOLOGIC CHANGES IN THE POSTPARTUM

During the first hours and days after childbirth, the mother undergoes dramatic physiologic changes involving nearly every system of the body. Were changes of this magnitude to occur in a patient other than a postpartum woman, they would give cause for grave concern. For instance, the postpartum woman typically experiences weight loss of 15 to 17 lb. Most of this loss (10 to 12 lb) is the result of the delivery of the infant, placenta, and amniotic fluid; in addition, 5 lb of excess fluid is lost through diuresis, and there is a blood loss of 500 ml or more. Fluid loss of this degree through diuresis and other mechanisms would likely pose a significant risk of hypovolemic shock to a nonmaternity patient. However, most postpartum women experience relatively little discomfort related to these physical findings.

Vital Signs

- Oral temperature of the postpartum woman within 24 hours of delivery may be as high as 100.4°F (38°C) resulting from muscular exertion or dehydration; after 24 hours she should be afebrile.
- Temperature elevation over 100.4°F on any of 2 of the first 10 postpartum days may suggest puerperal sepsis, urinary tract infection, endometritis, mastitis, or other infection.
- Temperature elevations on the second or third postpartum days should not persist longer than 24 hours without follow-up.

Cardiovascular Changes

- Dramatic maternal changes in the postpartum period involve the cardiovascular system.
- Substantial blood loss at delivery can be sustained because of the 40% increase in circulating blood volume during pregnancy. Blood losses up to 500 ml in a vaginal birth and 700 ml to 1000 ml in a cesarean section are not uncommon.
- Blood pressure (BP), and pulse, and respirations should remain at normal limits.

Urinary Changes

- Bladder tissue is edematous, congested, and hypotonic immediately postpartum and may result in overdistention, incomplete emptying, and collection of residual urine. Many of these effects are diminished by 24 hours.
- Excess fluid accumulation in tissue during pregnancy is eliminated by diuresis that begins within 12 hours after delivery accounting for as much as a 5-lb weight loss.

Gastrointestinal Changes

- Re-establishment of normal bowel function takes about one week because of decreased bowel motility, fluid loss, and bowel discomfort.
- By the end of the first week, as the woman's appetite and fluid intake increases, normal bowel function returns.

Musculoskeletal Changes

- Due to stretching, the abdominal muscles are often soft, weak, and flabby.
- Sensation in the lower extremities may be decreased the first 24 hours after delivery if regional anesthesia was used for the birth.
- Predisposition to thrombophlebitis results from decreased activity and increased prothrombin levels.
- Vigorous exercise to regain muscle tone is not recommended until complete healing has taken place.

Breast Changes

- Breast milk (colostrum) production begins around the third postpartum day.
- Initial engorgement occurs, and the breasts become larger, firmer, tender, and painful to touch.
- Prolactin secretion initiates the let-down, which is stimulated by suckling of the infant.
- Continued breastfeeding will decrease engorgement and increase milk production.

Uterine Changes

- The fundus is palpable 1 cm above the umbilicus at 12 hours postdelivery (see Table 10-1).
- Uterine contractions continue after delivery of the placenta. In primiparas uterine tone is high and the uterus remains firm. In multiparas periodic uterine contractions, known as "after pains," are common and may continue for 2 to 3 days postdelivery.
- Postdelivery lochia is red (lochia rubra) for 2 to 3 days; it progresses to a brownish color (lochia serosa), and is followed by a yellowish whitish color (lochia alba) by the seventh to tenth day (see Table 10-2).
- The pelvic floor, uterine ligaments, vaginal walls, and abdominal wall regain most of their tone during the postpartum period.

Table 10-1 Stages in Uterine Involution

Time Since Delivery	Position of Fundus	Uterine Weight (gram)	Lochia
1–2 hours	Midway between umbilicus and symphysis on midline	1000	Rubra
12 hours	1 cm above or at umbilicus		Rubra
3 days	3 cm below umbilicus (continues descent at 1 cm/day)		Serosa
9 days	Not palpable above symphysis	500	Alba
5–6 weeks	Not palpable above symphysis; slightly larger than in mullipara		Not present

Table 10-2 Characteristics of Lochia

Name	Approximate Time Since Delivery	Normal Discharge	Abnormal Discharge
Lochia Rubra	Days 1 to 3	Bloody with clots Fleshy odor Increase in flow upon rising, with breastfeeding, with exertion	Numerous large clots Foul smell Saturated perineal pad
Lochia Serosa	Days 4 to 9	Pink or brown with a seroanguinous consistency Fleshy odor	Foul smell Saturated perineal pad
Lochia Alba	Day 10	Yellow to white Fleshy odor	Foul smell Saturated perineal pad Persistent lochia serosa Return to pink or red discharge Persistent discharge over 2 to 3 weeks

PSYCHOLOGICAL CHANGES: RUBIN'S MATERNAL PHASES

Taking In: A Period of Dependent Behavior

- Focus on self
- Verbalization of need for sleep and food
- Reliving of birth experience
- Passive and dependent behavior

Taking Hold: Moving Between Dependence and Independence

- Widening of focus to include activities
- Independence in self-care activities
- Verbalized concern about body functions of self and infant
- Openness to instruction about care of self and infant
- Lack of confidence (mother is easily discouraged by caretaking skills)

Letting Go: Taking on New Role Responsibilities

- Increasing independence in care of self and infant
- Recognition of infant as separate from self
- Grief for relinquished roles, expectations
- Adjustment of family relationships to accommodate infant

NURSING ASSESSMENT

Nursing assessment of the postpartum family should include a review of the prenatal and intrapartal records, assessment of the mother's condition, and psychosocial assessment of the family members.

Medical record review will identify pre-existing and prenatal health problems, type of labor and its progress, fetal response to labor, use of medications and analgesia or anesthesia, and family response to labor and delivery.

Postpartum Assessment

- Assess uterine tone, position, and height by abdominal palpation at regular intervals.
- Gently palpate the uterus of a cesarean birth mother to assess

the surgical dressing for drainage or bleeding, and check the degree of pain being experienced.

- Determine the amount of lochia, its color, odor, and presence of clots, and question mother about the numbers of sanitary napkins being used and their degree of saturation.
- Palpate the breasts to determine their firmness and tenderness to assess engorgement.
- Inspect the perineum and rectum to assess for REEDA: redness, edema, ecchymosis, discharge, and approximation of wound edges.
- Measure urinary intake and output to identify potential urinary retention until normal function returns.
- Observe the woman for nausea and vomiting, question her regarding flatulence or bowel movements, and listen for bowel signs twice daily.
- Inspect the lower extremities for sensation, strength, edema, and signs of thromboembolism or thrombophlebitis.
- Inquire about the amount of rest and sleep the mother is getting.
- Regularly monitor the mother's mood and allow her to express her feelings about the birth experience and her infant.

NURSING INTERVENTION

Early Postpartum Care (first 6 hours)

- Monitor BP, pulse, skin color, and uterine tone every 15 minutes for the first hour.
- Massage the fundus as needed and observe lochial flow; a boggy uterus may indicate the need for oxytocin infusion.
- Instruct the patient on how to assess bleeding and uterine tone and how to perform fundal massage.
- Apply ice pack to the maternal perineum for the first 8 to 12 hours to reduce edema, bruising, and to promote maternal comfort.
- Encourage lying flat on the abdomen when discomfort due to uterine contractions or "afterpains" occurs; administer analgesia as indicated.
- Encourage early and frequent voiding, and assist the mother to the bathroom to expedite voiding when she is able.
- Encourage liberal fluid intake, as much as 2000 ml/12 hours, and diet as desired.
- Assist with breastfeeding and infant care as desired in the first 1 to 2 hours.

Ongoing Postpartum Care (6 hours to 3 days)

- If lochial flow appears excessive (more than one sanitary napkin saturated from end to end in 1 hour) or if flow increases after a progressive decrease, begin to count the sanitary napkins used and initiate closer monitoring to allow early identification of postpartum hemorrhage.
- Encourage cool to cold sitz baths the first day; warm sitz baths thereafter.
- Encourage warm showers and breast massage to stimulate circulation, promote let-down of breast milk, and decrease engorgement in nursing mothers.
- Apply ice packs to the breasts of nonbreastfeeding mothers; encourage them to wear a tight bra or binder; and administer analgesics as needed.
- Encourage rest, sleep, and relaxation.
- Prevent maternal constipation by encouraging liberal fluid intake and intake of foods such as fresh fruits and vegetables that are high in fiber; stool softeners may be administered when necessary.
- Facilitate early parent–infant interaction, and encourage parents to take advantage of available classes and demonstrations in infant care.
- Institute discharge teaching plan that includes both parents and covers the following information:
  - Expected changes in lochia and warning signs
  - Suggested exercise and activity level
  - Need for rest
  - Emotional aspects of the postpartum
  - Sexual relations and contraception
  - Breast and perineal care
  - Dietary recommendations
  - Need for follow-up care of mother and baby

Self-Care Teaching: Changes in Lochia to Report

Report the following signs:

- Foul-smelling lochia: suggests endometritis
- Heavy lochia: suggests uterine atony, retained placental fragments, or vaginal/cervical laceration

- Lochia rubra after the third postpartum day: suggests late postpartum hemorrhage
- Presence of clots: suggests retained placental fragments or hemorrhage.

BREASTFEEDING

The advantages of breastfeeding are well recognized, and breastfeeding is enjoying increasing popularity in the United States. Mothers frequently require information and support in their efforts to establish breastfeeding, and the nurse in the postpartum setting plays an especially important role in this process.

The Let-Down Reflex

The let-down reflex, a reflex from the breast to the hypothalamus, causes the release of oxytocin by the posterior pituitary gland. The infant's sucking, and even its cry or mere presence, can elicit the let-down reflex in the mother and release the flow of milk.

Nursing Assessment of the Breastfeeding Mother

- Determine how the mother feels about breastfeeding, whether she was taught to prepare her breasts prenatally, whether she was supported or discouraged to breastfeed by her family, and how she arrived at her decision to breastfeed. The success or failure of the process of breastfeeding hinges on these issues.
- Assess the breasts. Breast size and shape have little effect on lactation, and mothers with small breasts should be assured that they will be able to breastfeed and will produce sufficient quantities of milk.
- Examine the nipples and aerolae. This is especially important in detecting inverted or flat nipples, which make breastfeeding difficult (ideally this occurs during the prenatal period in anticipation of breastfeeding).
- Explain to mothers with retracted nipples who desire to nurse that they can wear plastic nipple shields to correct inverted nipples. Tell the mother that milk leaking into the shield is not to be fed to the baby.
- Encourage mothers wearing breast shields to keep the shields clean and dry to prevent rapid growth of bacteria.

Nursing Interventions for Promotion of Breastfeeding

Nursing interventions for the promotion of breastfeeding in the postpartum period center on teaching specific techniques of breastfeeding and general principles of lactation management to the couple.

- Diet
    - Avoid intentional weight loss while breastfeeding.
    - Maintain an additional 500 kcal in the diet for milk production.
    - Include foods from all four major food groups. (See Chapter 5 for a detailed discussion of nutritional needs during lactation.)
    - Drink 2 quarts of fluid per day, such as water, milk, and unsweetened juice.
    - Avoid cigarette smoking, caffeine, alcohol, and drugs, which may enter breast milk and be harmful to the infants. (See Appendix D-2, Medications in Breast Milk)

- Rest
    - Encourage the mother to rest or nap while the baby is asleep.
    - Limit visitors and allow others to do household chores.
    - Elicit the father's support in encouraging relaxation, rest, diet; in limiting family activities; and in assisting the mother in the infant's care.

- Care of the breasts and nipples
    - Discuss the use of a nursing bra; many women feel more comfortable with its support and convenience.
    - Nipple pads can protect clothing from stains from leaking milk. Instruct the woman to change them frequently and to keep the nipple from being continually damp.
    - Advise the mother to wash the breasts and nipples with warm water daily (soap on the nipple may be excessively drying and can cause the nipple to crack).
    - Advise buffing the nipples for a few seconds while drying them to help decrease their sensitivity and increase tolerance of the newborn's strong initial sucking.
    - Encourage the mother to expose her nipples to air for 5 minutes after each feeding to promote drying and healing of any earlier irritation.
    - Advise the mother to avoid putting any substances on the areolae or nipples that may irritate the skin; vitamin E, lanolin, or aloe vera may be used in small amounts if nipples seem dry but must be removed prior to nursing.

Self-Care Teaching: Breastfeeding

- Make sure the baby has as much of the areola as possible in its mouth during feeding.
- Change nursing positions often to vary points of maximum sucking pressure.
- Avoid the use of soap or other drying agents on the nipples.
- Apply small amount of nipple ointment (*e.g.*, anhydrous lanolin) to the nipple and areola after nursing if nipples are excessively dry. Avoid covering milk duct opening, or they may become clogged.
- Wash the nipples with clear water frequently to avoid the thickening and drying of milk on them.
- Expose the nipples to air as much as possible.
- Use the correct technique for removing the baby from the breast (insert fingers at the side of the baby's mouth to release suction).
- Nurse at the less sore breast first.
- Avoid engorgement.

If engorgement occurs, observe the following procedures:

- Nurse more frequently.
- Express milk to soften the areola before nursing.
- Massage firm breast area gently when nursing.
- Use a correctly fitted nursing bra that supports the breasts separately, does not bind, and encloses all of the breast tissue within the cups.
- Take frequent warm showers or baths or apply wet packs to the breasts to relieve discomfort and promote milk flow.
- If necessary, use oxytocin nasal spray to initiate let-down until this reflex is well established.
- Promptly report any symptoms of mastitis.
- Wean very gradually giving up one feeding every week, beginning with the one when the breasts are least full.

EARLY POSTPARTUM DISCHARGE

With the advent of alternative birth centers and more flexible hospital policies, healthy mothers and their newborns may now be discharged within the first 24 hours after birth. Most settings have specific criteria, such as the following for early discharge:

- Uncomplicated pregnancy
- Uncomplicated labor and vaginal delivery

- Vital signs within normal limits
- Firm uterus with moderate lochia
- Voiding without difficulty
- Maternal hemoglobin and hematocrit within normal limits
- Absence of nausea and vomiting
- Healthy newborn
- Positive parent–infant interaction
- Availability of home visit in the first 5 days by a nurse or a representative of a community agency

POSTPARTUM COMPLICATIONS

Nursing Objectives in Postpartum Complications

- To review and assess the health of the patient during the prenatal period
- To review the course of labor and delivery, assessing any deviations from the norm
- To initiate early intervention to help decrease the severity of the complication
- To closely monitor and give nursing support to the patient during her postpartum hospitalization
- To keep the spouse or partner informed of the patient's progress and be sensitive to his concerns
- To teach the patient how to care for herself and her infant prior to discharge
- To provide a list of resources from which help is available if it is needed

Possible Nursing Diagnoses Related to Postpartum Complications

- Alteration in reticuloendothelial system related to increased production of white blood cells and alteration of the immune response
- Alteration in cardiac output (decreased) related to serious illness or postpartum conditions such as puerperal infection, thromboembolic disease, or postpartum hemorrhage
- Alteration in comfort (pain) related to an infectious process or medical intervention

- Anxiety related to postpartum complications and their possible effects on the infant or family

---

Modern advances in health care have decreased the widespread morbidity and mortality of earlier decades, but recovery from childbirth is never routine. An uneventful puerperium cannot be taken for granted; each women's response to the awesome changes that have occurred in her body during pregnancy and birth is unique. The woman's body is vulnerable at this time, and prompt diagnosis and treatment is essential for her welfare and the welfare of her family.

Because the course of the puerperium is usually benignly progressive, it is particularly important for the nurse to use her powers of observation to assess subtle changes of affect or physical recovery in the postpartum woman.

NURSING INTERVENTIONS

Self-Care Teaching: Postpartum Complications

- Take antibiotics at the specified time, and complete the course of the drug even though symtoms have disappeared. Stop the drug if an allergic reaction occurs, and call the physician.
- Maintain a high fluid intake to keep the body well hydrated.
- Eat a well-rounded diet, and do not skip meals. If you have any prenatal vitamins left, continue taking one tablet per day.
- Maintain good hygiene when caring for the breasts and perineum. Handwashing should be routine before touching the breasts or the baby.
- Maintain good bowel habits and include roughage and fluids in the diet to prevent constipation.
- Get plenty of rest; nap when the baby is asleep. If possible, let other helpers do the cooking and housework.
- Exercise to get back in shape. A regular exercise regimen of walking or routine postpartum exercise is especially helpful. Strenuous exercise should not be done until after a normal 6-week postpartum check-up.
- Treat yourself to an occasional outing without the baby. Get a babysitter and plan a day away from home doing something you enjoy; have a special dinner with your spouse or partner; visit with friends; or pursue your favorite hobby. You will return home relaxed and refreshed.

Puerperal Infection

Predisposing Factors in Puerperal Infections

- Improper aseptic technique
- Emergency delivery outside the hospital
- Cesarean delivery after rupture of the membranes
- Prolonged rupture of the membranes
- Labor prolonged for more than 24 hours
- Trauma from obstetric interventions
- Manual removal of the placenta
- Lacerations or hematoma of the vagina and perineum
- Hemorrhage
- Improper perineal care

The most common puerperal infections are covered in Table 10-3. Antibiotic drugs used in treatment of puerperal infections are discussed in Table 10-4; anticoagulants for puerperal thromboembolic disease are discussed in Table 10-5.

Self-Care Teaching: The Patient With Thrombophlebitis

- Avoid periods of prolonged sitting at work or while traveling or watching television. Getting up to walk around every half-hour or every hour prevents pooling in the legs by increasing circulatory return to the heart.
- Avoid pressure under the knees, such as propping with pillows.
- Elevate the foot of the bed to promote venous drainage.
- Avoid crossing the legs while seated, which decreases circulation to the leg because of pressure on the popliteal space behind the knee.
- Elevate the legs when sitting whenever possible.
- Use correct method for putting on support (Jobst) stockings: lie flat with legs elevated and roll on stockings.
- Wear loose clothing.
- Do not wear garters or other tight restrictions around the legs.
- Reduce gastric distress caused by daily dose of anticoagulant by dividing it or taking it with food.
- Avoid possible Coumadin interaction with over-the-counter preparations, such as those containing acetylsalicylic acid formulations (aspirin-based products), and check with your physician about the interactive effects of other prescribed drugs.
- Do not use a straight razor or a safety razor. Use an electric razor that does not nick or scrape or depilatories.

(*text continues on pg. 375*)

Table 10-3 Treatment and Nursing Interventions for Puerperal Infections

Infection/Symptoms	Treatment and Nursing Interventions
Perineal Infection	

• Acute infection: chills and fever to 104°F (40°C)
• Low-grade infection: temperature 101°F (38.5°C) pulse 100/min
  • Leukocytosis
  • Localized pain, erythema at lesion site, ecchymosis, purulent drainage, induration
	• Keep the patient warm with extra blankets and hot water bottle if chills occur; provide cool sponge baths and antipyretic when the temperature is high.
	• Episiotomy infection requires removal of sutures to enhance drainage.
	• Perineal wound is assessed daily noting degree of redness, presense of pain, and type of discharge.
	• Provide sitz bath and perineal lamp 2 to 3 times daily.
	• Change perineal pads frequently and give analgesia as ordered.

Metritis and Endometritis	
• Temperature elevation 101°F to 102°F (33.8°C to 38.9°C) • Rapid pulse rate (100 to 140 bpm) • Vague malaise, anorexia, abdominal tenderness • Elevated WBC • Uterine subinvolution	• Palpate abdomen and uterus daily to assess pain and involution. • Patient may be discharged with instructions for home care. • Encourage bedrest with bathroom privileges for 1 week. • Stress importance of following drug regimen. • Instruct patient to refrain from intercourse and douching. • Encourage fluid intake and nutrients high in protein and vitamins. • Encourage a return appointment in 1 week.

Parametritis

• Symptoms appear 24 hours after delivery • Spiking fever of 103°F to 104°F (39.4°C to 40°C) • Tachycardia, tachypnea • Exquisite uterine and cervical motion tenderness • Palpable abscess formation in the vagina or rectum • Elevated WBC to 15,000 to 30,000/mm^3	• Maintain bedrest in the semi-Fowler's position • Give cool sponge bath to decrease fever and assess for dehydration • Check temperature, respirations, pulse and BP every 4 hours • Check perineal pad and perineum for heavy, foul, or nonfoul lochia (foulness indicates anaerobic infection). • Check for evidence of hematoma or abscess. • Maintain fluid intake at 3000 to 4000 ml • Administer antibiotics and analgesics as ordered. • Provide the patient with an opportunity to discuss her feelings and ask questions if surgical intervention becomes necessary.

Peritonitis

• Chills and fever to 105°F (40.5°C) • Rapid, weak pulse to 140 bpm; rapid, shallow breathing • Loss of fluids through vomiting and diarrhea; excessive thirst • Decreased urinary output • Paralytic ileus with paroxysmal pain and abdominal distention	• Keep the patient warm and give antipyretic as ordered. • Maintain flow of oxygen to increase oxygen supply and decrease intestinal anoxia. • Maintain IV infusion for antibiotic administration and to maintain hydration. • Record fluid intake and urinary output; closely monitor nasogastric tube and central venous pressure. • Note bowel sounds and presence of abdominal distention. • When the infecting organisms is beta-hemolytic streptococci, the mother will be isolated and unable to breastfeed. When the threat of infections is passed, the mother can resume breastfeeding.

(*continued*)

Table 10-3 Treatment and Nursing Interventions for Puerperal Infections (*continued*)

Infection/Symptoms	Treatment and Nursing Interventions
Deep Vein Thrombophlebitis	
• Minimal fever • Skin warm to touch but without visible or palpable lesions • Positive Homans' sign • Deep vein tenderness and spasm of calf muscles • Dull ache, frank pain in calf, or aching in the leg • Swelling in the extremities due to venous obstruction	• Check vital signs every 4 hours. • Maintain strict bedrest for 1 to 2 weeks. • When diagnosed, anticoagulant therapy begins and continues for about 6 weeks. • Elastic stocking or Ace-type bandages should be applied from ankle to knee with the affected limb elevated to optimize venous drainage. • Apply warm, moist packs to the affected limb several times daily to dilate the blood vessels and decrease lymphatic congestion. • Check for bleeding gums, hematuria, epistaxis, and occult blood while anticoagulants are being used. • When inflammation subsides, allow the patient to walk while wearing elastic stockings. (See self-care teaching for anticoagulant therapy and thrombophlebitis, this Chapter.)
Thromboembolic Disease	
• Swift and wide variations in body temperature (96°F to 105°F; 35.5°C to 40.5°C) • Severe abdominal pain (cardinal sign)	• Arrange for diagnostic studies, including chest x-ray and lung scan, complete blood count (CBC), coagulation studies, ultrasound Doppler flow detection studies to ascertain impaired

• Drop in BP with a pulse rate exceeding 120 bpm • Severe chills, pale skin • Cyanosed lips and fingers	blood flow ahead of the thrombus, electrocardiogram (ECG), and blood cultures. • Assist with placement of IV heparin in the early stage of anticoagulant therapy (see Table 10-5). • Closely monitor vital signs to ensure against shock; monitor patient response to therapy. • Supply oxygen as needed; maintain antibiotic infusion. • Stay with the patient as much possible to promote comfort and permit swift action in the event of increasing illness. • Explain to the patient the need to temporarily discontinue breastfeeding; help patient to pump her breasts to maintain milk supply.
Urinary Tract Infections	
Cystitis: Lower Tract Infection • Symptoms appear within 48 hours • Dysuria, frequency, urgency • Suprapubic pain • Hematuria, bacteriuria • Slight or absent temperature elevation	• Obtain a urine specimen for urinalysis and culture. • Encourage spontaneous urination in the patient to aovid catheterization. • Insert an indwelling catheter as ordered when the patient is unable to void spontaneously; leave it in place for 24 hours to prevent recurrence of urinary retention. • Encourage the woman to void frequently. • Provide antibiotic therapy as ordered. • Repeat urine culture 1 week after completion of drug therapy to ensure adequate treatment.

(continued)

Table 10-3 Treatment and Nursing Interventions for Puerperal Infections (*continued*)

Infection/Symptoms	Treatment and Nursing Interventions
Urinary Tract Infections	
Pyelonephritis: Upper Tract Infection	
• Signs and symptoms of cystitis • Temperature elevation, chills • Nausea and vomiting • Flank pain in area of one or both kidneys • Tenderness of the costovertebral angle • Foul-smelling, cloudy urine	• Monitor vital signs every 2 to 4 hours. • Collect urine for urinalysis and culture. • Obtain a white blood count (WBC). • Administer IV antibiotic therapy. • Measure intake and output to assess kidney function. • Encourage fluid intake of 3000 to 4000 ml per day. • Monitor patient's diet and fluid intake to ensure adequacy. • Encourage the mother to breastfeed when the drugs she receives for treatment are not harmful to the baby. • Teach the mother how to prevent subsequent bladder or kidney infections.
Mastitis	
• Symptoms occur about 1 week postpartum • Sore, cracked nipple • Body aches, malaise, fever, chills • Redness and warmth of skin over infection site, palpable lumps	• Obtain culture and sensitivity test on breast milk. • Apply heat to the breast to encourage milk flow and reduce congestion. • Empty the breasts by manual expression or by use of a hand or electric pump to help relieve stasis.

• Possible abscess formation • Temperature elevation 103 to 104°F (39.5 to 40.0°C), increased pulse rate	• Provide analgesics as ordered. • Prepare the patient for incision and drainage when an abscess occurs. • Discontinue breastfeeding when fever is high and the breast milk contains pus. • Maintain the woman's breastfeeding ability by routinely having her pump her breasts; discard the milk. • Assure the mother that when she becomes afebrile for 24 hours she may resume breastfeeding.

Complications of Puerperal Infections

• Maternal death • Hemorrhage • Subinvolution • Thrombophlebitis • Neonatal Infection • Sterility
• Chronic kidney disease • Pulmonary embolism • Septic shock • Disseminated intravascular coagulation

(See Table 10-6 for Other Puerperal Complications)

Table 10-4 Antibiotic Drugs Commonly Used to Treat Puerperal Infection

Drug	Dosage	Potential Side-Effects	Nursing Implications
Ampicillin (Amcill)—penicillin group	Orally: 250 to 500 mg qid IM or IV: 250 mg to 2 g every 6 hours	Allergic reaction as seen in penicillin hypersensitivity: rash, nausea, vomiting, dermatitis, anaphylactic reaction	Drug is not used in patients with penicillin allergy. 30% of hospital strains of *Escherichia coli* are resistant to penicillin drugs. Drug appears in breast milk.
Carbenicillin (Geopen)—synthetic penicillin	IM or IV; 4 to 40 g daily in divided doses	Allergic reactions as seen in penicillin hypersensitivity; vein irritation at point of injection	Unpleasant taste and dry mouth may occur; mouth care needed. Advise patient to report any change in urine quantity or quality.
Cefoxitin (Mefoxin)—semisynthetic and related to penicillin	IM or IV; 1 to 2 g every 6 to 8 hours	Pain, tenderness, induration at IM injection site; thrombophlebitis at IV site; rash, fever, allergic reaction	Drug is not used in patients sensitive to penicillin or cephalosporins.

Clindamycin (Cleocin)	Orally: 150 to 450 mg every 6 hours; IM or IV: 300 to 600 mg every 6 to 8 hours, up to 2400 mg/day	Loose stools, diarrhea, nausea, vomiting, abdominal cramps, colitis, rash; abnormal liver function test following rapid IV injection	Drug is reserved for serious infections where less toxic antimicrobials are ineffective. It is the drug of choice in treating *Bacteroides fragilis*, a normal inhabitant of genital tract that causes severe infection when blood clots or necrotic tissue are present.
Chloramphenicol Palmitate	Orally: 50 to 100 mg/kg/day in four equally divided doses	Bone marrow depression, gastrointestinal disturbances, nausea, vomiting, bad taste in mouth	Shake medicine well. Drug is to be taken with water on an empty stomach 1 to 2 hours before or after a meal.
Chloramphenicol, Sodium Succinate	IV use only: 50 mg/kg body weight in equally divided doses every 6 hours	Neurotoxicity: headache, mental depression, confusion; optic effects: visual disturbances, contact conjunctivitis; hypersensitivity, fever, rash, topical itching	Patientis hospitalized for close observation and lab tests. Observe closely for signs of toxicity. Patient should report sore throat, fatigue, petechiae, bleeding. Check temperature every 4 hours.

(*continued*)

Table 10-4 Antibiotic Drugs Commonly Used to Treat Puerperal Infection (*continued*)

Drug	Dosage	Potential Side-Effects	Nursing Implications
Metronidazol (Flagyl)	IV or anaerobic infection: loading dose 15 mg/kg infused over 1-hr period; maintenance dose 7.5 mg/kg IV or orally every 6 hours	Anorexia, nausea, vomiting, diarrhea, epigastric distress, bad taste in mouth; possible carcinogenic, teratogenic, and mutagenic changes found in animal studies	Do not mix with another drug. Drug is contraindicated in patients with blood dyscrasias. Alcoholic beverages should not be consumed (drug is used in antiabuse therapy).
Streptomycin Sulfate aminoglycoside	IM: 1 to 4 g daily in divided doses every 6 to 12 hours	Ototoxicity: labyrinth damage, auditory change; neurotoxicity: parasthesia, headache, inability to concentrate, muscular weakness; hypersensitivity	Drug is administered deep in to large muscle mass to avoid irritation. Injections are painful. Avoid direct contact with drug—sensitization can occur. Advise patient to report unusual symptoms (esp. ear symptoms). Monitor intake and output.

Kanamycin Sulfate—aminoglycoside	IM: 15 mg/kg in two to four equally divided doses; IV: not to exceed 15 mg/kg body weight in two to three equal doses	Gastrointestinal effects: nausea, vomiting, diarrhea; nephrotoxicity: hematuria, proteinuria; ototoxicity: deafness, vertigo, tinnitus; neurotoxicity: paresthesia, optic or peripheral neuritis; hypersensitivity: pruritus, rash; changes in many blood studies	Drug is administered IM deep into upper-outer quadrant of buttock. Keep patient well hydrated (sufficient amount to produce 1500 ml urine/day). Postoperative patients should be monitored for respiratory and neuromuscular depression.
Gentamicin (Garamycin)—aminoglycoside	IM or IV: 3 to 5 mg/kg/day in three divided doses every 8 hours	Ototoxicity, nephrotoxicity; allergic reactions: rash, pruritus, fever, burning sensation of skin, local irritation of skin	Observe closely for signs of ototoxicity (headache, dizziness, nausea, ataxia, tinnitus). Monitor intake and output. Drug is not to be mixed with any other drug.
Tobramycin (Nebcin)—aminoglycoside	IM: 3 mg/kg/day, three equal doses every 8 hours	Ototoxicity (ear), nephrotoxicity (kidney), rash, headache, nausea, vomiting, tremor, paresthesia	Observe closely for signs of toxicity. Keep patient well hydrated. Monitor urinary intake and output.

Table 10-5 Anticoagulants Commonly Used in Puerperal Thromboembolic Disease

	Coumadin Derivatives	
Heparin Sodium	*Warfarin Sodium (Coumadin, Panwarfin)*	*Dicumarol (Acenocoumarol)*
Dose		
IV, SC: 5000 to 30,000 U May be ordered as a drip over 24 hours Prophylactic dose: 5000 U SC every 12 hours	IM, IV: 50 mg per vial with diluent; orally: 2.5, 5, 7.5, 10, 25 mg tablets	Initial, oral: second day: 200 mg; subsequent days: as indicated by prothrombin time Maintenance dose: 25 to 100 mg/day orally
Mechanism of Action		
Inhibits conversion of prothrombin to thrombin Decreases agglutination of platelets Prolongs clotting time Has no effect on existing clots but prevents extension of old clots and formation of new ones	Inhibits prothrombin synthesis in liver by interfering with the action of vitamin K Acts more quickly than dicumarol, but effects last for a shorter time	Suppresses activity of liver in formation of prothrombin Prolongs clotting Takes 12 to 14 hours to take effect Action persists 24 to 72 hours after drug is discontinued Slower-acting but more prolonged in effect than heparin Used for maintenance

Therapeutic Uses for Postpartum Patients		
Lowering prothrombin time until slower-acting oral anticoagulants can take effect Prophylaxis and treatment of venous thrombosis and its extension Prophylaxis and treatment of pulmonary emboli	Prophylaxis and treatment of pulmonary thrombosis Prophylaxis and treatment of extension of venous thrombosis	Treatment of thrombophlebitis and pulmonary embolism (especially valuable in treatment of thrombosis and embolism)
Contraindications		
Not to be used in patients sensitive to heparin Not to be used in patients with any uncontrolled bleeding Not to be used in patients who cannot be supervised Incompatible with many antibiotics: check before use No IM injections because of risk of hematoma formation	Not to be used in patients with history of coumadin sensitivity Not to be used in patients with any bleeding conditions Not to be used in patients who cannot be supervised Must be used with caution in patients at risk for occupational injury	Same as warfarin sodium

(*continued*)

Table 10-5 Anticoagulants Commonly Used in Puerperal Thromboembolic Disease (*continued*)

	Coumadin Derivatives	
Heparin Sodium	*Warfarin Sodium (Coumadin, Panwarfin)*	*Dicumarol (Acenocoumarol)*
Nursing Implications		
Monitor patients constantly for bleeding. Coagulation time determinations should be checked frequently (normal prothrombin time is 11–13 sec; levels above this are set for individual patients by physician). Rotate administration sites and check for hemorrhage. Avoid massaging IV site. Observe women for hemorrhage during postpartum period. Breastfeeding may continue: heparin does not appear in breast milk.	Monitor patients constantly for bleeding. Significant decreases in coagulant activity occur in patients taking estrogens, barbiturates, and oral contraceptives. Abdominal or lumbar pain may be due to hemorrhage and thus should be promptly reported. Hemorrhage may be treated with vitamin K or whole blood. Clotting status is monitored by prothrombin time.	Vitamin K should be available as an antidote. Frequent dose adjustments are necessary in first 2 weeks of therapy (drug absorption is variable). Patients on maintenance doses may be checked semiweekly, weekly, or at 2- to 4-week intervals, depending on response to drug.

Table 10-6 Other Puerperal Complications

Problem/Symptoms	Treatment and Nursing Implications
Postpartum Hemorrhage	
Early Hemorrhage • Usually results from uterine atony, genital lacerations, and hematoma formation • Excessive uterine bleeding during the first hour after delivery	• Review the patient's chart to identify risk factors. • Maintain close contact with the patient during the first hour postpartum. • Check vital signs and palpate the uterus every 15 minutes or more often if necessary. • Urge the patient to void frequently as a full bladder pushes the uterus into the abdomen making massage difficult and exacerbating bleeding. • Maintain oxytocin infusion when bleeding is heavy. • Call the physician when uterine atony and heavy bleeding continue despite massage. (See Appendix C-4, Oxytocic Drugs Used to Control Postpartum Atony and Hemorrhage)
Late Postpartum Hemorrhage • May occur as late as 8 weeks after delivery due to retention of placental tissue, subinvolution or infection of the placental site, hematoma of the broad ligament, vagina or vulva • Decreasing blood pressure; weak, rapid pulse, cyanosis of lips, fingers	• Hospitalization is swift due to heavy bleeding. • Obtain a blood sample for crossmatching and typing. • Prepare for blood transfusion and IV oxytocin. • Administer antibiotics as ordered. • Keep the patient warm and be alert to possible shock when the patient's BP decreases, and her pulse is weak and rapid. • Prepare the patient when necessary for surgical repair of genital lacerations or curettage for removal of placental fragments.

(*continued*)

Table 10-6 Other Puerperal Complications (*continued*)

Problem/Symptoms	Treatment and Nursing Implications
Hematoma	
• Hematomas of differing sizes and seriousness may occur in the vagina, vulva, and broad ligament. Signs and symptoms include: • Swelling and blue-black discoloration • Severe pain out of proportion to the trauma of delivery • Pallor, tachycardia, and hypotension when large amounts of blood are lost • Dislocation of the uterus to one side • Pressure to the perineum, vagina, urethra, bladder, and rectum • Urinary retention from pressure on urethra	• Apply ice packs to the area to decrease swelling and increase comfort. • Assess location, quality, and amount of pain, and note rate of enlargement. Administer analgesics as ordered. • Obtain and record vital signs every 4 hours or as necessary. • Obtain serial blood counts when bleeding is excessive. • Prepare for blood replacement when hypovolemia and anemia occur. • Assess uterine position and record and report any deviation. • Prepare the patient when necessary for surgical excision of large hematomas, removal of blood clots, and ligation of bleeding sites. • Perform catheterization when necessary to relieve urinary retention.

Subinvolution of the Uterus	

• Common causes of subinvolution are retained placental fragments that cause endometritis, cesarean delivery, and uterine fibroids.
• Possible chills and fever
• Pelvic or back pain
• Prolonged, excessive flow of lochia or bleeding
• Infection
• Loss of body fluids from nausea and vomiting
	• Palpation of the uterus reveals a soft, boggy uterus that is larger than normal.
	• Prepare the patient for D and C when retained placental fragments are identified as the cause of subinvolution.
	• Check vital signs frequently to assess increasing infection.
	• Encourage rest in bed to speed resolution of infection.
	• Facilitate collection of culture specimens when appropriate.
	• Maintain antibiotic treatment in hospitalized patients, and administer analgesics as ordered.
	• Ensure adequate IV hydration and electrolyte balance.
	• (See Nursing Interventions for endometritis).
	• In the absence of infection the following regimen is used:
	  • Inform the patient that Methergine 0.2 mg is given every 3 to 4 hours for 2 to 3 days to reduce uterine size.
	  • Explain that the medication will cause uncomfortable uterine cramping but will control bleeding and restore the uterus to normal size. Encourage bed rest as much as possible.
	  • See patient in 2 weeks to assess uterine involution.

(continued)

Table 10-6 Other Puerperal Complications (*continued*)

Problem/Symptoms	Treatment and Nursing Implications
Postpartum Emotional Disturbances	
Postpartum Blues • Behavioral change beginning about 24 hours after delivery: mood swings, sobbing, fatigue, insecurity, irritability, feeling of being overwhelmed, decreased self-image • Expression of concerns, *e.g.*, ambivalence about the baby, lifestyle changes, finances; for working women, concerns about change in status, loss of wages, self-esteem, and opportunities for career promotion	• Talk with patient about her concerns; provide her the opportunity to express her unhappiness without fear of being "different." • Allow the patient to ventilate her feelings. • Reassure patient that sad feelings will pass and that many women feel the same in the early postpartum. • Encourage patient to talk to her partner about her concerns. Often partner has similar concerns; discussing them together may lead to some resolutions.

Anticoagulant Therapy

- Discuss with the nurse or other health care provider the action mechanism of anticoagulants and possible length of therapy.
- Take the medication at the same time each day.
- Keep follow-up appointments to allow care providers to monitor clotting time and adjust medication.
- Do not take or stop taking other medications without your physician's approval.
- Be aware of signs of overdose, such as bloody stools, hematomas, widespread bruising, bleeding gums, bleeding into joints. If symptoms occur, discontinue the drug and call the physician.
- Avoid trauma or injury that might cause bleeding, such as brushing teeth, contrast sports, shaving the legs (use an electric razor).
- Avoid marked changes in eating habits or lifestyle.
- Avoid aspirin. It inhibits platelet adhesiveness and increases the antiocoagulant effect of heparin.
- Explain that stools may change color to pink, red, or black as a result of coagulant use.
- Wear a Medic-Alert bracelet or necklace indicating the anticoagulant drug being used.
- Rare, sporadic, or heavy menstrual periods may occur. Heavy menses are never a contraindication for anticoagulant treatment. If anemia occurs, iron supplementation is given.

Other Puerperal Complications

Table 10-6 lists other puerperal complications along with treatment and nursing interventions.

NOTES

11
Nursing Assessment and Care of the Normal and High-Risk Neonate

Nursing Objectives in Newborn Assessment

- To evaluate the neonate's physiologic status in the immediate postbirth period and the adequacy of adaptation to extrauterine life in the first 6 to 8 hours
- To observe and document physical characteristics of the neonate
- To estimate the gestational age of the neonate
- To assess the behavioral capabilities of the neonate
- To use the newborn assessment to teach parents about their newborn

The nurse is often the first health care professional to perform a thorough assessment of the newborn. Although immediate evaluation is made by the birth attendant, the nurse is usually responsible for monitoring the infant during the 6- to 8-hour transition period and for completing the initial assessment.

NURSING ASSESSMENT

Neonatal History

It is essential that the nurse have as comprehensive a knowledge of the pregnancy, labor, and delivery history as possible to understand the significance of findings and to modify initial care to the neonate. The physical and behavioral state of the neonate is affected by medical and obstetric complications of pregnancy, drugs administered to the mother during labor, and the degree of birth asphyxia. Data that is significant to include in the neonatal history are described in Table 11-1. See the neonatal history form used in your facility.

Table 11-1 Essential Elements of the Neonatal Health History

Major Categories of Data Obtained	Specific Elements of Health History
Maternal Prenatal Care	Extent of prenatal care: Number of visits Degree of compliance with care plan Type of facility (clinic, health department, private practice)
Maternal Prenatal History	Last menstrual period (LMP) Estimated due date (EDC) Weight gain in pregnancy Obstetric complications Medical complications Types of treatment received Types of medication received History of hospitalization
Maternal Blood Type and Rh Factor	History of isoimmunization (Rh or ABO incompatibilities) Antibody titers
Maternal Screening Test Results	Rubella titer Hepatitis antigen screening Chlamydia screening VDRL Gonorrhea cultures Herpes cultures Other screening test results
Labor History	Onset of labor Length of labor Length of gestation at time of labor Obstetric complications Medication administration Types and amount Time of last medication Anesthesia received in labor
Rupture of Membranes	Length of time between rupture of membranes and onset of labor Amount of fluid Presence of meconium
Fetal Monitoring Record	Indication for monitoring Internal or external monitoring Abnormal FHR patterns Evidence of fetal distress

(*continued*)

Table 11-1 Essential Elements of the Neonatal Health History (*continued*)

Major Categories of Data Obtained	Specific Elements of Health History
	Fetal scalp sampling Blood gas analysis results

Delivery History	Length of second stage
	Type of delivery
	  Vaginal
	  Cesarean
	Place of delivery
	  Delivery room
	  Alternate birthing room
	  Labor room
	  Home birth
	    Planned
	    Unplanned
	  Other locations
	Anesthesia administered
	Medication administered
	Use of forceps/vacuum extractor
	Fetal heart rate pattern in second stage
	Fetal position at birth
	  Shoulder dystocia
	  Compound presentation
	Breaks in sterile technique

Postnatal History	Delay in cord clamping
	Respiratory effort at birth
	  Assisted
	  Unassisted
	Need for resuscitation
	  Type and extent of 1- and 5-minute Apgar scores
	Medications administered to neonate
	Parent-infant interaction
	  Quality
	  Extent
	Evidence of birth injury
	Evidence of narcosis
	Passage of urine or stool
	Other significant physiologic or behavioral responses
	Other significant procedures performed
	  Gastric aspiration

Table 11-1 Essential Elements of the Neonatal Health History (*continued*)

Major Categories of Data Obtained	Specific Elements of Health History
	Laryngoscopy and tracheal suctioning
	Others
Significant Social History	Family structure
	Anticipated versus actual birth experience
	Presence of significant others at birth
	Evidence of social support system
	Significant cultural variables
	Ethnic background
	Primary language
	Religious practices related to infant care
	Plans for infant feeding
	Plans for rooming-in
	Anticipated length of hospital stay
	Early discharge
	Traditional length for recovery
	Significant social problems
	Lack of social support system
	Language barrier
	History of substance abuse
	Lack of adequate housing
	Financial distress
	Others

Vital Signs and Measurement

After the neonatal history and inspection of the infant, the nurse proceeds to take vital signs and obtains important measurements. Table 11-2 outlines the techniques used to assess the normal neonate.

Physical Assessment

A detailed physical assessment gives the nurse important information about the neonate's progress in adapting to extrauterine life and about the infant's particular capabilities and level of maturity. Table 11-3 summarizes normal and unusual physical findings in the neonatal assessment.

(*text continues on pg. 402*)

Table 11-2 Vital Signs and Measurements of the Normal Neonate

Newborn Assessment	Assessment Techniques
Respiratory Rate	
Normal rate ranges from 30 to 60 breaths per minute.	Count respirations for 1 full minute by observing the abdomen.
Heart Rate	
Normal rate ranges from 120 to 160 bpm. Rate may drop to 100 bpm during sleep and rise to 180 bpm with crying.	Auscultate the heart rate for 1 full minute over the cardiac apex, which is normally located below third or fourth intercostal space.
Temperature	
Normal temperature ranges from 97.5°F to 99°F (36.4°C to 37.2°C)	Use axillary measurement if possible; there is a risk of traumatizing or perforating rectal mucosa when rectal temperature is taken. Hold thermometer in axillary fold for 5 minutes. If rectal measurement is needed, insert thermometer no further than 0.25 to 0.5 inch into rectum. Hold in place for 5 minutes. Hold infant's legs to prevent dislodgement or breakage.

Weight	
Average full-term weight is 3400 g (7 lb 8 oz); 95% of newborns weigh between 2500 g and 4250 g.	Weigh infant at same time each day, preferably before feeding. Undress infant completely, including diaper, and place on scale in supine position. Place protecting hand just above infant while reading weight.
Length	
Average full-term length is 49.5 cm (19.5 inches).	Measure length from bregma (anterior fontanelle) to heel. Place the infant on flat surface and take care to extend legs fully before measureing length.
Head Circumference	
Average head circumference is 35.5 cm. Normally it is approximately 2 cm larger than chest.	Place tape measure above eyebrow, over top of ears and around fullest part of occiput.
Chest Circumference	
Average chest circumference is 33 cm. It is approximately 2 to 3 cm smaller than head.	Place tape measure across lower border of scapulae and over nipples.
Blood Pressure	
Average blood pressure at birth is 80/46.	May not be routinely measured.

Table 11-3 Physical Findings in the Assessment of the Neonate*

Normal Findings and Common Variations	Unusual Findings and Significant Deviations	Possible Causes and Potential Problems
Integument		
General Appearance and Texture		
Skin smooth and pliant, with good turgor and visible layer of adipose tissue below Superficial peeling after first 24 hours Rarely, visible veins Milia over nose, chin, and forehead Vernix only in skin creases or absent	Skin thick and leathery, cracked with generalized peeling Long nails	Postmaturity
	Skin thin and transparent with minimal adipose tissue and many visible veins Thick layer of vernix or lanugo Nails thin and incompletely developed	Prematurity
Lanugo patchy or absent Nails soft and pliant but well formed	Skin wrinkled with poor turgor and minimal adipose tissue Umbilical cord thin Skin, unbilical cord, and nails stained with meconium	Intrauterine growth retardation Chronic maternal malnutrition
	Generalized edema	Severe erythroblastosis fetalis

Color		
Skin pink, with incomplete pigmentation in dark-skinned races at birth Acrocyanosis	Pallor	Anemia Asphyxia Shock Sepsis Hypothermia Congenital heart disease
Mottling Harlequin's sign Jaundice (after first 24 hours)	Cyanosis	Asphyxia Anoxia Congenital heart anomaly Hypoglycemia
	Plethora	Polycythemia
	Jaundice (within first 24 hours)	Blood incompatibilities Sepsis Biliary obstruction Drug reactions
Integrity		
Skin intact, with petechiae over presenting part	Lacerations or punctures	Accidental incision of skin with surgical scalpel during cesarean delivery Application of fetal scalp electrode during labor Fetal scalp sampling
	Generalized petechiae	Clotting disorders Sepsis

(continued)

Table 11-3 Physical Findings in the Assessment of the Neonate* (*continued*)

Normal Findings and Common Variations	Unusual Findings and Significant Deviations	Possible Causes and Potential Problems
Integument		
Ecchymosis secondary to application of forceps	Ecchymosis secondary to birth trauma or manipulation during delivery of infant	Cephalopelvic disproportion Shoulder dystocia Breech presentation at birth Precipitous delivery
Rashes		
Erythema toxicum Diaper rash	Skin pustules	Staphylococcal or beta-hemolytic streptococcal skin infection
	Vesicles	Congenital syphilis Herpesvirus infection
	Perianal eruptions Spreading diaper-rash-like skin eruption	Yeast infection (*Candida albicans*) Congenital rubella
	Generalized scaling	Genetic disorders
Vascular and Pigmented Nevi		
Nevus vasculosis	Nevus vasculosis	Genetic disorders (Sturge-Weber syndrome)

	Nevus flammeus	
	Cavernous hemangiomas	Genetic disorders
Mongolian spots	Café-au-lait spots	Neurofibromatosis
	Hypopigmentation	Genetic disorders
Head		
Size		
(See Table 11–2)	Microcephaly	Intrauterine growth retardation Genetic disorders Fetal alcohol syndrome
	Macrocephaly	Hydrocephalus
Shape		
Head rounded, with mild to moderate molding	Severe molding	Cephalopelvic disproportion
Plagiocephaly		
Caput succedaneum	Brachycephaly with flat occiput	Down syndrome
	Cephalhematoma	Head trauma secondary to labor dystocia, cephalopelvic disproportion, or forceps application
	Craniotabes	Postmaturity

(continued)

Table 11-3 Physical Findings in the Assessment of the Neonate* (*continued*)

Normal Findings and Common Variations	Unusual Findings and Significant Deviations	Possible Causes and Potential Problems
Head		
Fontanelles		
Anterior fontanelle diamond-shaped, 3 to 4 cm by 2 to 3 cm wide (Closes by 12 to 18 months)	Bulging, tense fontanelle	Hydrocephalus Meningitis
Posterior fontanelle triangular-shaped May be closed at birth due to molding (Closes by 8 to 12 weeks)	Abnormally large, flat open fontanelle	Hypothyroidism Intrauterine growth retardation Prematurity
	Depressed fontanelle	Dehydration
Sutures		
Sutures slightly separated or overlapping at birth due to molding	Widely separated sutures	Hypothyroidism Hydrocephalus Prematurity Intrauterine growth retardation
	Premature closure of sutures (craniosynostosis)	Genetic disorders

Hair		
Hair silky, may be curly or kinky based on familial and racial traits	Fine and wooly, sparse Coarse, brittle	Prematurity Endocrine disorders Genetic disorders Intrauterine growth disorders
	Lowset hairline, low forehead	Genetic disorders
Eyes		
Appearance and Position		
Eyes symmetrically spaced, less than 3 cm apart, clear, with transient discharge secondary to chemical conjunctivitis	Agenesis (failure to develop)	Genetic disorders Teratogenic injury
	Hypertelorism (abnormal width in eye spacing)	Genetic disorders
Pseudostrabismus	Persistent purulent discharge	Ophthalmia neonatorum Chlamydia conjunctivitis
Cornea and Lens		
Eyes clear, without clouding	Large or uneven cornea Corneal ulcerations Clouding or opacity of lens	Congenital glaucoma Herpesvirus infection Cataracts (rubella infection)

(continued)

Table 11-3 Physical Findings in the Assessment of the Neonate*

Normal Findings and Common Variations	Unusual Findings and Significant Deviations	Possible Causes and Potential Problems
Eyes		
Sclera and Conjunctiva		
Sclera white or has faint blue tinge	True blue sclera	Osteogenesis imperfecta
Icteric after first 24 hours	Icteric within first 24 hours	Pathologic jaundice
Chemical conjunctivitis	Persistent purulent eye discharge	Ophthalmia neonatorum Chlamydia conjunctivitis
Subconjunctival hemorrhage		
Iris		
Iris slate gray or brown	Pink iris	Albinism
	Colobomas (lesions or clefts in structures)	May be benign or may be associated with genetic disorders
	Brushfield's spots	Down syndrome
Pupils		
Pupils equal and reactive to light	Anisocoria (unequal pupil size) Nonreactive, fixed	Neurologic injury

Retina		
Presence of red reflex	Absence of red reflex	Congenital cataracts
Eyelids and Lacrimal Glands		
Eyelids close completely	Eyelids fused closed	Genetic disorders
Transient edema		Severe prematurity
Transient erythema and petechiae	Ptosis	11th cranial nerve injury
Epicanthal folds in Oriental infants and in 15 to 20% of non-Oriental infants	Shortened palpebral fissures	Fetal alcohol syndrome
	Epicanthal folds in non-Oriental infants	Down syndrome in conjunction with other physical findings
Eyelashes	Absence of eyelashes	Genetic disorders
Absence of tears, scant tearing	Excessive tearing	Plugged lacrimal duct
Neuromuscular Function		
Transient tracking and fixation ability	Persistent strabismus	Neuromuscular disorder
Transient strabismus	Vertical nystagmus	Seizure disorder
Doll's eye movement	Setting sun sign	CNS injury/disorders
Glabellar (blink) reflex	Blink reflex absent	CNS injury
		Neuromuscular disorder

(continued)

Table 11-3 Physical Findings in the Assessment of the Neonate* (*continued*)

Normal Findings and Common Variations	Unusual Findings and Significant Deviations	Possible Causes and Potential Problems
Ears		
Ears normally placed with pinna at or above level of line drawn from canthus of eye	Low-set ears	Genetic abnormalities
Ears well-formed and firm with good recoil if folded against head	Soft, unformed ear with little cartilage	Prematurity
Auricular skin tags	Preauricular sinus	Failure of embryonic closure of branchial cleft, may lead to infection
Nose		
Nose in midline with wide flat bridge	Short, upturned with hypoplastic philtrum	Fetal alcohol syndrome
Infant is obligate nose breather	Nasal flaring, grunting	Nasal obstruction, choanal atresia
Scant nasal discharge	Copious nasal discharge	CNS anomalies Infection
Occasional sneezing	Frequent sneezing Snuffles	Drug withdrawal Congenital syphilis

Mouth and Chin		
Mouth moist and pink with scant saliva production	Fusion of lips, atresia, or agenesis of oral structures	Genetic disorders Teratogenic injury
Symmetrical movement with crying and sucking	Asymmetry of mouth with sucking or crying	Facial nerve injury
Inclusion cysts, Epstein's pearls		
Lips intact, labial tubercles present	Cleft lip	Genetic disorders Teratogenic injury
Tongue mobile with short frenum	Macroglossia (hypertrophied tongue)	Genetic disorders Prematurity
Sucking fat pads in cheeks	White plaques on tongue, gums, buccal cavity	*Candida albicans* infection
	Hypertonic suck	Drug withdrawal
	Weak, discoordinate suck	Prematurity, Neuromuscular disorders Asphyxia
Palates intact	Cleft palate Uvula not in midline	Genetic disorder Teratogenic injury
Presence of rooting, sucking, swallowing, gagging reflexes	Absence of reflexes	Prematurity Asphyxia CNS injury/disorders
Vigorous cry	High-pitched cry	CNS disorders
	Crowing cry	Laryngeal disorder
	Natal teeth	Potential for aspiration if dislodged

(continued)

Table 11-3 Physical Findings in the Assessment of the Neonate* (*continued*)

Normal Findings and Common Variations	Unusual Findings and Significant Deviations	Possible Causes and Potential Problems
Neck and Shoulder		
Neck short, in midline, with head maintained in midline	Abnormally short	Genetic disorders (Turner syndrome)
	Deviation from midline Lateral flexion	Congenital torticollis
Range of motion normal	Limited range of motion Nuchal rigidity	Meningitis
Ability to raise head momentarily	Inability to control head Severe head lag	Prematurity Asphyxia CNS injury Neuromuscular disorders
Trachea in midline Thyroid not palpable	Trachea deviated Enlarged thyroid	Neck mass Hyperthyroidism Hypothyroidism
	Lump or crepitus over clavicle	Fracture of clavicle
Chest		
Lung		
Normal respiratory rate (See Table 11–2)	Tachypnea	Sepsis Respiratory distress

		Hypothermia Hypoglycemia
Symmetrical respiratory excursion	Seesaw breathing Retractions Grunting	Diaphragmatic hernia Respiratory distress Prematurity
Breath sounds clear and equal bilaterally Transient rales at birth	Rales Rhonchi	Atelectasis Meconium aspiration
	Decreased breath sounds	Atelectasis Pneumothorax
	Hyperresonance	Air trapping
Shape		
Chest rounded, symmetrical Transient breast engorgement and nipple discharge (nonpurulent)	Asymmetrical chest Unilateral chest bulging	Pneumothorax Air trapping
	Supernumerary nipples	Benign finding, but potential cosmetic concern in later life
Heart		
Heart rate normal (See Table 11–2)	Tachycardia	Prematurity Anemia Shock Sepsis Congenital heart anomalies

(continued)

Table 11-3 Physical Findings in the Assessment of the Neonate* (*continued*)

Normal Findings and Common Variations	Unusual Findings and Significant Deviations	Possible Causes and Potential Problems
Chest		
Sinus rhythm with transient arrhythmias	Persistent arrhythmias	Congenital heart anomaly
Transient murmurs	Persistent murmur	Persistent fetal circulation Congenital heart anomaly Fluid overload
Quiet precordium	Active precordium	Persistent fetal circulation Congenital heart anomaly Fluid overload Congestive heart failure
Back, Hips, and Buttocks		
Back straight, spine intact, posture slightly flexed	Pilonidal dimple	Potential CNS anomaly
	Pilonidal sinus	Potential CNS anomaly Potential infection
	Hairy nevus at base of spine	Potential CNS anomaly
	Meningomyelocele	CNS anomaly
	Hip clicks	Congenital hip dysplasia
Symmetrical buttock folds	Asymmetrical buttock folds	Congenital hip dysplasia

Mongolian spots on buttocks		
Transient ecchymosis of buttocks after breech delivery		
Anus patent	Absence of stools after 24 hours	Imperforate anus, GI obstruction
	Anal fissures	Potential infection
Abdomen		
Abdomen full, rounded, and soft	Scaphoid abdomen	Diaphragmatic hernia
	Flat abdomen with horizontal wrinkles	Intrauterine growth retardation Chronic malnutrition
Bowel sounds	Hyperactive bowel sounds	Drug withdrawal Bowel obstructions
	Visible peristaltic waves	Pyloric stenosis
	Hypoactive bowel sounds	Sepsis
	Abdominal distention at birth	Abdominal masses GI obstruction Malrotation of bowel Hydronephrosis
	Development of abdominal distention after birth, no passage of stools	GI obstruction Meconium plug Meconium ileus Hirsprung's disease Imperforate anus

(continued)

Table 11-3 Physical Findings in the Assessment of the Neonate* (*continued*)

Normal Findings and Common Variations	Unusual Findings and Significant Deviations	Possible Causes and Potential Problems
Back, Hips, and Buttocks		
	Presence of fecal smears in diaper without passage of stool through anus	Rectovaginal fistula
Liver palpable 1 to 2 cm below left costal margin	Hepatosplenomegaly	Intrauterine infection
Linea nigra		
Umbilical cord white with Wharton's jelly	Thin, meconium-stained cord	Fetal distress Intrauterine growth retardation
	Urine drainage around umbilical cord	Patent urachus
	Oozing of blood at base of cord	Premature detachment of cord stump Trauma to base of cord
	Purulent discharge at base of cord, foul odor, red streaking from base of cord across abdomen	Omphalitis
Two arteries, one vein	One artery, one vein	Congenital heart anomaly
	Intestine palpated in abdominal area at base of umbilical cord	Umbilical hernia

	Protrusion of abdominal contents on surface of abdomen at umbilicus	GI anomaly (omphalocele)
	Protrusion of abdominal contents on surface of abdomen, but not involving umbilicus	GI anomaly (gastroschisis)
	Bladder distention	Meatal stenosis
Genitals		
Female		
Labia majora large (may be slightly edematous), covering clitoris and labia minora	Ambiguous genitalia	Genetic disorder
Transient mucoid vaginal discharge		
Pseudomenstruation		
Hymen tag visible		
First void within 24 to 48 hours	Absence of full stream	Meatal stenosis
	Absence of urination	Meatal stenosis Renal disorder
Uric acid crystals present		
Male		
Penis with foreskin intact (if no circumcision)	Ambiguous genitalia	Genetic disorder

(continued)

Table 11-3 Physical Findings in the Assessment of the Neonate* (*continued*)

Normal Findings and Common Variations	Unusual Findings and Significant Deviations	Possible Causes and Potential Problems
Genitals		
Foreskin covers glans	Inability to retract foreskin to any degree	True phimosis
Meatus in center of glans at tip of penis	Meatus located on dorsal surface of penis	GU anomaly (Epispadias)
	Meatus located on ventral surface of penis	GU anomaly (Hypospadias)
Full urine stream	Spurts or dribbling of urine	Meatal stenosis
Glans clean, erythematous, with nonpurulent serous membrane post circumcision	Purulent discharge and foul odor	Infection
Uric acid crystals present in urine		
Scrotum large, pendulous, well-rugated	Small, shiny scrotum with few or absent rugations	Prematurity
Testes descended	Testes undescended	Cryptorchidism Prematurity Genetic disorder
Transient edema of scrotal sac after birth		
	Fluid in testes	Hydrocele
	Presence of intestine in inguinal canal	Inguinal hernia

Extremities		
Arms		
Posture of flexion at rest	Extension of arm from shoulder or elbow	Brachial plexus injury
Symmetrical movement	Asymmetrical movement of arms or guarding of extremity	CNS injury Fracture of long bone Brachial plexus injury
	Repetitive rowing motions	Seizure disorder
Strong muscle tonus and good recoil with extension of arm	Weak or absent tonus	Prematurity CNS injury Neuromuscular disorder Genetic disorder
Palpable brachial and radial pulses	Bounding pulses	Fluid overload
	Absence of radial pulse	Congenital absence Spasm or obstruction
Hands and Fingers		
Fingers flexed at rest	Hand relaxed	CNS injury
Strong grasp reflex	Absence of grasp reflex	Neuromuscular disorder Brachial nerve injury
Symmetrical hand movement	Asymmetrical hand movement	Fracture, soft tissue injury, CNS injury
Multiple palmar creases	Simian crease	Down syndrome (in conjunction with other findings)
Five fingers, flexed but straight and separate	Polydactyly	Familial trait
	Syndactyly	Familial trait Genetic disorder

(continued)

Table 11-3 Physical Findings in the Assessment of the Neonate* (*continued*)

Normal Findings and Common Variations	Unusual Findings and Significant Deviations	Possible Causes and Potential Problems
Extremities		
	Incurving of little finger	Down syndrome
Nails firm, pliant, well-formed	Thin, incompletely formed nails	Prematurity
	Meconium-stained nails	Fetal distress
Moro reflex symmetrical	Asymmetrical Moro	CNS injury Brachial nerve injury Fracture of long bone or calvicle
Legs		
Legs well flexed at rest.	Amelia or phocomelia	Genetic disorder Teratogenic injury
Slightly bowed appearance	Shortened long bones	Genetic disorder (dwarfism or achondroplasia
Muscle tonus strong with good recoil when legs are extended	Weak or absent muscle tone	Prematurity Neuromuscular disorder CNS injury
	Asymmetrical movement or guarding of extremity	Fracture of long bone Soft-tissue injury CNS injury
Femoral pulses palpable	Differential between pulses in upper and lower extremities	Coarctation of aorta
	Blanching of one extremity	Thrombosis, arterial spasm

Feet and Toes		
Feet have fat pad on sole	Rocker-bottom soles	Genetic disorder
Sole crease over at least anterior two-thirds of foot	Absence of creases or few sole creases	Prematurity
Ankle mobile, with full range of motion	Abnormal positioning or rigid fixation of ankle or heel	Congenital clubfoot (talipes deformity)
	Deformity of arch of foot	Congenital clubfoot (talipes deformity)
Pedal pulses palpable	Differential in pulses between upper and lower extremities	Coarctation of aorta
Five toes	Polydactyly	Familial trait
	Syndactyly	Familial trait
		Genetic disorder
Toenails well formed	Thin, poorly developed nails	Prematurity
Presence of plantar grasp	Absence of grasp	CNS injury
Positive Babinski sign	Negative Babinski sign	Neuromuscular disorder

This table summarizes normal and unusual physical findings in the neonatal assessment. Normal variations are rarely charted in the neonatal record but should be explained to parents if they have questions or concerns. The nurse should note any unusual findings and ascertain if they have been recorded by other examiners in the neonate's chart. If not, the nurse should chart her findings according to that setting's protocol, and bring the findings to the physician's attention.

Neuromuscular Assessment: Neonatal Reflexes

Although several reflexes may already have been elicited during the assessment, a complete evaluation of reflexes should be done at this time. Table 11-4 lists the neonatal reflexes and how they are elicited.

Gestational Age Assessment

- *Premature infant.* An infant born before 37 weeks gestation
- *Mature (full-term) infant.* An infant born between 38 and 42 weeks
- *Postmature infant.* An infant born after 42 weeks gestation
- *Small-for-gestational-age (SGA) infant.* A newborn whose weight is below the tenth percentile for estimated week of gestation or two standard deviations below the mean
- *Appropriate-for-gestational-age (AGA) infant.* A newborn whose weight falls between the tenth and 90th percentiles for estimated gestational age or within two standard deviations from the mean
- *Large-for-gestational-age (LGA) infant.* A newborn whose weight is above the 90th percentile for estimated gestational age or two standard deviations above the mean

Behavioral Assessment

The Brazelton Neonatal Behavioral Assessment Scale is a tool that helps evaluate newborn behavioral competencies. It is recommended that the test be performed on the third day after delivery and takes approximately 30 minutes to perform. The examiner must complete training in the use of the tool before performing the assessment. The behaviors on the Brazelton assessment scale are divided into the following six categories:

- *Habituation.* The ability of the newborn to diminish his or her response to a sound, light, or pinprick to the heel. A normal newborn will startle but shut the sensation out when it is repeated. Immature neonates and those with central nervous system (CNS) problems may respond in an erratic fashion.
- *Orientation.* The newborn's ability to attend to visual and auditory stimuli. Alert newborns will attend to voices and fixate and follow visual stimuli. Preterm infants may have a limited ability to orient and a limited attention span and response to visual stimuli.
- *Motor maturity.* Reflected in the newborn's ability to control and coordinate motor activities. Normal newborns demonstrate

(*text continues on pg. 408*)

Table 11-4 Assessment of Neonatal Reflexes

Reflex	Category	How Elicited	Normal Response	Abnormal Response	Duration of Reflex
Rooting and sucking	Feeding	Touch cheek, lip or corner of mouth with finger or nipple.	Infant turns head in direction of stimulus, opens mouth and begins to suck.	Weak or absent response. Seen with prematurity, neurologic deficit or injury, or CNS depression secondary to maternal drug ingestion (*e.g.*, narcotics).	Diminished by fifth to sixth month. Disappears by 1 year
Swallowing	Feeding	Place fluid on back of tongue.	Infant swallows in coordination with sucking.	Gagging, coughing, or regurgitation of fluid. Possibly associated with cyanosis secondary to prematurity, neurologic deficit, or injury. Often seen after laryngoscopy.	Does not disappear

(continued)

Table 11-4 Assessment of Neonatal Reflexes (*continued*)

Reflex	Category	How Elicited	Normal Response	Abnormal Response	Duration of Reflex
Extrusion	Feeding	Touch tip of tongue with finger or nipple.	Infant pushes tongue outward.	Continuous extrusion of tongue or repetitive tongue thrusting. Seen with CNS anomalies and seizures.	Disappears by about fourth month
Moro	Postural	Change infant's position suddenly or place on back on flat surface.	Bilateral symmetrical extension and abduction of all extremities, with thumb and forefinger forming characteristic "C", followed by adduction of extremities and return to relaxed flexion.	Asymmetrical response. Seen with peripheral nerve injury (brachial plexus) or fracture of clavicle or long bone of arm or leg. No response with severe CNS injury.	Diminished by fourth month. Disappears by sixth month.

Stepping	Postural	Hold infant in upright position and touch one foot to flat surface.	Infant will step with one foot and then the other in walking motion.	Asymmetrical response. Seen with CNS or peripheral nerve injury or fracture of long bone of leg.	Disappears within 1 to 2 months
Prone Crawl	Postural	Place infant on abdomen on flat surface.	Infant will attempt to crawl forward with both arms and legs.	Asymmetrical response. Seen with CNS or peripheral nerve injury or fracture of long bone.	Disappears within 1 to 2 months
Tonic Neck or "Fencing"	Postural	Turn infant's head to one side when infant is resting.	Extremities on side to which head is turned will extend and opposite extremities will flex. Response may be absent or incomplete immediately after birth.	Persistent response after fourth month. May indicate neurologic injury. Persistent absence in CNS injury, neuromuscular disorders.	Diminishes by fourth month

(continued)

Table 11-4 Assessment of Neonatal Reflexes (*continued*)

Reflex	Category	How Elicited	Normal Response	Abnormal Response	Duration of Reflex
Startle	Protective	Expose infant to sudden movement or loud noise.	Infant abducts and flexes all extremities and may begin to cry.	Absence of response may indicate neurologic deficit or injury. Complete, consistent absence of response to loud noises may indicate deafness. Response may be absent or diminished during deep sleep.	Diminishes by fourth month
Crossed Extension	Protective	Place infant in supine position and extend one leg while stimulating bottom of foot.	Infant's opposite leg will flex and then extend rapidly as if trying to deflect stimulus to other foot.	Weak or absent response. Seen with peripheral nerve injury or fracture of long bone.	Disappears by fourth to sixth month
Glabellar "Blink"	Protective	Tap bridge of infant's nose	Infant will blink with first four	Persistent blinking and failure	

		when eyes are open.	or five taps.	to habituate. Suggestive of neurologic deficit.	
Palmar Grasp	Social	Place finger in palm of infant's hand.	Infant's finger will curl around object and hold momentarily.	Diminished response with prematurity. Asymmetry with peripheral nerve damage (brachial plexus) or fracture of humerus. No response with severe neurologic deficit.	Diminishes by fourth month
Plantar Grasp	Social	Place finger against base of toes.	Infant's toes will curl downward.	Diminished response with prematurity. No response with severe neurologic deficit.	Diminishes by fourth month
Babinski	Not categorized	Stroke one side of foot upward from heel and across ball of foot.	Infant's toes will hyperextend and fan apart from dorsiflexion of big toe.	No response with CNS deficit.	Disappears by 1 year

smooth, free movements while preterm infants or those with nervous system problems may move their extremities unevenly and frequently jerkily.

- *Self-quieting ability.* The ability of newborns to utilize their own resources to quiet and comfort themselves, such as hand-to-mouth movements, sucking on fist, or attending stimuli. Infants with neurologic problems may be unable to engage in self-quieting activities and require comfort from caregivers.
- *Social behaviors.* The extent to which infants need and respond to cuddling and how often they smile. Some infants enjoy being held, while others, such as the neurologically damaged infant, may resist any form of cuddling.
- *Sleep/awake states.* Include two sleep states and four awake states. Recognizing these states and their patterns is critical to understanding the infant's behavioral capacities. These sleep/awake states include deep sleep, light sleep, drowsy state, quiet-alert state, eyes-open state, and crying state.

NURSING INTERVENTIONS IN CARE OF THE NORMAL NEWBORN

Nursing interventions can focus on acquainting parents to the unique behavioral qualities of their infant.

Nursing Objectives in Well-Newborn Care

- To prevent potential complications of the neonatal period
- To promote parent-infant interaction and acquaintance
- To support parental caregiving behaviors

Possible Nursing Diagnoses Related to Care of the Well Newborn

- Potential for ineffective airway clearance related to mucous obstruction
- Potential for impaired gas exchange related to cold or stress
- Alteration in comfort (pain) related to heel stick
- Potential alteration in parenting related to lack of knowledge related to infant care

Nursing Care During the First 5 to 8 Hours of Life

Once the nurse has completed assessment of the neonate and has identified any problems, a nursing care plan is initiated that meets the needs of each infant.

Vital Signs

- Temperature, apical heart rate, and respiratory rate are recorded and reassessed at least every 30 minutes for the first hour, then once an hour for the next 3 to 6 hours.
- Record information about the course of labor, maternal illness, drugs administered during labor and delivery, type of delivery, and evidence of asphyxia at birth when assessing the infant, and the infant's 1- and 5-minute Apgar scores.

Temperature Control

- The infant's body and head should be carefully dried to prevent heat loss through evaporation.
- The infant is double-wrapped in warm, dry blankets, and a stockinette cap is placed on its head.
- The infant's temperature is taken at admission and at least every 4 to 6 hours after that.
- A hypothermic infant (temperature below 97.5°F (36.4°C) should be temporarily placed in a radiant warmer or isolette.

Pulmonary Function Support

- The infant's airway is kept free from mucous obstruction by use of a bulb syringe to clear the nose and mouth, and an 8 or 10 French catheter attached to suction is used to clear the airway.
- The newborn is placed in Trendelenburg's position to facilitate drainage of fluids. When stable, the infant is positioned on its side, never on its back, to prevent aspiration when unattended.

Cardiac and Circulatory Support

- Uncompromised temperature control and a mucous-free respiratory system is necessary to support circulatory and cardiac adaptation.
- The cord clamp should be checked for bleeding, and the infant's pulses should be palpated frequently; the skin on the infant's

trunk and extremities should be blanched periodically for assessment of central and peripheral capillary fill and indirect evaluation of tissue perfusion.
- Apical heart rate should be auscultated for evidence of murmurs or abnormal rate or rhythm.

Forestalling Potential Neonatal Complications

It is the responsibility of the nurse caring for neonates to be informed and aware of the signs of potential complications in the infant and to act quickly to forestall problems.

Prevention of Aspiration

If the infant begins to gag or choke or becomes suddenly cyanotic:

- Turn the infant on his or her side or abdomen with the head slightly lower than the feet (10 to 15 degree angle).
- Pat the infant firmly on the back to encourage drainage of fluids from the mouth and nose.
- Insert a bulb syringe or suction catheter attached to wall suction (on low pressure) into the mouth first and remove all secretions.
- Be sure to compress the bulb first before placing the tip of the bulb syringe into the infant's mouth or nares.
- Suction both nares *after the mouth is cleared.*
- If the infant is apneic or remains cyanotic after secretions are removed from the mouth and nose, apply 100% oxygen by resuscitation bag and mask apparatus until color improves and breathing is resumed.

Prevention of Infection

- To prevent ocular infection, administer either silver nitrate solution or erythromycin ophthalmic ointment several hours after birth.
- Special care of the umbilical cord to prevent omphalitis involves the application of antibiotic ointment or solution or swabbing the cord with alcohol at each diaper change.
- Each person who comes in contact with the newborn must observe principles of sepsis. *Handwashing is the single most important preventive measure.*
- Guidelines established to restrict personnel with infections, diarrhea, open wounds, infectious skin rashes, herpesvirus, or other communicable diseases must be adhered to.
- Encourage frequent contact with mother and breast feeding to provide maternal immune factors.

Prevention of Hypoglycemia

- Hypoglycemia is defined as a blood glucose level under 30 mg/dl whole blood during the first 72 hours of life in the full-term infant.
- Blood glucose levels may be monitored during the critical 4 to 6 hours after birth.
- Early feeding and prevention of cold stress reduces risk of hypoglycemia.
- When hypoglycemia is diagnosed, a slow IV bolus of 10% to 25% glucose followed by administration of a continuous IV infusion of 10% glucose is administered until levels are stabilized.

Prevention of Hemorrhagic Disease

- An infant who experiences a transient deficiency in vitamin K is at risk for hemorrhage on the second or third day of life.
- A 0.5-mg to 1-mg dose of vitamin K (phytonadione) is administered intraumuscularly (IM) after birth to prevent bleeding.

Prevention of Hyperbilirubinemia

Nursing care is directed at reducing the incidence and severity of neonatal physiologic jaundice and is achieved by:

- Prevention of cold stress that can cause buildup of unconjugated serum bilirubin
- Initiation of early and frequent feedings to promote peristalsis and the passage of stools, preventing enteric reabsorption of conjugated bilirubin from the stool. Early introduction of milk also provides the infant with nutrients and calories required to produce bilirubin-binding proteins.
- Promotion of adequate hydration to prevent hemoconcentration and facilitate urinary excretion of acid metabolites
- Be alert for danger signs in the neonate (Table 11-5).

Facilitation of Parent-Infant Interaction

- During the first hour after birth the infant is awake and alert to visual and auditory stimuli. This is an ideal time for the nurse to foster parent-infant interaction.
- The first few hours after birth may be a particularly sensitive period for the formation of bonds between parents and the infant through skin-by-skin contact, rooming in, and extended periods of contact throughout the day.

(text continues on pg. 414)

Table 11-5 Danger Signs in the Neonate

Affected System	Presenting Signs	Potential Neonatal Disorder
Central Nervous System	Jitteriness Diaphoresis Abnormal cry Excessive irritability Twitching Convulsions Hypotonia	Hypoglycemia Chromosomal anomalies Asphyxia Intracranial hemorrhage Brain edema Neuromuscular anomalies Sepsis Chronic intrauterine infection
	Bulging fontanelle, small head size Large head size	Chromosomal anomalies Fetal alcohol syndrome Hydrocephalus
Cardiovascular and Respiratory Systems	Apnea Rapid slow, or irregular pulse Cyanosis Rapid respiration, chest retraction	Congenital heart anomaly Persistent fetal circulation Hypoplastic lung Respiratory distress sydnrome (type 1 or type II)
	Grunting Flaring Stridor	Meconium aspiration syndrome Tracheal malacia Aspiration

	Pallor	Pneumothorax
	Plethora	Polycythemia
	Single umbilical artery	Congenital heart anomaly
Gastrointestinal System	Vomiting	Gastrointestinal obstruction
	Abdominal distention	Gastrointestinal obstruction
	No meconium stool (beyond 48 hours after birth)	Imperforate anus, gastrointestinal obstruction
	Diarrhea	Sepsis
	Jaundice (within first 24 hours of life)	Hemolytic disease of newborn, biliary atresia
	Excessive salivation	Tracheo-esophageal fistula
Genitourinary System	Delayed/inadequate voiding (beyond 48 hours after birth)	Genitourinary anomalies, renal failure secondary to hypoxia
Musculoskeletal System	Hypotonia	Congenital neuromuscular anomaly
	Uneven thigh or buttock folds	Congenital hip dysplasia
	Facial asymmetry with crying	Facial nerve injury
	Limited movement of arm	Brachial palsy
Integumentary System	Purulent discharge from cord	Omphalitis
	Skin pustules	Staphylococcal skin infection
	Rash	Congenital rubella, congenital syphilis
Hematologic System	Bleeding or oozing from cord, petechiae	Hemorrhagic disease of newborn
Immunologic System	Hypothermia	Sepsis
	Fever	Intracranial hemorrhage

Daily Care of the Newborn

It is the nurse's responsibility to evaluate the newborn's adjustments to extrauterine life until the infant is discharged.

- Weigh the infant at the same time each day. (See Appendix B-5, Weight Conversion Table (Pounds and Ounces to Grams)
  - The infant may lose between 5% to 10% of its body weight in water during the first 3 or 4 days of life; reassure parents that this is normal.
  - When infant nutrition is adequate, a 1-oz or 30-g weight gain occurs each day thereafter.
- Elimination patterns vary, but urinary output slowly increases so that at the end of the first week of life the neonate may void as freqently as 2 to 30 times a day.
  - Within 2 to 3 days of birth the thick, greenish meconium stool is replaced by a yellowish green transitional stool: the absence of a stool, presence of blood or mucus, or diarrhea is abnormal and must be investigated.
- After 2 or 3 days of milk or formula ingestion, screening for phenylketonuria (PKU) should be performed.

Parent Teaching

Most postpartum settings have organized parent teaching procedures, including classes, demonstrations, and discharge teaching guides. Parents can also obtain additional information from child-care reference books, community health nurses, and parent education groups. The nurse should have general knowledge of the institutional and popular literature of infant care and of community resources for parent education and support.

Common Concerns of Parents

- Bathing
- Cord care
- Diapering and clothing the infant
- Taking the infant's temperature
- Feeding techniques
- Formula preparation
- Safety considerations
- Elimination patterns
- Signs and symptoms of illness
- Crying
- Circumcision care
- Care of the uncircumcised infant
- Treatment of diaper rash

Self-Care Teaching: Practical Tips for Care of the Newborn

- Avoid startling the newborn when picking him or her up by putting your hands under its body for a moment or two before lifting.
- Wrapping the baby securely can help meet the baby's need for contact comfort and provide a relaxing arrangement for sleep.
- Burp the baby occasionally during feeding to allow swallowed air to escape from the stomach.
- Clean the umbilical cord with a small amount of rubbing alcohol several times a day and keep the diaper folded so that it does not rub against the cord. Within 7 to 10 days the cord will dry and fall off.
- Diapers should be checked often and changed when wet, cleansing the area with warm water. Soap and water washings are necessary when the infant has passed stools. A & D ointment may be applied after cleansing if the infant's skin is especially sensitive.
- Be aware that the infant cries frequently, especially when hungry or wet, and may cry on an average of 2 hours per day. The infant should be comforted and picked up often; the baby will not become "spoiled" by this practice.
- Bathing the baby daily is not always necessary, especially during the winter months when skin is likely to become dry. When a complete bath is not given, the face, neck, genitalia, and perianal area should be washed daily.
- Recognize signs and symptoms of illness such as:
  - Lethargy. Difficulty in waking the baby
  - Fever. Temperature above 100°F (32.2°C)
  - Vomiting. Spitting up of a large part or all of a feeding two or more times
  - Diarrhea. Three or more green, liquid stools in succession
  - Loss of appetite. Refusal of two feedings in a row

CARE OF THE HIGH-RISK NEONATE

Nursing Objectives in Care of the High-Risk Neonate

- To identify prenatal, intrapartum, and postnatal variables that place the neonate at risk for injury or illness
- To prepare for appropriate monitoring and support of the high risk neonate

- To recognize signs in the neonate that indicate injury or illness
- To prepare and give emotional support to parents of a high-risk or sick infant

---

Possible Nursing Diagnoses Related to Care of the High-Risk Neonate

- Alterations in cardiac output related to decreased output
- Alterations in respiratory functions related to impairment of gas exchange
- Alterations in nutrition less than body requirements related to sucking or swallowing difficulties
- Fluid volume excess related to excessive fluid intake or obstruction
- Fluid volume deficit related to excessive urinary output
- Alterations in sensory perception related to sensory overload, sleep and rest imbalance, or immature nervous system

---

Nursing Assessment

Identification of Risk Factors

Prenatal Risk Factors

It is estimated that approximately 60% of infants requiring special care and treatment at birth can be identified through careful evaluation of the mother's prenatal history. Table 11-6 lists examples of prenatal maternal conditions and obstetric complications that place the fetus at risk for increased morbidity and mortality.

Intrapartal Risk Factors

It is not possible to predict from the prenatal history alone which infants will require special assistance and care after birth. Approximately 10% to 20% of all women who have experienced normal pregnancies will develop problems intrapartally that place the infant at increased risk for neonatal complications. Table 11-7 lists major intrapartal factors that contribute to neonatal complications.

Nursing Interventions

Management of Neonatal Resuscitation and Ongoing Support Measures: See Appendix C-5, Drugs Used in Neonatal Resuscitation

Table 11-6 Prenatal Risk Factors and Potential Fetal and Neonatal Complications

Risk Factors	Potential Complications
Demographic Factors	
Maternal age:	
Under 16 or over 35 years	Small for gestational age (SGA); genetic abnormalities
Primigravida over 30 years	Labor dystocia; birth trauma
Parity:	
Grand multiparity (Over five pregnancies)	Fetal malposition
Substance Abuse:	
Drug addiction	SGA; neonatal withdrawl syndrome
Alcoholism	Fetal alcohol syndrome
Smoking	SGA; polycythemia
Maternal Nutritional Status	
Maternal malnutrition	
Weight less than 100 pounds	SGA
Weight more than 200 pounds	SGA, LGA
Previous Pregnancy Complications	
Fetal loss at over 28 weeks of gestation	Fetal loss
Premature delivery	Prematurity
Abnormal fetal position	Fetal malposition and potential birth trauma
Bleeding in second or third trimester	Recurrent bleeding in subsequent pregnancy
Pregnancy-induced hypertension	Recurrent hypertension
Rh sensitization	Erythroblastosis
Fetal distress of unknown origin	Fetal distress
Birth of an infant with anomalies	Congenital anomalies
Birth of infant over 10 pounds	Birth of large-for-gestational age (LGA) infant
Birth of postterm infant	Postterm infant; intrauterine growth retardation (IUGR)
Neonatal death	Neonatal death

(continued)

Table 11-6 Prenatal Risk Factors and Potential Fetal and Neonatal Complications (*continued*)

Risk Factors	Potential Complications
Central Nervous System Disorders	
Hereditary CNS disorders	Inherited CNS disorder
Seizure disorders requiring medication	Congenital anomalies (as a result of Dilantin use)
Cardiovascular Disease	
Chronic hypertension	IUGR; asphyxia
Congenital heart disease with congestive heart failure	Prematurity; inherited defects
Hematologic Disorders	
Anemia (Under 10 g)	Prematurity; low birth weight
Sickle cell disease	IUGR; fetal demise
Hemaglobinopathies	IUGR; inherited hemoglobinopathies
Idiopathic thrombocytopenic purpura (ITP)	Transient ITP
Renal Disease	
Chronic glomerulonephritis	IUGR; SGA; prematurity; asphyxia
Renal insufficiency	IUGR; SGA; prematurity; asphyxia
Reproductive Disorders	
Uterine malformation	Prematurity; fetal malposition
Cervical incompetence	Prematurity
Metabolic Disorders	
Diabetes	LGA; hypoglycemia and hypocalcemia; anomalies; respiratory distress syndrome
Thyroid disease	Hypothyroidism; CNS defects Hyperthyroidism, goiter
Current Pregnancy Complications	
Pregnancy-induced hypertension	IUGR; SGA
Maternal infections:	
TORCH infections	IUGR; SGA; active infection; anomalies

Table 11-6 Prenatal Risk Factors and Potential Fetal and Neonatal Complications (*continued*)

Risk Factors	Potential Complications
Sexually transmitted disease	Ophthalmia neonatorum; Congenital syphilis
Acute cystitis, pyelonephritis	Prematurity
Hepatitis	Hepatitis
Multiple gestation	Prematurity; asphyxia; IUGR; SGA
Fetal malposition	Prolapsed cord; asphyxia; birth trauma
Rh sensitization	Erythroblastosis fetalis
Prolonged pregnancy	Postmaturity; meconium aspiration; IUGR; asphyxia

Apgar score evaluation begins with the assignment of the Apgar score. Guidelines to assist in determining appropriate interventions based on the 1-minute Apgar score are shown in Table 11-8.

Positioning

- When not contraindicated, neonates are positioned on their sides to facilitate drainage of fluids from the mouth and nares.
- Sick infants may be placed in a supine position on an open bed to facilitate administration of IV fluids through the umbilical artery or the performance of procedures such as chest x-rays and ultrasonography.

Airways Management

- The infant is initially placed on a flat surface in Trendelenberg's position to facilitate drainage of mucus.
- The infant is placed in the "sniffing position" to fully open the airway for laryngoscopy. This procedure allows visualization and suctioning of meconium and mucus from the airway and is necessary for placement of an endotracheal tube if ventilation is required.
- A bulb syringe is adequate only for removing secretions from the mouth and nose.
- A suction catheter with mucous trap is used if there is respiratory depression or meconium in the airway and deeper suction is needed using a No. 5 to No. 10 French catheter.
- Deep suctioning requires sterile technique and should last no longer than 10 seconds on a low-pressure setting (less than 50 mm Hg).
- The infant's heart rate must be monitored during suction be-

Table 11-7 Intrapartal Risk Factors and Potential Fetal and Neonatal Complications

Risk Factors	Potential Complications
Umbilical Cord	
Prolapsed umbilical cord	Asphyxia
True knot in cord	Asphyxia
Velamentous insertion	Intrauterine blood loss; shock; anemia
Vasa previa	Intrauterine blood loss; shock; anemia
Rupture or tearing of cord	Blood loss; shock; anemia
Membranes	
Premature rupture of membranes	Infection; RDS; prolapsed cord; asphyxia
Prolonged rupture of membranes	Infection
Amnionitis	Infection
Oligohydramnios	Congenital anomalies
Polyhydramnios	Congenital anomalies; prolapsed cord
Placenta	
Placenta previa	Prematurity; asphyxia
Abruptio placentae	Prematurity; asphyxia
Placental insufficiency	IUGR; SGA
Abnormal Fetal Presentations	
Breech delivery	Asphyxia; birth injuries (CNS, skeletal)
Face or brow presentation	Asphyxia; facial trauma
Transverse lie	Asphyxia; birth injuries; cesarean delivery
Labor Dystocias	
Prolonged labor	Asphyxia; birth trauma; infection
Uterine inertia	Complications of prolonged labor
Uterine tetany	Asphyxia
Precipitate labor	Asphyxia; birth trauma

Table 11-7 Intrapartal Risk Factors and Potential Fetal and Neonatal Complications (*continued*)

Risk Factors	Potential Complications
Delivery Complications	
Forceps-assisted delivery	CNS trauma; cephalhematoma; asphyxia
Vacuum extraction	Cephalhematoma
Manual version or extraction	Asphyxia; birth trauma; prolapsed cord
Shoulder dystocia	Asphyxia; brachial plexus injury; fractured clavicle
Precipitate delivery	Asphyxia; birth trauma (CNS)
Undiagnosed multiple gestation	Asphyxia; birth trauma
Administration of Drugs	
Oxytocin	Complications of uterine tetany (asphyxia)
Magnesium sulfate	Hypermagnesemia; CNS depression
Analgesics	CNS and respiratory depression
Anesthetics	CNS and respiratory depression; bradycardia

cause bradycardia can occur due to stimulation of the vagus nerve.

Chest Percussion and Drainage

- Chest percussion and postural drainage is another method of facilitating drainage of mucus and maintaining a patent airway.
- A dome-shaped cupping device is used manually to percuss the infant's chest over lung tissue to loosen pulmonary secretions.
- Postural drainage, in which the infant's position is changed frequently, is used to prevent stasis of lung secretions.

Ventilating the Neonate

- The nurse must ventilate using the correct rate, pressures, oxygen concentration, and equipment.
- The normal ventilation rate is 30 to 50 times per minute, but with severe meconium aspiration higher rates may be necessary for the adequate exchange of gas.

(*text continues on pg. 424*)

Table 11-8 Management of Neonatal Resuscitation Based on the Infant's Condition and Assigned Apgar Score

Apgar Score	Infant's Condition	Management
7 to 10 (no evidence of asphyxia)	Pink, active, responsive to stimuli, crying, heart rate over 100 bpm	Suction mouth and nares. Dry thoroughly, including head. Maintain body temperature. Perform brief physical examination. Unite with parents. Assign 5-minute Apgar score.
4 to 6 (mild to moderate asphyxia)	Cyanotic, moving with decreased muscle tone, breathing shallow, respirtory effort poor, heart rate below 100 bpm	Suction mouth, nares and larynx if amniotic fluid is meconium-stained. Dry quickly. Maintain body temperature. Provide 100% oxygen via bag and mask. Call for help if alone. Continue ventilating at 30 to 50 times per minute until heart rate is above 100 bpm, color is pink, and spontaneous respirations begin. As soon as possible, assign someone to support parents.

0 to 3 (severe asphyxia)	Deeply cyanotic, no muscle tone, absent respiratory effort or periodic gasps, heart rate slow or absent	Clear airway quickly; call for help. Insert endotracheal tube. Initiate bag ventilation with 100% oxygen at 40 to 60 breaths per minute at pressures great enough to move chest wall. Perform cardiac massage at a rate of 100 to 120 times per minute. If heart rate is under 100 bpm despite 2 minutes of adequate ventilation and cardiac massage, insert umbilical venous catheter and administer drugs. As soon as additional personnel arrive, ensure maintenance of body temperature. Assign someone to support parents.

Adapted from Avery M, Taeusch HW: Shaffer's Diseases of the Newborn, 5th ed. Philadelphia, WB Saunders, 1984

- Ventilation pressures are initially high to effectively inflate the lungs, but subsequent pressures of 25 cm H_2O to 35 cm H_2O or lower should be sufficient.
- When the infant is sick it may require intubation and use of a mechanical ventilator.

Administering Oxygen to the Neonate

- During initial resuscitation efforts, a 100% oxygen concentration is administered.
- After stabilization of the infant's condition, oxygen concentration is adjusted to maintain the P_aO_2 within acceptable limits to avoid irreparable damage to the retinal vessels and injury to the lung tissue.
- Oxygen masks are used only as a temporary method for delivery of oxygen to the neonate during resuscitative efforts.
- In a moderately depressed infant, oxygen is administered through a tight-fitting mask designed for infants. Care must be taken to prevent pressure on the infant's eyeballs, which may cause tissue ischemia and blindness.
- Severely depressed infants are oxygenated through an uncuffed endotracheal tube attached to a ventilating bag or mechanical ventilator when extended ventilatory assistance is required.

Initiation and Support of Cardiac Function

- External cardiac massage is initiated when the heart beat is absent or remains under 60 bpm after breathing has been established.
- The infant is placed in a supine position on a flat, firm surface. The index and middle fingers are placed on the middle third of the sternum, which is depressed to 2 cm at a rate of 100 to 120 times per minute.
- The effectiveness of massage is evaluated by palpating the femoral pulse or umbilical cord.
- Adjunctive drug therapy is administered through an umbilical vein when a spontaneous heart rate of at least 100 bpm has not been established after 5 minutes of cardiac massage.

Major Danger Signals of Neonatal Morbidity

Central Nervous System Signs

- Lethargy (listlessness, difficulty in rousing for feedings)
- High-pitched cry
- Jitteriness
- Seizure activity (nystagmus, repeated blinking, sucking mo-

tions, tongue thrusting, rhythmic rowing movements of upper extremities, bicycling motions of lower extremities, assumption of rigid posture)
- Abnormal fontanelle size or bulging fontanelles

Respiratory Signs

- Apnea (frequently preceded by "periodic breathing," which is a cyclic pattern of regular breathing for 10 to 15 seconds followed by a similar period with no breathing, resulting in *no* cyanosis or heart rate change, with an average respiratory rate of 30 to 40/min.)
- Tachypnea (rapid respiratory rate)
- Nasal flaring
- Chest retractions
- Asynchronous breathing movements (flattening of chest and protrusion of abdomen with each inspiration: seesaw respirations)
- Expiratory grunting

Cardiovascular Signs

- Abnormal rate and rhythm
- Murmurs (frequently associated with other cardiovascular findings)
- Alterations and differentials in pulses (variations in rate, regularity, amplitude, volume, rhythm, symmetry)
- Changes in perfusion and skin color

Gastrointestinal Signs

- Refusal of two or more feedings
- Absent or uncoordinated feeding reflexes (uncoordinated suck, swallow, or gag reflexes)
- Vomiting (projectile, occurring at any time, resulting in significant losses of body fluids and electrolytes)
- Abdominal distention (protuberant abdomen; taut, shiny skin; prominent superficial veins)
- Changes in stool patterns (diarrhea, absence of stools, bloody stools)

Metabolic Alterations

- Hypoglycemia
- Hypocalcemia
- Hyperbilirubinemia and jaundice
- Temperature instability

Nursing Care of the Sick Infant

Intravenous Therapy in the Sick Infant

- IV therapy may be instituted to meet the infant's basic fluid requirements when oral intake is limited.
- During the first few days of life fluid requirements are about 60 to 70 ml/kg/day and may be adjusted upward when necessary.
- The infant must be carefully monitored for signs of dehydration or fluid overload during IV therapy.
- Peripheral veins are also used for the infusion of fluid and electrolytes, and their use is preferred over other IV methods because risk of serious complications is lower.
- Infants requiring prolonged IV therapy or hyperalimentation may require insertion of a special central IV catheter.

Metabolic Process: Prevention of Hyperbilirubinemia and Kernicterus

The sick or compromised infant is at greater risk for developing hyperbilirubinemia and jaundice. The goal of nursing care for these infants is prevention of kernicterus and encephalopathy, which result from deposition of unconjugated and unbound bilirubin in brain cells.

- Sick preterm infants who weigh less than 1500 g seem to be at greatest risk for developing kernicterus and sustaining permanent neurologic damage. Other factors that contribute to its development are hypothermia, asphyxia, acidosis, sepsis, and hypoalbuminemia.
- When the infant develops pathologic jaundice, the nurse supports the conjugation and excretion of bilirubin with the following measures:
  - Preventing hypothermia
  - Reducing energy expenditures by placing the infant in a neutral thermal environment
  - Supporting frequent feedings to facilitate adequate hydration and excretion of wastes (if oral feeding is not contraindicated)
  - Supporting adequate caloric intake to meet energy requirements and maintain adequate serum albumin levels
  - Initiating phototherapy when ordered by the physician
  - Preparing the infant for exchange transfusion when necessary, assembling the equipment, and monitoring the infant's physiologic response during and after the procedure

Nursing Care of Neonates with Major Complications

Nursing intervention for high-risk and sick neonates focuses on supporting life processes, preventing complications, and promoting healthy family adaptation. Table 11-9 outlines the major complications of the neonate.

The Neonate with Infection

The neonate is susceptible to infection as a result of immature immunologic functioning at birth. This susceptibility is increased when the infant is preterm or is suffering from other complications such as asphyxia or trauma. Infection can result from:

- Maternal disease during pregnancy such as rubella, syphilis, chlamydia
- Contact during delivery with pathogens within the birth canal, such as herpesvirus, gonococci, or B-hemolytic streptococci
- Increased use of invasive procedures and diagnostic tests that put the infant at risk for iatrogenic infection during the neonatal period

Signs of Infection

- Early signs of infection may be nonspecific and include lethargy, refusal to eat, and vomiting.
- Temperature instability and hypothermia may be indicators.
- Subtle color changes that include cyanosis, mottling or grayish tone may be noted.
- Apnea may occur as a sign of infection.

Signs that Indicate the Location of Infection

- Jitteriness and seizure activity with disease of the central nervous system
- Respiratory distress with pulmonary infection
- Diarrhea associated with intestinal infection

Signs of Viral Infection During the Prenatal Period

- Growth retardation
- Microcephaly
- Mental Retardation
- Heptosplenomegaly
- Cerebral calcification
- Small for gestational age

The types of neonatal infection are outlined in Table 11-12.

(*text continues on pg. 448*)

Table 11-9 Major Complications of the Neonate

Complication/Symptoms	Treatment and Nursing Interventions
Birth Asphyxia	
• A variety of maternal, fetal and neonatal conditions can lead to asphyxia of the infant at birth: it is characterized by hypoxemia, hypercarbia, and acidosis. • Potential cardiopulmonary compromise	• Quickly dry, stimulate, and clear the infant's airway within 60 seconds of birth. • Evaluate the infant's heart rate, respiratory effort, color, muscle tone, reflex irritability, grunting, retracting, and decreased blood pressure (BP). • Monitor vital signs every half-hour for 2 hours, then every hour for 4 to 6 hours or until the infant is stable. • Supply oxygen, ventilate, and perform cardiac compression when the infant is severely depressed. An Apgar score of 7 or under indicates the need for ongoing intensive life support.
• Potential hypoglycemia	• Observe infant for signs of jitteriness, lethargy, irritability, tremors, hypotonia. Perform Dextrostix on admission, then every half-hour for 2 hours, then as appropriate until stable.
• Temperature instability	• Take infant's temperature every half-hour for 2 hours, then every hour for 4 to 6 hours.
• Potential hyperbilirubinemia	• Observe the infant's color every 8 hours, and notify the physician of jaundice present in the first 24 hours. • Transfer the infant to the special care unit for stabilization as necessary.

Nervous System Injuries	
Intracranial Hemorrhage	
• Rupture of cerebral vessels resulting in intracranial hemorrhage is one of the most serious complications and may result in permanent neurologic impairment or death. • Extent of neurologic damage depends upon its location. • Signs of intracranial pressure: seizures; decreased or absent reflexes; hypotonia; bulging fontanelles; enlarged head circumference; "setting sun eyes"; high, shrill cry; hypothermia; and episodes of apnea or bradycardia	• Intracranial hemorrhage is confirmed by computed tomography (CT) scan. • Nursing care is aimed at supporting vital functions and reducing the neonate's energy requirement to a minimum. • Place the infant in a neutral thermal environment. • Observe vital signs by use of a cardiorespiratory monitor. • Elevate the head slightly above the hips, and measure its circumference daily to determine enlargement. • Maintain a patent airway, correctly align the extremities, and turn the infant routinely when flaccidity or paralysis is evident. • Maintain IV therapy when depressed reflexes and responsiveness are demonstrated. • Keep an accurate intake and output report. • Administer anticonvulsants to control seizure activity as ordered. • Support the parents by keeping them informed and allowing them to participate in some care of the infant.
Other Nervous System Injuries	
Brachial Plexus Injury	
• Nerves in this plexus innervate muscles of the arm and upper extremities. Trauma to them may cause:	

(continued)

Table 11-9 Major Complications of the Neonate (*continued*)

Complication/Symptoms	Treatment and Nursing Interventions
Other Nervous System Injuries	
• *Erb-Duchenne Palsy*. Loss of motor function in upper arm; absence of Moro's reflex on the affected side; no loss of motor function • *Klumpke's Paralysis*. Loss of motor function in the muscles of the hand; absence of grasp reflex • *Complete Brachial Plexis Injury*. The entire brachial plexus may be damaged, and complete paralysis of the arm and hand results	• Prevent contractures of the affected muscles by placing the arm in a neutral position and performing passive range of motion exercises. • Immobilize in a natural position by pinning the sleeve to the shirt or by swaddling. • Initiate gentle passive range of motion exercises after 7 to 10 days. • Instruct the parents in correctly positioning the arm and in performing range of motion exercises prior to discharge
• *Phrenic Nerve Injury*. Paralysis of the diaphragm occurs when the phrenic nerve is injured. The diaphragm on the affected side is fixed. Lung tissue is displaced upward and fails to expand completely, resulting in diminished respiratory excursion on the affected side. Tachypnea and signs of respiratory distress occur, and atelectasis and pneumonia commonly occur.	• Care is aimed at alleviating respiratory distress. • Place the infant in a neutral thermal environment. • Enrich the oxygen atmosphere frequently as ordered. • Place the infant on the affected side to allow expansion of the opposite lung. • Gavage feed the infant initially, but bottle or breastfeeding can be initiated when the infant becomes stabilized. • Provide encouragement and support to the parents in their efforts to feed and care for the infant.

Hemolytic Disease of the Newborn

- A disorder in which the infant's red blood cells are destroyed or hemolyzed with resultant hyperbilirubinemia and jaundice, the two most common being Rh disease and ABO incompatibility

Rh Incompatibilty (Erythroblastosis Fetalis)

- Occurs when the mother's blood is Rh-negative and the fetus is Rh-positive. Has positive direct Coombs' test
- *Hydrops fetalis* is a severe form of the disease where the fetus becomes severely anemic
  - Hepatosplenomegaly evident at birth
  - Hydrothorax
  - Generalized edema
  - Cardiomegaly and hypoxia lead to cardiac failure and death if not treated

ABO Incompatibility

- Milder form of hemolytic disease and stillbirths and hydrops almost never occur. It involves group A or B infants born to group O mothers.

- When hyperbilirubinemia results from blood incompatibility and isoimmunization, follow the guidelines below for blood type and Rh factor when exchange transfusions are performed:
  - Rh incompatibility (mother Rh−; infant Rh+); group O, Rh-negative whole blood or packed cells. The RBCs in this type blood contains no Rh antigens and will not be hemolyzed by maternal antibodies remaining in the infant's bloodstream.

- Allow extended periods of rest for the anemic neonate who is hemolyzing RBCs and is jaundiced.
- Place the infant in a neutral thermal environment to reduce expenditure of energy.
- Monitor vital signs frequently; tachycardia is evident with severe anemia.
- Observe the infant's color every 4 to 8 hours.
- Begin phototherapy as ordered based on bilirubin levels; cover the infant's eyes with protective patches to prevent retinal damage from the light. (Remove and check eyes every 8 hours.)
- Place the infant nude into the isolette at a distance of 18 inches from the light source, and turn the infant every 2 hours.
- Offer the infant 5% dextrose in water or sterile water, 2 oz, between feedings.

(continued)

Table 11-9 Major Complications of the Neonate (*continued*)

Complication/Symptoms	Treatment and Nursing Interventions
Hemolytic Disease of the Newborn	• Prepare for exchange infusion as ordered. • ABO incompatibility (mother group O; infant group A, B, or AB): group O, Rh-specific whole blood with low titers of anti-A and anti-B antibodies. The RBCs in this type blood contain no antigens that will be hemolyzed by maternal antibodies.
Complications Related to Gestational Age	
The Preterm Infant	

• The preterm (premature) neonate is one who is born before 38 weeks gestation. See Table 11-10 for causes of prematurity. These infants suffer anatomic and physiologic immaturity in all systems. Problems may include:
  • Ineffective gas exchange because of immaturity and collapse of the air sacs due to minimal surfactant production
  • Respiratory Distress Syndrome Type 1 (hyaline membrane disease), which causes labored respiration; cyanosis; pallor;
	• Position the infant to maintain airway and facilitate drainage of mucus or regurgitated milk; suction as needed.
	• Monitor breathing and HR with cardiorespiratory monitor.
	• Prevent stomach distention by avoiding overfeeding and aspiration of air before gavage feedings, and administer correct amounts of formula.
	• Administer and monitor correct oxygen concentrations.
	• Obtain infant's daily weight and plot on growth chart.
	• Test all stools for presence of glucose or blood.
	• Check for hypoglycemia with a Dextrostix.
	• Strictly monitor intake and output, and test urine for *p*H and SG.
	• Maintain all IV infusions with IV infusion pumps.

retractions; nasal flaring, grunting, hypotonia, and episodes of apnea that may cause acidosis	• Minimize insensible water losses. • Observe optimal aseptic technqiue to avoid infant exposure to pathogens. • Prevent cold stress by placing the infant in a double-walled isolette and placing a cap on its head. • Encourage early and frequent visits by parents and keep them informed.
Small for Gestational Age Infant (SGA) • The SGA infant is one whose weight falls below the tenth percentile or is 2 standard deviations below the mean. *Intrauterine Growth Retardation* (IUGR) • Symmetrical IUGR. Occurs with early and prolonged nutritional deprivation related to maternal factors, resulting in deficient numbers of body cells; small head and body; diminished brain size and permanent mental retardation • Asymmetrical IUGR. Occurs from nutritional deficits and placental insufficiency in late pregnancy, resulting in appropriate number of cells that are diminished in size; disproportionately large head in relation to body; long, emaciated body with muscular	• Nursing care of the SGA infant is aimed at supporting physiologic adaptations after birth and preventing major complications associated with this disorder • Position the infant to maintain airway and facilitate chest expansion, and suction as needed • Administer ultrasonic mist therapy or aerosol via oxygen hood, and perform percussion and drainage of the chest • Monitor respirations with cardiorespiratory monitor and administer and monitor correct oxygen concentrations • Administer formula as ordered in small frequent feedings; avoid stomach distention; discontinue oral feedings at the first sign of respiratory distress, and position the infant on its right side or abdomen after feeding • Prevent cold stress by placing the infant in a double-walled isolette, use a heat shield over the infant's body, and warm hands before handling the infant; place a cap on the infant's head. • Use a skin temperature probe to monitor skin temperature variations

(*continued*)

Table 11-9 Major Complications of the Neonate (*continued*)

Complication/Symptoms	Treatment and Nursing Interventions
Complications Related to Gestational Age	
wasting; widely separated cranial sutures; birth weight below tenth percentile, but normal head size; excellent potential for normal intellectual functioning (Factors associated with IUGR are shown in Table 11-11.)	
Large for Gestational Age Infant (LGA)	
• LGA infants weigh over 4000 g and are above the 90th percentile or 2 standard deviations above the mean in size with potential for: • Hypocalcemia • Hypoglycemia • Birth trauma or injury: cephalohematoma, bruising, fracture of calvicle, CNS trauma • Parental anxiety due to trauma of delivery	

• *Infant of the diabetic mother (IDM).* Is often LGA as a result of high levels of maternal glucose crossing the placenta during pregnancy and the effect of hyperinsulinism on cell growth: • High blood sugar levels present at birth drop before the first feeding. • Hypoglycemia rapidly ensues. • Hypocalcemia may relate to depressed parathyroid function in the neonate. • Hyperbilirubinemia and jaundice may result from increased prematurity of the LGA infant. • Respiratory distress syndrome type II may be related to the IDM's decreased surfactant production. • Potential for polycythemia. • Potential for congenital anomaly.	• Assess the infant for signs of hypoglycemia such as jitteriness, tremors, hypotonia, lethargy, irritability, sweating, apnea seizures. • Check Dextrostix every hour for 30 minutes × 4; every hour until feedings begin; then before feedings until stable. • Notify physician when Dextrostix is less than 45 mg/dL. • Begin formula or breastfeeding as soon as possible. • Observe for signs and symptoms of hypocalcemia (indistinguishable from hypoglycemia); Check calcium level if ordered. • Prepare the infant for transfer to the ICN for IV administration of calcium when indicated. • Observe for development of jaundice and check the bilirubin level as ordered; report symptoms to the physician. • Closely observe respiratory status and check vital signs every four hours. Check for tachypnea, grunting, flaring, retraction, breath sound changes, and cyanosis. • Observe for plethora; check heelstick hematocrit as needed. • Carefully assess the infant for the presence of physical anomalies, especially cardiac and neural tube defects.
• Parental anxiety.	• Keep the parents apprised of the infant's condition and explain the need for Dextrostix and other laboratory diagnostic studies. Carefully explain the infant's treatment and rationale. Allow them ample time with their infant. • Infants of Class A, B, and C diabetic mothers are frequently LGA. • Check Dextrostic regularly; hypoglycemia may result from stress of LGA delivery.

(*continued*)

Table 11-9 Major Complications of the Neonate (*continued*)

Complication/Symptoms	Treatment and Nursing Interventions
Complications Related to Gestational Age	
	• Assess the infant for signs of birth trauma or injury (see Nervous System Injuries). • Discuss with parents the birth sequelae affecting their infant. Explain that nerve palsies are usually transient and resolve within a few days; describe the infant's treatment.

The Postterm Neonate
• The postterm infant is born after 42 weeks gestation and is at risk for developing complications related to compromised utero-placental perfusion and hypoxia
  • Infant is long, thin, and appears wasted.
  • Skin is thick, wrinkled, and parchment-like, with generalized pealing.
  • Skin, hair, nails, and umbilical cord are meconium stained.	

- Meconium aspiration syndrome (MAS) may occur at birth when a hypoxic post-term infant takes its first breath, causing meconium plugs to enter the alveolus resulting in air trapping.
  - Chemical pneumonitis occurs.
  - Polycythemia may occur.
  - Hypoglycemia may result from depletion of liver glycogen stores.

- Assist at birth with suctioning of the trachea to remove any meconium present in the airway.
- Assist the pediatrician with passing an endotracheal tube and deep tracheal sunctioning.
- Swaddle the infant's chest to prevent the infant from taking the first breath until the airway is clear as ordered.
- (See nursing interventions for respiratory care of the SGA infant.)
- Obtain a hematocrit immediately after birth to determine if polycythemia is a complicating factor: a partial exchange transfusion may be necessary to prevent hyperviscosity.
- Do serial glucose determinations to monitor glucose levels; early feedings may be initiated if not complicated by respiratory problems.
- Place the infant in a neutral thermal environment.

Table 11-10 Causes of Prematurity

Obstetric Factors	Medical Factors	Socioeconomic Factors
Uterine malformation	Maternal diabetes	Absence of prenatal care
Multiple gestation	Chronic hypertensive disease	Low socioeconomic status
Incompetent cervical os	Urinary tract infection	Malnutrition
Premature rupture of membranes and chorioamnionitis	Other acute illness	Early adolescent pregnancy
Pregnancy-induced hypertension		
Placenta previa		
History of previous premature birth		
Rh isoimmunization		

Table 11-11 Maternal Factors Associated with Intrauterine Growth Retardation

Socioeconomic Factors	Environmental Factors	Medical Complications	Obstetric Complications
Low socioeconomic status	Poor living conditions	Heart disease Renal disease	History of infertility
Maternal age (extremes of youth and age) Absence of prenatal care Marital status (single)	High altitude Use of therapeutic drugs: Antimetabolities Anticonvulsants Substance abuse Alcohol Drugs Cigarettes Malnutrition	Chronic hypertension Sickle cell disease Phenylketonuria Diabetes mellitus (class D, E, F, or R) Other chronic diseases	History of abortions Grand multiparity Pregnancy-induced hypertension

Table 11-12 Types of Neonatal Infection

Description	Effects on the Neonate
Bacterial Infections	
• Acquired from passage through the birth canal and birth; bacterial infections account for 10% to 20% of infant mortality	• The neonate is colonized with the microorganism during labor and delivery and may develop neonatal infection. • Preterm infants are at greater risk for developing this infection, although it may occur in apparently healthy full-term neonates.
Group B Beta-Hemolytic Streptococcus Infections	
• *Early Onset.* Develops within the first 24 hours of life and is often fatal	• Effects on the neonate: • Hypotonia, hypothermia • Acute respiratory distress, pneomonia • Cardiovascular collapse may cause death within hours of the first indication of infection
• *Late Onset.* Develops after the first 2 weeks of life as a meningeal infection; associated with a much lower mortality rate than early onset strep infection	• Effects on the neonate: • Fever, lethargy • Signs of increased intracranial pressure such as bulging fontanelle, nuchal rigidity, high-pitched cry • Permanent neurologic disability secondary to meningitis • Both forms of the disease are treated with IV antibiotics such as gentamicin, ampicillin, or penicillin.

Listeria	
• A gram-positive organism, the Listeria is an intracellular parasite recently implicated in the etiology of neonatal sepsis. As with the strep infection, early and late onsets have been demonstrated.	• The neonate contacts the disease during passage through a birth canal colonized with the organism.
• *Early onset*. Infection develops within a day or two of birth,	• Effects on the neonate: • Diffuse granulomatous skin papules over the trunk and on the pharynx • The infant appears very ill and may experience respiratory distress and cyanosis
• *Late onset*. Infection develops around the second week of life.	• Effects on the neonate: • Manifests as a meningitis that appears to be associated with a different strain of the organism (Type IV B) • Both forms of the disease are treated with drugs such as ampicillin gentamicin, and kanamycin.
Escherichia coli	
• A strain of E. coli (K1 antigen-positive) is a virulent organism that is a major cause of neonatal meningitis and septicemia.	• The neonate is colonized with microorganism during labor and delivery, or from nursery personnel harboring the organism • Infants suceptible to this organism may have decreased circulating antibodies against E coli K1 antigen. Treatment consists of IV antibiotic administration.

(continued)

Table 11-12 Types of Neonatal Infection (*continued*)

Description	Effects on the Neonate
Bacterial Infections	
Neisseria gonorrhoeae	

• A severe infection of the conjunctiva, ophthalmia neonatorum, is caused by this bacterium.	• The mother who has gonorrhea transmits the organism to her infant as it passes through the birth canal during labor and delivery.
	• Initial treatment consists of instillation of 1% silver nitrate solution or erythromycin ointment into the neonate's eyes.
	• An untreated neonate will exhibit signs of eye infection by the third or fourth day of life:
	  • Copious purulent eye discharge
	  • Corneal ulceration and blindness rapidly occur if appropriate treatment is not initiated
	• Therapy consists of saline eye irrigations followed by topical and systemic administration of penicillin.

Viral and Protozoan Infections	
• Over a dozen known viral infections may be contacted by the neonate either in utero or postnatally. TORCH is an acronym for the following virulent infections:	

Toxoplasmosis	
• A protozoan infection acquired by eating raw infected meat or contact with infected cat feces	• Infection may be "silent" in the mother and when undiagnosed or treated, placental transmission of the organism occurs with serious disease resulting in the neonate such as microcephaly, cerebral calcifications, chorioretinitis, hepatosplenomegaly, and jaundice. Treatment consists of drug therapy that may limit further central nervous system injury but that does not reverse prenatal damage already sustained by the neonate.
Syphilis	

• Transmission of Treponema pallidum, the organism responsible for syphilis, can occur during the second half of pregnancy.	• When the infected mother receives no treatment, the neonate will be born with congenital, usually infectious, syphilis.
	• Effects on the neonate:
	  • Intrauterine growth retardation
	  • Ascites, persistent rhinitis
	  • Jaundice, anemia hepatosplenomegaly, and lymphadenopathy
	  • A copper-colored rash may develop over the face, palms, and soles of the feet during the first week of life
	• Immediate treatment with procaine penicillin G for 10 to 14 days is initiated

(*continued*)

Table 11-12 Types of Neonatal Infection (*continued*)

Description	Effects on the Neonate
Viral and Protozoan Infections	
Rubella	

• Rubella is a virus that attacks the fetus in utero. Severity of damage to the neonate born with congenital syphilis reflects the length of intrauterine infection and the time of first exposure.	• Approximately 30% to 50% of fetuses who acquire rubella during the first gestational month suffer cardiac anomalies.
	• Other signs of rubella infection in the neonate include:
	  • Neural deafness, congenital cataracts, glaucoma
	  • Microphthalmia, blindness
	  • IUGR, hepatosplenomegaly: signs of chronic infection
	  • Microcephaly and mental retardation: reflects CNS involvement
	• The neonate born with congenital syphilis is highly infectious and should be isolated. The infant may shed virus for as long as a year.
	• No specific drug therapy is effective in limiting the disease postnatally.

Cytomegalovirus (CMV)	

• CMV disease is poorly understood. The infection causes severe central nervous system injury when acquired prenatally.	• The neonate is born with a constellation of signs that are characteristic of other intrauterine viral infections.
	  • Microcephaly; cerebral calcification
	  • IUGR, hepatosplenomegaly
	• Many neonates who harbor the virus are asymptomatic but develop central nervous system injury later in childhood.
	• There is no effective prevention or treatment of CMV at present.

Herpesvirus Type 2	

• Prenatal infection is rare, but risk of developing a neonatal infection after vaginal delivery when the mother has an active lesion is as high as 60%.	• Infants born to mothers with primary herpes infections may develop a more severe, systemic form of the disease that includes:
	  • Hepatitis, pneumonia
	  • Encephalitis, disseminated intravascular coagulopathy
	  • Death may occur within hours of birth; mortality approaches 50% to 60%.
	• Infants born to mothers with recurrent infections often have a milder disease and experience vesicular skin lesions, lethargy, hypothermia, and hypotonia.
	• The infant is highly contagious and is isolated. Treatment with antiviral drugs is limited.
	• Life support is employed in care of the critically ill infants and intensive nursing care is required 24 hours a day.

Hepatitis B	
• Transmission of hepatitis B virus and surface antigen (HBsAg) occurs transplacentally during pregnancy, and during passage through the birth canal when mothers have chronic or acute hepatitis infection. • Most infants who become HBsAg-positive due to transmission of the virus in the pre-	• Neonates rarely present with classic signs of the disease, but prematurity and low birth weight are common. • Usually after 4 to 6 weeks jaundice, hepatomegaly, abdominal distention, and poor feeding habits develop. • Infants at risk for developing hepatitis B include those born to mothers who are IV drug users, and who are refugees from Southeast Asia and the Far East. • Current prophylaxis for the neonate born to a mother with posi-

(continued)

Table 11-12 Types of Neonatal Infection (*continued*)

Description	Effects on the Neonate
Viral and Protozoan Infections	
natal period suffer from the chronic (carrier state) form of the disease and may never demonstrate signs and symptoms of the disease.	tive hepatitis B antigen consists of intramuscular administration of 0.5 ml of hyperimmune hepatitis B globulin at birth and at one month. • The neonate is bathed once with a bactericidal agent such as a hexachlorophene soap when its condition has stabilized. • The infant is not isolated and may remain with its mother. • All nurseries should have a clearly outlined procedure for care of neonates born to mothers with hepatitis B.
Chlamydia	
• Chlamydia is an intracellular parasite found in the vaginas of 2% to 13% of women. It has recently been identified as a causative agent in neonatal infection. It is the most	• Neonatal conjunctivitis, pneumonia, and otitis media occur, and the genital tract of the infant may be infected. • Prenatal diagnosis is possible, and screening of the pregnant woman is recommended to prevent infection in the neonate.

common sexually transmitted disease in the United States today (3 times greater than gonorrhea). It is transmitted to the infant during delivery through an infected cervix.	• Chlamydial conjunctivitis (Inclusion Blennorrhea), an infection of the neonate's eyes, results in inflammation of the conjunctiva, edema of the eyelids, and copious purulent discharge.
	  • A pseudomembrane may form over the eyes bilaterally.
	  • Treatment consists of topical application of erythromycin ointment or tetracycline combined with systemic administration of oral erythromycin.
	  • This infection is highly contagious, and the nurse must observe scrupulous aseptic technique.

• *Chlamydial Pneumonia* Chlamydial infection of the lung results in late onset pneumonia.	• The infant is usually afebrile, presenting with a severe, often paroxysmal cough. • Diffuse lung involvement is common, and rales can often be heard. • Pneumonia is frequently preceded by chlamydial conjunctivitis that was ineffectively treated by topical antibiotics alone. • Treatment with systemic antibiotics, including erythromycin, is recommended. Recovery may take up to two months.

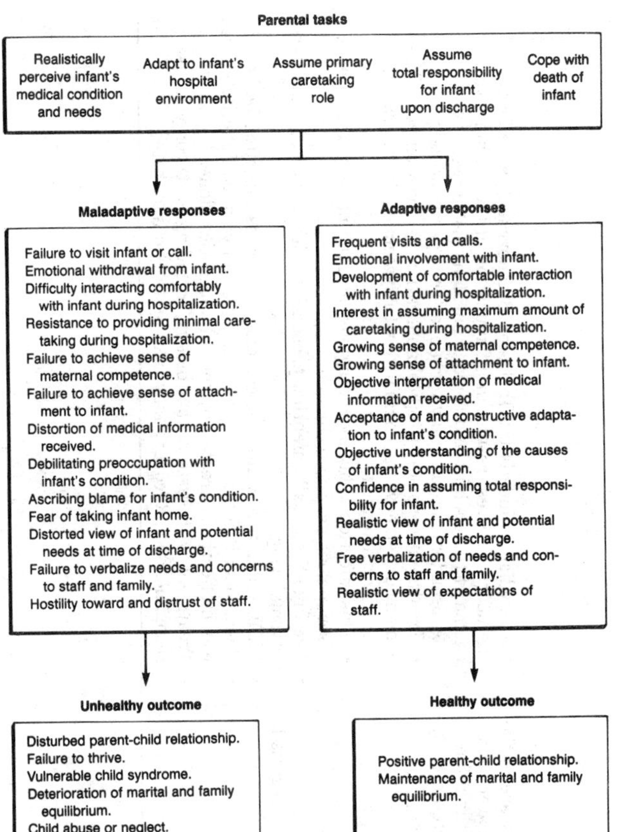

Figure 11-1 Parents may show either adaptive or maladaptive responses to the tasks of parenting a high-risk newborn. The nurse should assess the quality of parental adaptation so that effective and appropriate intervention can be implemented. (Grant P: Psychosocial needs of families of high-risk infants. Fam Commun Health 11:93, 1978).

Nursing Care of the Family with a High-Risk Neonate

The parent-infant acquaintance process is seriously threatened when the infant is ill at birth. Parental visiting may be difficult or impossible. The nurse caring for the infant must have an understanding of current theory regarding parental responses to the birth of a sick or defective infant before she attempts to facilitate the acquaintance process.

The nurse caring for a high-risk neonate must also assess and diagnose the parents' response to their infant. Many factors impinge on the parents as they struggle with the grieving process. Figure 11-1 shows parental tasks that may lead to either adaptive of maladaptive behavior in response to their infant's illness.

NOTES

12 Procedures and Medical Tests*

ALPHA-FETOPROTEIN SCREENING (Lab)

An alpha-fetoprotein (AFP) screening blood test has been developed to identify possible neural tube defects in the unborn infant. It can be used in women who have been informed and agree to testing. Many states now require that all pregnant women who enter the health care system before 16 to 18 weeks gestation have the opportunity to be tested.

Alpha-fetoprotein is produced by liver cells of the fetus, and when the neural tube is incomplete, an abnormal amount leaks into the amniotic fluid and passes into the mother's blood. Its collection at 16 to 18 weeks gestation ensures an adequate AFP blood concentration.

Elevated levels of AFP are predictive, but initial test results should be confirmed by a second test, and amniocentesis and ultrasound should be performed where indicated.

AMNIOCENTESIS (MD)

When indicated, amniocentesis is performed on pregnant women at 16 to 18 weeks from the last menstrual period (LMP) to obtain 12 to 24 ml of amniotic fluid for study. In conjunction with the use of ultrasound, a needle is inserted through the abdomen into the uterus, and amniotic fluid is withdrawn for use in diagnostic studies. The procedure can only be performed after 15 weeks gestation when sufficient fluid has been produced to supply an adequate specimen. Procedure-related fetal loss is estimated at about 1%. Indications for use of amniocentesis can be either diagnostic or therapeutic.

*To designate the health professional who can perform these tests or procedures, the letters in parentheses apply:
(MD) MD
(RN) RN
(Lab) Laboratory
(Rad) Radiologist

Diagnostic Indications

- Prenatal diagnosis of congenital disorders or infections (for women who have had a previous defective child, or a family history of birth defects, or for women over 35 years of age)
  - Chromosomal disorders (*e.g.*, Down Syndrome)
  - Enzyme deficiencies (*e.g.*, Tay-Sachs disease)
  - Sex-linked disorders (*e.g.*, hemophilia)
  - Metabolic disorders (*e.g.*, cystic fibrosis)
- Studies of fetal well-being
  - Alpha-fetoprotein
  - Color of amniotic fluid (meconium-stained)
  - Bilirubin determination (hemolytic disease)
- Estimation of Fetal Maturity
  - Cytologic staining of fat cells
  - Creatinine concentration
  - Bilirubin (in the absence of hemolytic disease, should decrease as pregnancy progresses)
  - Osmolarity: Increased fetal urine in the amniotic fluid causes the fluid to become hypotonic.

Therapeutic Indications

- Relief of hydramnios
- Intrauterine transfusion
- Therapeutic abortion (second trimester)

Complications

- Maternal complications
  - Hemorrhage and hematoma formation from puncture of a uterine vessel
  - Uterine contractions and premature labor
  - Amniotic fluid leak (usually benign)
  - Syncope from supine hypotension
- Fetal Complications
  - Fetomaternal bleeding with potential isoimmunization (sensitization of an unsensitized Rh-negative mother)
  - Infection
  - Spontaneous abortion
  - Hemorrhage (puncture of a fetal vessel or placenta)
  - Fetal puncture

AMNIOGRAPHY (MD)

Amniography is the injection of radiopaque agents into the amniotic sac. The sac becomes opaque and makes possible the identification of certain characteristics of the fetus, placenta, and amniotic fluid such as:

- An abnormal amount of amniotic fluid
- An abnormal location of the placenta
- Soft-tissue silhouette of the fetus
- Visualization of the fetal gastrointestinal tract a few hours after ingestion of the radiopaque agent

AMNIOSCOPY (MD)

During late pregnancy amnioscopy may be performed by direct visualization of the amniotic fluid through the membranes using a cone-shaped hollow tube placed through a dilated cervix. It is used to identify meconium-stained amniotic fluid that may be associated with maternal hypertension, prolonged pregnancy, suspected fetal intrauterine growth retardation (IUGR), previous unexplained stillbirth, lack of fetal descent, or lack of expected cervical dilatation.

Associated risks include:

- A closed cervix that makes passage of the amnioscope impossible
- An inaccessible cervix
- Accidental rupture of the membranes
- Introduction of infection to the mother or fetus

Use of amnioscopy is unpopular in the United States. It is contraindicated with known or suspected placenta previa.

AMNIOTOMY (MD)

Amniotomy is the artificial rupture of the amniotic membrane, and although controversial in some settings, it is routine practice in others. Amniotomy is performed by insertion of an amniotic hook into the amniotic sac and tearing the membrane.

Presumed benefits are to:

- Speed the process of labor
- Induce labor
- Detect meconium-stained amniotic fluid
- Allow placement of a fetal scalp electrode

- Permit insertion of a pressure catheter into the uterine cavity for internal electric monitoring
- Obtain fetal scalp blood for acid-base evaluation

Possible risks are:

- Failure to induce or speed the process of labor
- Cord prolapse
- Ascending infection to the mother and fetus, especially after multiple vaginal examinations
- Increased incidence of caput succedaneum
- Increased incidence of early fetal heart decelerations
- Occlusion of the fetal umbilical vessels

Contraindications include high presenting part, unripe cervix, abnormal fetal heart rate patterns, and other than vertex position.

APT TEST (MD, Lab)

Vaginal bleeding may be of fetal origin (resulting from rupture of fetal or placental vessel such as in vasa previa). The Apt test is based on the principle that fetal hemoglobin is alkaline stable, while adult hemoglobin is not.

The test is performed by mixing 5 ml of water with about 1 ml of blood from the vagina to make a pink solution. After filtering this solution, 1 ml of 1% sodium hydroxide solution is added. Test results:

- Bleeding of maternal origin: the pink solution turns brownish yellow within 2 minutes.
- Bleeding of fetal origin: the pink color of the solution remains unchanged within a 2 minute period.

A small amount of maternal hemoglobin in the fetal blood will not significantly alter the color of the test.

BASAL BODY TEMPERATURE (MD, RN)

The temperature of the body when at complete rest is called the basal body temperature (BBT). Indications for its use in women's health include:

- Infertility workup to assess ovulatory status
- Natural family-planning method to calculate fertile days
- An indicator for initiation of drugs in the treatment of dysmenorrhea

An oral or rectal temperature is taken for 2 to 5 minutes immediately upon awakening in the morning, and before any activity has occurred (any type of activity will elevate the base temperature). A BBT thermometer is used for easy reading since it has larger numbers to indicate degrees of temperature. The early morning temperature is recorded on a BBT calendar. Notations should be made on the calendar when illness, menses, coitus, or use of medications have occurred, all of which may affect the temperature reading. The body temperature drops slightly 24 to 36 hours after ovulation, then rises abruptly. Progesterone produced by the ovary after ovulation causes an elevation of the BBT of 0.5°F to 0.7°F. The temperature elevation continues until the end of the menstrual cycle and indicates ovulation. The BBT calendar should be kept over a period of months to demonstrate a temperature pattern. A biphasic curve usually indicates ovulation and can be helpful in predicting when ovulation will occur. A monophasic curve usually indicates anovulatory cycles.

BIOPSIES

Chorionic Villi Biopsy (MD)

Chorionic villi sampling is a recent development in prenatal diagnosis. During the first trimester it permits testing for chromosomal and biochemical disorders. Performed at 8 to 10 weeks LMP, it involves the passage of a plastic catheter through a metal obturator into the uterus. Under ultrasonic guidance, a small sample of chorionic villi is aspirated under negative pressure. The chorionic villi are rapidly dividing cells, and test results can be obtained within ten days, and often as soon as 1 to 2 days.

Advantages

- Performed in first trimester
- First trimester pregnancy termination is an option when fetal abnormality exists

Disadvantages

- Risk to the woman and her pregnancy have not yet been quantified.
- The technique is being researched and has not yet been proved to be as safe, reliable, or accurate as amniocentesis.

- Septic shock may possibly be a complication of the procedure.
- Testing for AFP cannot be done routinely as with amniocentesis.

Cone Biopsy (Conization) (MD)

Conization of the cervix is the surgical excision of a cone of cervical tissue surrounding the external os with the apex of the cone extending into the endocervical canal. Dilatation and curettage (D and C) may be performed in conjunction with this procedure.

Indications:

- A deep-seated cervical infection
- Discrepancy between the cytology report, the colposcopic findings, or the biopsy report
- When limits of the lesion cannot be seen colposcopically
- When microinvasive cancer is suspected or present
- When patient follow-up may be difficult

Endometrial Biopsy (MD)

Endometrial biopsy is a direct histologic examination of the endometrial tissue. It may be performed with a cutting instrument such as a biopsy forceps or by passing a hollow endometrial biopsy curet into the uterine cavity and using a suction syringe to aspirate endometrial fragments into the curet. In addition to its use for cancer detection, this test is an important component of infertility testing. A histologic endometrial specimen can be tested to determine the adequacy of secretory tissue and to determine whether the endometrium is in harmony with the woman's phase of menstruation. When the endometrial lining does not show the amount of secretory tissue that would be expected for the day of the woman's menstrual cycle, the adequacy of the luteal phase and progesterone production is in doubt.

BISHOP SCORE (MD, RN)

When labor induction of a pregnant woman is being considered, maternal readiness in terms of cervical status and fetal position should be assessed. This can be accomplished by means of the Bishop score. Each parameter is assigned a score from 0 to 3, and a total score is calculated. The higher the total score, the higher the likelihood of successful induction. Scores of 6 or more suggest a high probability (95%) of successful induction.

Bishop Score for Assessing Readiness for Induction

	Assigned Value			
Factor	*0*	*1*	*2*	*3*
Cervical dilatation	0	1–2 cm	3–4 cm	5 cm or more
Cervical effacement	0%–30%	40%–50%	60%–70%	80% or more
Fetal station	−3	−2	−1, 0	+1, +2
Cervical consistency	Firm	Moderate	Soft	
Cervical position	Posterior	Midposition	Anterior	

Adapted from Bishop EH: Pelvic scoring for elective induction. Obstet Gynecol 24:266, 1964

COLPOSCOPY (MD)

The colposcope is an optical instrument with a magnification of 10 to 20 times that is used for examining the cervix and vagina. It enables three-dimensional visualization of areas of cellular dysplasia or vascular abnormalities. During pregnancy, directed biopsies made of possible malignant lesions have been shown to be safe and reliable, eliminating the need for conization in most cases. Other indications for use of colposcopy include:

- Evaluation of cytologic abnormalities
- Examination of the cervix when there is suspicion of malignancy but no obvious lesion
- Evaluation of abnormalities detected clinically
- Guiding the biopsy of suspicious lesions
- Evaluation and follow-up of DES daughters

CRYOSURGERY (MD)

A method of treatment for benign lesions, cryosurgery causes local tissue destruction by the application of subfreezing temperatures. Prior to treatment the lesion must be carefully diagnosed, since use of this technique for treatment of invasive cancer will have serious consequences. The most common genital lesions treated by this method are condyloma and chronic cervicitis.

Cryosurgery is performed by passing liquid refrigerant, such as nitrogen, Freon 22, carbon dioxide, or nitrous oxide, through a hollow probe that is placed on the affected tissue and left until the desired amount of freezing occurs. The tissue that has been frozen sloughs as healing takes place and new epithelium is formed. Anesthesia is usually unnecessary, postoperative bleeding is uncommon, and there is no scarring of the tissue in the healing process.

The woman will experience profuse leukorrhea for 2 to 3 weeks after treatment as the tissue continues to slough. Complete healing takes place within 6 weeks.

CULDOCENTESIS (MD)

Culdocentesis is aspiration of fluid from the rectouterine pouch by means of a needle inserted through the posterior vaginal fornix. This procedure may be done on an outpatient basis to identify bloody fluid that does not clot. This finding is compatible with the diagnosis of hemoperitoneum resulting from ectopic pregnancy. Other indications for its use include evaluating acute upper abdominal disorders; identifying peritoneal fluid, pus, or blood in the pelvis; and draining an abscess in the cul-de-sac.

Culdocentesis is of limited value, since it may not provide a diagnosis without the presence of other clinical findings.

EPIDURAL BLOCK

Caudal Epidural Block (MD)

1. The patient is positioned in a side-lying position and supported by the nurse.
2. The lower back and coccygeal area are scrubbed with antiseptic solution and draped for asepsis.
3. A skin wheal is raised by intradermal injection of local anesthetic over the area of the sacral hiatus of the last sacral vertebra (S-4). Using a longer needle the anesthetic solution is injected more deeply into the fascia over the sacral hiatus.
4. An 18-gauge needle is directed toward the sacral hiatus and through the sacrococcygeal membrane and inserted approximately 3 cm into the caudal canal. The syringe should be aspirated; if cerebrospinal fluid or blood is found, the procedure should be discontinued because of the risk of incorrect needle placement into maternal soft tissue or the fetal head.
5. A test dose of anesthetic is administered; the nurse monitors maternal vital signs for indications of spinal block. If no indications are noted after 5 minutes, the caudal dose is administered by the physician or anesthetist.

If continuous caudal anesthesia is desired, steps 1 through 4 above are followed by:

5. A plastic catheter is advanced through the needle for a distance of 5 cm, and the needle is withdrawn. The catheter is taped securely in place. A test dose is administered as above. If no

adverse signs are noted after 5 minutes, the caudal dose is administered. The catheter is then closed off, and the nurse continues close monitoring of maternal blood pressure, pulse, respiration, and anesthetic level. Additional doses of anesthetic may be administered by the physician or anesthetist as needed.

Lumbar Epidural Block (MD)

1. The patient is positioned on her left side with shoulders aligned and legs slightly flexed. Spinal flexion is not recommended, since it stretches the dura and increases the possibility of puncture and inadvertent spinal block. A sitting position may be necessary for patients when the lumbar interspaces are small.
2. The nurse verifies patency of the intravenous infusion, and provides reassurance and support to the patient.
3. The lower back is scrubbed with antiseptic solution and draped for asepsis.
4. A skin wheal is raised by intradermal injection of local anesthetic at the proposed injection site.
5. A short 18-gauge beveled needle is introduced into an interspace between L-2 and L-4 and advanced to the ligamentum flavum. This landmark is noted by resistance to injected fluid or air; injected substance will rebound back into the syringe.
6. The needle is then advanced another millimeter into the peridural space; this is noted by loss of resistance to injected air or fluid. The syringe is aspirated for cerebrospinal fluid or blood. If cerebrospinal fluid or blood is aspirated, the needle is withdrawn and insertion is attempted at another site.
7. A test dose of anesthetic agent is injected. Signs of inadvertent spinal anesthesia (onset of anesthesia after the test dose) are monitored for 5 minutes. The nurse begins assessment of maternal blood pressure, pulse, and respiration every 1 to 2 minutes at this point.
8. If the test dose produces warmth and tingling in lower extremities, but no anesthesia, the needle is judged to be properly placed in the peridural space, and the appropriate amount of anesthetic agent is administered.

If continuous lumbar anesthesia is desired, steps 1 through 6 above are followed by:

7. A plastic catheter is threaded through the needle into the peridural space and advanced 3 to 5 cm beyond the needle tip. The needle is then removed. (Note: The catheter should not be retracted through the needle because the soft catheter may be shredded or broken off in the peridural space.) Transient hyper-

esthesia (increased cutaneous sensitivity) may occur in the back, leg, or hip if the catheter touches a nerve in the peridural space.

8. A test dose is administered and is monitored as in steps 7 and 8 above.
9. The catheter is closed off and taped in place, allowing for additional injections by the anesthetist or physician (not the labor nurse) as needed.

FERN TEST (CERVICAL MUCUS ARBORIZATION TEST) (MD, RN, Lab)

The fern test is a qualitative microscopic slide test used to assess secretion in women by examination of endocervical mucus. Ferning of the mucus (a fernlike pattern on a dried smear) indicates a high level of estrogen that occurs during the proliferative phase of the menstrual cycle and reaches a maximum at ovulation when estrogen peaks. Indications for this test include:

- Determining the presence or absence of ovulation
- Determining the time of ovulation
- Monitoring the induction of ovulation
- Assessing corpus luteum function (progesterone secretion)
- Use as a parameter of an infertility workup
- Use during labor to determine premature rupture of the membranes

The test is performed by spreading endocervical mucus on a glass slide and allowing it to dry for 10 to 20 minutes. The slide is then examined microscopically to assess arborization (fernlike pattern) of the mucus. When the test is positive, ferning and crystallization are seen on the slide, which indicate a predominant estrogenic effect. When the test is negative, no ferning or crystallization occurs, indicating no estrogenic effects (Fig. 12-1). Within 24 to 72 hours after ovulation, ferning disappears due to the effect of progesterone.

FETOGRAPHY (MD)

In fetography a solution of iodinated lipid is injected into the amniotic sac. It adheres to and outlines the maturing fetus and provides information without the use of more intrusive measures such as amniotomy, diagnostic x-rays, invading the amniotic sac, and injection of potentially harmful chemicals.

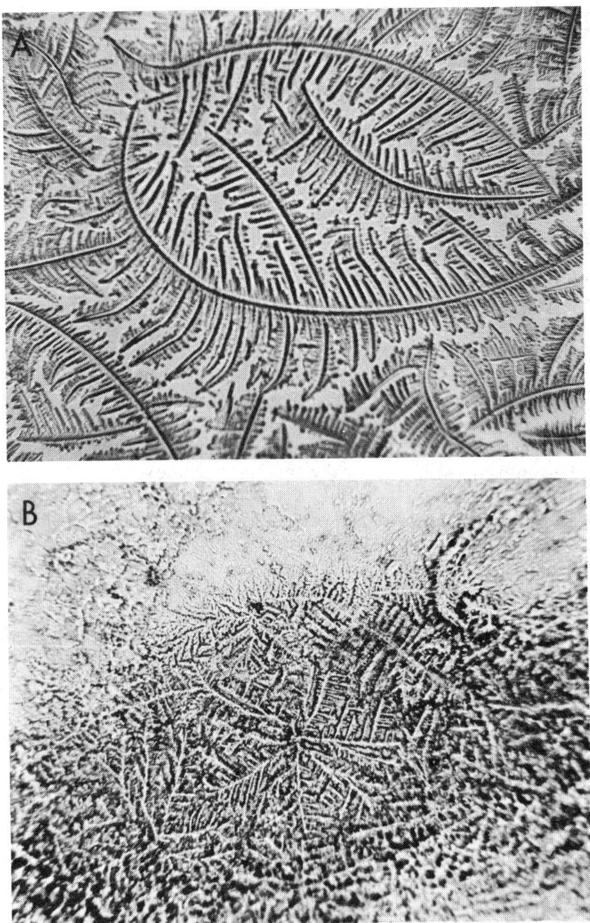

Figure 12-1 *(A)* Typical ferning of cervical mucus at midcycle. *(B)* Incomplete (atypical) ferning during early secretory phase of cycle. (Danforth DN [ed]: Obstetrics and Gynecology, 4th ed. Philadelphia, JB Lippincott, 1982)

FETOSCOPY (MD)

Fetoscopy allows direct visualization of the fetus and placenta in utero and collection of specimens from them by means of a fetoscope that is introduced into the uterus through an abdominal incision. This procedure is primarily in the research stage because of its limitations and increased risk to the mother and fetus.

GLUCOSE INTOLERANCE OF PREGNANCY (MD, Lab)

All women 25 years of age and older should be screened for diabetes in pregnancy, as should those women under 25 with the following risk factors:

- Family history of diabetes, including parents, siblings, aunts, uncles
- History of a previous stillborn infant
- Prior infant who weighed over 9 pounds (4000 g)
- Prior unexplained fetal death
- Obesity (over 200 pounds or 15% of nonpregnant ideal body weight)
- Glycosuria
- Polyhydramnios
- Poor reproductive history with more than 3 spontaneous abortions in the first or second trimester
- Chronic hypertension
- Recurrent urinary tract infections

Oral Glucose Tolerance Test

- For three days prior to the oral glucose tolerance test (OGTT), the patient should be instructed to eat a 200-g minimal carbohydrate diet. This can be achieved by advising the patient to eat a candy bar daily for 3 days.
- Fasting is necessary from after dinner the night before the test until the OGTT is completed the next morning.
- A fasting blood sugar is obtained, after which a glucose load of 100 g glucose dissolved in 400 ml water is ingested within a 5-minute period.
- Blood sugar levels are then drawn at 1, 2, and 3 hours. Urine spot checks are also obtained to detect glucosuria.

Normal Glucose Levels

	Fasting	1:Hr	2:Hr	3:Hr
Whole blood	90	165	145	125 mg/dl
Plasma or serum	100	180	160	140 mg/dl

The test is considered abnormal when two or more values are elevated. If one value is elevated, the test is considered normal. Women at high risk should be tested in early pregnancy and again at 30 weeks gestation. Test results that are considered "borderline" should be repeated.

GONORRHEA SMEAR (MD, RN)

The gonorrhea smear is the most common method of diagnosing gonorrheal infection in women. Use of a gram-stained slide in diagnosis is not adequate. Culture specimens should be obtained from the endocervix and inoculated on Thayer-Martin (TM) culture plates. (Holding media may also be used for transfer of the specimen to the laboratory where it will be inoculated on TM). The combination of a positive oxidase reaction of colonies, and gram-negative diplococci grown on medium provides sufficient criteria for diagnosis of gonorrhea.

Microscopic Gram stain evaluation of penile drainage in the male is possible for diagnosis of male disease. Pharyngeal or anal cultures may also be collected for evaluation.

HYPERREFLEXIA (MD, RN)

Hyperreflexia is determined by deep tendon reflexes (DRTs) on a 0 to 4+ scale:

- 0: No response
- 1+: Low normal or somewhat diminished
- 2+: Normal, average
- 3+: Above average briskness
- 4+: Very brisk, hyperactive; also associated with clonus (a series of convulsive ankle movements that occurs when the foot is dorsiflexed)

Assessing Deep Tendon Reflexes and Clonus

Hyperreflexia reflects increased central nervous system (CNS) irritability. Intrapartal patients with preeclampsia or eclampsia should be frequently evaluated for increasingly brisk DTRs, as this finding suggests worsening of their condition and the possibility of seizure activity. In assessing DTRs, begin with the arms and move to the legs, comparing the reflex responses on left and right sides. Note and record any asymmetry. Place the limb to be tested in a relaxed, semiflexed position; a brisk tap places additional tension on the respective tendon and elicits the reflex response.

Biceps Reflex

- Palpate for the tendon of the biceps in the bend of the elbow; place your thumb over it.
- Tap your thumb briskly with the pointed end of the reflex hammer; note the reflex movement of the biceps muscle and flexion of the lower arm.

Quadriceps Reflex

- Position the patient's legs so they are slightly flexed.
- Supporting the leg under the knee with one arm, palpate the patellar tendon just below the patella; strike it briskly with the pointed end of the reflex hammer, noting the reflex extension of the lower leg.

Ankle Clonus

- If DTRs are increased, assess for ankle clonus. Position the patient so the knee is slightly flexed.
- Support the leg under the knee with one arm. With the other hand, grasp the foot, dorsiflex it quickly, and maintain this position. Observe for the rhythmic, repetitive jerks or beats of clonus, and chart the number of beats.

HYSTEROSALPINGOGRAPHY (MD, Rad)

Hysterosalpingography is an outpatient radiologic examination for visualization of the endocervix, uterine cavity, and fallopian tubes. The procedure allows immediate visualization of the genital organs by monitoring spread of the contrast medium under fluoroscopy.

The test is most commonly used for fertility workup to provide more explicit information than is available from other tests. The greatest weakness of the test is that it does not show the condition of the tubal fimbriae and peritubal area. The test is performed 1 week after the menstrual period to prevent reflux of endometrial cells into the tubes and peritoneum. Sedation may be necessary for some patients, and if severe pain occurs, the procedure should be discontinued.

Indications:

- Evaluation of tubal patency
- Identification of congenital anomalies, deformities, or adhesions of the genital organs
- Identification of polyps, leiomyomas, hydatidiform moles, and extrinsic pressure

To perform the test, 1 to 10 ml of contrast medium is instilled in small increments into the cervix under low pressure. Films are taken after each injection and again at 45 minutes after completion of the test to assess spillage of the medium into the peritoneum (indicating tubal patency). A repeat film is taken in 24 hours to evaluate peritubal adhesions. Fluoroscopic viewing of the contrast medium entering the cervix and uterus at the time of the procedure may provide the physician more immediate data. Complications include pain; hemorrhage; shock; endometriosis (peritoneal reflux of endometrial cells); allergic reaction to the medium; intravascular injection of the medium into the blood stream; uterine perforation; and possible exposure to radiation.

KEGEL EXERCISES (MD, RN)

Kegel exercises are a series of exercises for women whose pubococcygeal muscles are so slack that the women lose urine when they cough or sneeze. This may be a problem for both older women who lack muscle tone and postpartum women. Regular practice of the Kegel exercises can restore muscle tone in about 6 weeks. The pelvic floor muscles contract during orgasm, and like any other muscle, they work better when they are in well toned. Thus, there is a sexual benefit when muscle tone improves.

The steps for the Kegel exercises are as follows:

1. Locate the muscles surrounding the vagina by sitting on the toilet and starting and stopping the flow of urine.
2. Test the baseline strength of the muscles by inserting a finger in the opening of the vagina and contracting the muscles.
3. Exercise A. Sequeeze the muscles together and hold the squeeze for 3 seconds. Relax the muscles. Repeat.
4. Exercise B. Contract and relax the muscles as rapidly as possible 10 to 25 times. Repeat.
5. Exercise C. Imagine sitting in a pan of water and sucking water into the vagina. Hold for 3 seconds.
6. Exercise D. Push out as during a bowel movement, only with the vagina. Hold for 3 seconds.
7. Repeat exercises A, C, and D ten times each; repeat exercise B once. Repeat the entire series three times a day.

Additional benefits from the Kegel exercises are increased vaginal lubrication during sexual arousal, stronger gripping of the base of the penis during intercourse, relief of constipation, and increased flexibility of episiotomy scars.

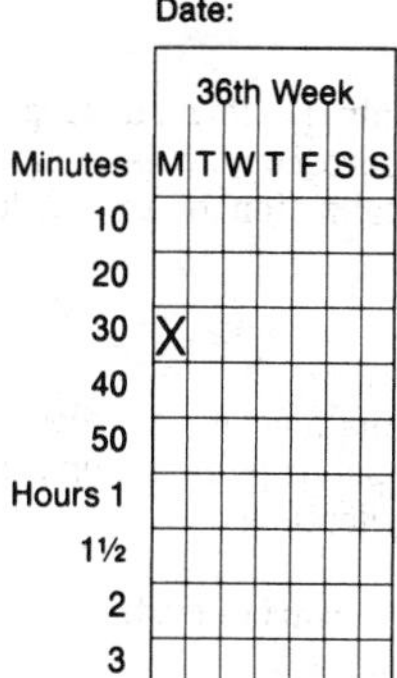

Date:
36th Week
Minutes
M T W T F S S
10
20
30
X
40
50
Hours 1
1½
2
3

KICKS COUNTS (RN, MD)

An easy way to check the health of the baby is through kick counting. The woman is instructed in how to count and is given a chart on which to record the number of kicks. Instructions for the patient are as follow:

- At the same time each day, after you have eaten, record the amount of time it takes for your baby to kick ten times. For example, on Monday you begin to count your baby's kicks at 10:00 AM. By 10:30 AM your baby has kicked ten times. You fill in the chart like this:
- Remember that each baby has sleep times and active times. If you start counting and the baby is not kicking, stop, walk around for 5 minutes, then count again. (Hint: Count baby's kicks after you have eaten.)
- If your baby has not kicked ten times at the end of 3 hours, call the delivery room at the hospital.

KLEIHAUER-BETKE TEST (MD, Lab)

This test is a more precise, quantitative assessment of fetal–maternal blood admixture (as opposed to the Apt test). The test is based on the difference in solubility of fetal and maternal hemoglobin. A fresh blood smear is fixed and exposed to a phosphate buffer that is dried and stained with eosin. Test results:

- Fetal red cells appear red.
- Maternal red cells appear as "ghosts" without hemoglobin staining.

LAPAROSCOPY (MD)

The second most commonly performed surgical procedure for gynecologic diagnosis is laparoscopy. It is an endoscopic procedure performed to permit visualization of the abdominal and pelvic organs. Its uses include:

- Infertility workups
- Evaluation of genital malformations, possible ectopic pregnancy, adnexal masses, pelvic pain, endometriosis, pelvic infections, postsurgical complications
- Biopsy
- Aspiration of physiologic ovarian cysts
- Lysis of peritubal adhesions
- Extraction of an IUD located within the abdomen
- Tubal ligation

Prior to insertion of the laparoscope through an umbilical stab incision, a pneumoperitoneum (injection of carbon dioxide into the abdomen) is performed to force the bowel upward to protect it from trauma. The laparoscope, with its telescopic lens, is introduced into the abdomen and provides a 180 degree view of the abdominal and pelvic organs. Ancillary instruments for performing biopsy, tubal ligations, lysing of adhesions, and for photographing the structures can be used by insertion through the cannula of the laparoscope. Hospitalization and general anesthesia are usually necessary.

DETERMINATION OF LECITHIN-SPHINGOMYELIN RATIO (MD, Lab)

The lecithin-sphingomyelin (L/S) ratio is tested by sampling the amniotic fluid during pregnancy. The L/S ratio gives an indication of fetal lung maturity, which helps prevent respiratory distress syndrome (RDS) in the neonate. Pulmonary surfactant, which normally prevents collapse of the lung alveoli, contains lecithin and sphingomyelin. Measurement of the ratio of these two substances (2 : 1) in the amniotic fluid surrounding the fetus gives an indication of its lung maturity.

In high-risk pregnancies where optimum fetal well-being is desired, early delivery may be necessary, and the state of the fetal lung must be assessed. Amniocentesis is performed to obtain a sample of amniotic fluid to be used for L/S ratio and other tests. High-risk pregnancies that may need early delivery include erythroblastosis fetalis, maternal diabetes, preeclampsia/eclampsia, and hypertension. (Also see Shake test.)

NONSTRESS TEST (MD, RN)

The least invasive test of fetal well-being, the nonstress test, is done to assess the integrity of the fetal CNS and the reflex responses that control the fetal heart rate. The fetal response to spontaneous contractions or fetal activity is an indication of the health of the infant and how well the infant will tolerate the stresses of labor. A fetal heart rate increase of 20 beats per minute indicates fetal homeostasis. If results of the nonstress test are equivocal, a contraction stress test may be indicated.

OXYTOCIN CHALLENGE TEST OR CONTRACTION STIMULATION TEST (MD with RN)

The oxytocin challenge test (OCT), also known as the contraction stimulation test (CST), evaluates fetal heart rate response to the stress of uterine contractions (either spontaneous or induced with oxytocin). This test has largely been replaced by the nonstress test that does not use medication to induce contractions and is equally reliable. Indications are hypertension; diabetes; intrauterine growth retardation (IUGR); previous stillbirth; prolonged pregnancy; preelampsia; and maternal heart disease.

The procedure is performed by placing a fetal monitor on the patient and monitoring a "baseline strip" for 30 minutes. When no contractions are observed for 30 minutes, oxytocin is used. The oxytocin infusion is begun at 0.5 mU/min and increased by 0.5 mU/min every 15 minutes until contractions are achieved. The goal is to achieve three contractions within 10 minutes that reach a peak intensity of at least 50 mm Hg.

Results:

- *Positive:* consistent and persistent late deceleration of the FHR
- *Negative:* a minimum of 3 contractions in 10 minutes that last 40 seconds and that are not identified with late decelerations of the FHR
- *Suspicious:* inconstant late deceleration that does not persist with subsequent contractions
- *Hyperstimulation:* uterine contractions occurring more frequently than every 2 minutes and lasting longer than 90 seconds;

persistent uterine hypertonus suspected; late deceleration does not necessarily indicate uteroplacental disease
- *Unsatisfactory:* frequency of contractions is less than 3 in 10 minutes or the tracing is of poor quality

PAPANICOLAOU SMEAR (MD, RN)

The Papanicolaou (PAP) smear is the cytologic screening of cells collected from the cervix. It is used specifically to detect cervical cancer; it is an inappropriate screening method for detecting endometrial or ovarian cancer.

Considerations Prior to Specimen Collection

- The optimum time for collecting the Pap smear is 5 days after the last menstrual period.
- No douching or use of vaginal medications should have occurred 24 hours prior to the test.
- The smear should not be collected during menstruation, since the presence of red blood cells interferes with cytologic interpretation.
- Lubricating jelly should not be used on the speculum before insertion because it causes distortion of the cells.
- During pregnancy the cervix is friable, and vigorous scraping may induce heavy bleeding and invalidate the test.
- Pregnancy causes changes in the cervical cells, making it difficult for the cytologist to identify cells from the squamocolumnar junction.

The frequency with which a Pap smear should be obtained is now under debate, but the American College of Obstetrics and Gynecology still recommends a yearly Pap smear for all women. Risk for cervical cancer may be associated with the following:

- Personal history of cervical or uterine cancer
- Previous abnormal Pap test
- Early age of first sexual intercourse
- Multiple sexual partners
- History of genital herpes infection or genital warts
- Women whose mothers took DES (diethylstilbesterol) during pregnancy
- Low socioeconomic status
- Prostatic or penile cancer in partner(s)

Classification of Pap Smear Results: Cervical Intraepithelial Neoplasia (CIN)

Finding	Designation	Interpretation
Normal squamous epithelium	Normal	
Mild dysplasia	(Grade I)	Lower third of the epithelium is replaced by immature, undifferentiated cells with frequent mitosis
Moderate dysplasia	(Grade II)	Involvement of the middle third of the epithelium
Severe dysplasia	(Grade III)	Involvement of the upper third of the epithelium, but still some maturation on the surface

PELVIMETRY (MD, RN)

Pelvimetry is the measurement of the dimensions and proportions of the bony pelvis. It is performed to assess whether the pelvis is large enough to accommodate the delivery of an infant. A normal delivery can occur only when the bony pelvis is large enough for the largest diameter of the infant, the head, to pass through it. Assessment of pelvimetry is subjective, and its accuracy depends upon the skill and experience of the examiner. Although precise measurements cannot be made, the adequacy of the pelvic dimensions can be quite accurately estimated. This examination has become less important as more women are allowed a trial of labor even though the pelvis may be considered borderline.

POSTCOITAL TEST (MD, RN)

The postcoital test, or Sims-Huhner test, provides information on the receptivity of the cervical mucus and the ability of sperm to reach and survive in it. It is an important part of an infertility workup.

Performing the Test

- The test is scheduled for the anticipated day of ovulation.
- The couple is instructed to have sexual intercourse at this time, after a 48-hour period of abstinence.
- The woman is examined within 8 hours of intercourse.
- A sample of cervical mucus is examined microscopically for characteristics that enhance sperm survival and for indications of adequate estrogen production.
- Normal ovulatory mucus reveals a ferning pattern and demonstrates *spinnbarkeit,* or the ability to stretch as much as 6 to 10 inches without breaking.
- Some sperm may be seen normally, but there is no agreement on what number of sperm constitutes a normal postcoital test.

PREGNANCY TESTS (MD, RN, Lab)

Immunologic Tests (Lab)

Use of immunologic tests is based on the ability of human chorionic gonadotropin (HCG) in the woman's urine or serum to stimulate antibody reduction, producing an antigen–antibody on a slide or in a tube. They are performed by mixing the woman's urine with a prepared serum containing antibodies to HCG. Then a carrier—either latex for the slide test or erythrocytes coated with HCG for the tube test—is added to the mixture.

- Slide Test: This test can be completed and reported in 2 minutes. It is easy to read but less sensitive than the tube test. It will be negative if performed before 42 days after the LMP. When negative at this time it should be repeated in 2 weeks in case of error in calculating the date of the LMP.
- Tube Test: This test requires 2 hours to complete and is sensitive to lower levels of HCG. It also has fewer false negative results.
- Test results
  - Positive reading: A cloudy suspension (indicating absence of agglutination [AI]
  - Negative reading: Presence of agglutination (clumping)

RADIOIMMUNOASSAY TEST (Lab)

The radioimmunoassay test (RIA beta-subunit HCG) is a highly specific and sensitive assay that can detect as little as 0.003 IU/ml of beta-HCG in the serum. It can detect pregnancy in the first week after conception (6 days) with almost 100% accuracy in 1 to 3 hours.

RADIORECEPTOR TEST (Lab)

The radioreceptor test (RRA) is the most recent addition to pregnancy testing. Biologically active HCG is detected even more accurately by this test than by the RIA. The test is currently available as a kit that permits measurement of HCG within 1 hour. Except for the beta-subunit RIA, the RRA is the most sensitive pregnancy test now available. These two tests are not available in all women's health care settings. Sophisticated equipment for interpreting the tests is available only in large hospitals or medical centers.

PHOSPHATIDYLGLYCEROL (Lab)

Continued research into the physiology of fetal lung maturity has uncovered many additional phospholipids and fatty acids. The presence of phosphatidylglycerol (PG) and phosphatidylinositol (PI) has been found to correlate reliably with fetal lung maturity. Preliminary studies have shown that prematurely born neonates without RDS have had PG isolated from gastric, pharyngeal, and tracheal aspirates within 4 hours after birth. Infants with RDS had no detectable PG.

PG is used in conjunction with the L/S ratio. If the L/S ratio is 2 and the PG is positive, there is strong evidence of fetal lung maturity. PG may provide stability that makes the infant less susceptible to RDS when experiencing hypoglycemia, hypothermia, or hypoxia.

Research continues using PI, and the presence of PI is also a reliable indicator of fetal lung maturity.

RUBIN TEST (MD)

The tubal insufflation test, or Rubin test, is used occasionally instead of the hysterosalpingogram. This test involves the injection of carbon dioxide into the uterus and tubes to determine patency. When the tubes are patent, the carbon dioxide flows from the ends of the tubes and collects in the abdomen. Abdominal sounds are produced that can be heard on auscultation, and referred shoulder pain is experienced by the patient. This test has a high rate of false-positive results and is painful to the patient. For these reasons the hysterosalpingogram is used more commonly.

SHAKE TEST (FOAM STABILITY TEST) (MD, Lab)

The shake test is a qualitative measurement of the amount of pulmonary surfactant contained in the amniotic fluid. The advantage of this test over the L/S ratio is that it is highly reliable and can be performed by a physician or technician.

It is performed by centrifuging the amniotic fluid, adding 95% alcohol, and shaking the specimen for 15 seconds. A ring of bubbles formed around the meniscus at 15 minutes is a positive test result, meaning that the risk of respiratory distress is very low. There are two problems with the test. First, test results may be markedly altered by slight contamination of the amniotic fluid, equipment, or errors in measurement. Second, false-negative readings are common.

SPINAL BLOCK (MD)

1. The patient is positioned in a sitting or side-lying position and supported by the nurse; the nurse verifies that the intravenous infusion is patent and provides reassurance throughout the procedure.
2. The lower back is scrubbed with an antiseptic solution and draped for asepsis.
3. A skin wheal is raised at the L3–4 interspace by intradermal injection of local anesthetic.
4. The patient is assisted to curve her back and neck forward, with arms between knees, and is supported in this position by the nurse.
5. A No. 20- or No. 21-gauge needle is introduced into the wheal and advanced into the interspinous ligament, the ligamentum flavum, and the epidural space.
6. A smaller gauge needle (No. 25 or No. 26) is then inserted into the larger needle and advanced through the dura into the subarachnoid space. The presence of spinal fluid in the needle hub verifies that placement is correct.
7. Appropriate amount of anesthetic is injected slowly, and both needles are removed.
8. The nurse assists the patient into the desired position (supine for anesthesia for cesarean birth; sitting for anesthesia for vaginal delivery) for 3 to 5 minutes and begins monitoring blood pressure, respiration, and pulse every 1 to 2 minutes for the first 10 minutes after administration.
9. The nurse observes for signs of toxic reaction or respiratory difficulty, which signals possible respiratory paralysis.

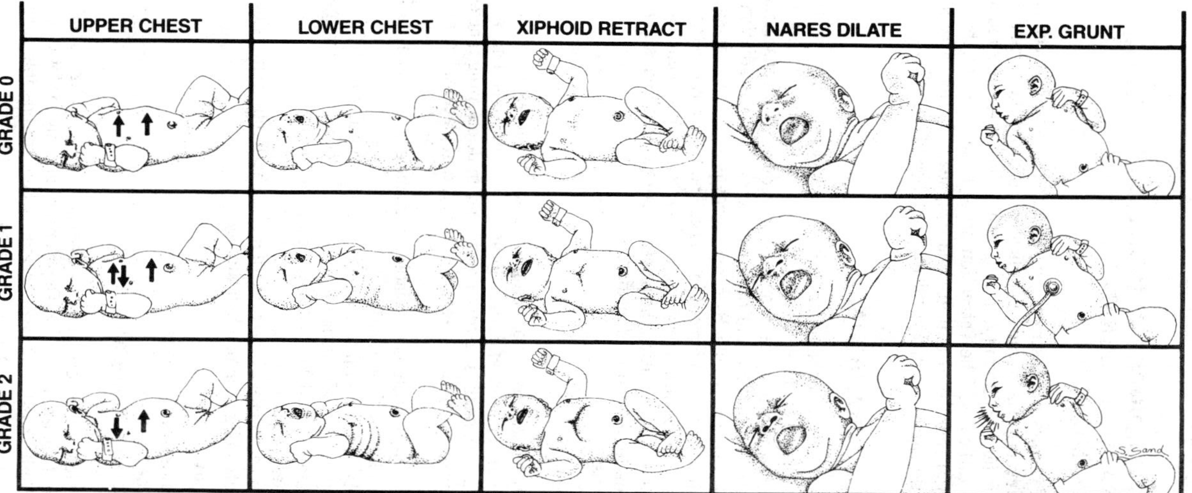

Figure 12-2 An index of respiratory distress is determined by grading each of five arbitrary criteria. Grade 0 indicates no difficulty; grade 1 indicates moderate difficulty; and grade 2 indicates maximum respiratory difficulty. The retraction score is the sum of these values; a total score of 0 indicates no dyspnea, whereas a total score of 10 denotes maximal respiratory distress.

SILVERMAN-ANDERSON INDEX OF NEONATAL RESPIRATORY DISTRESS (MD, RN)

An index of respiratory distress is determined by grading each of five arbitrary criteria. Grade 0 indicates no difficulty; grade 1 indicates moderate difficulty; and grade 2 indicates maximum respiratory difficulty. The retraction score is the sum of these values; a total score of 0 indicates no dyspnea, whereas a total score of 10 denotes maximal respiratory distress (Fig. 12-2).

ULTRASONOGRAPHY (MD)

Ultrasonography is a scanning procedure that uses sound waves to display two-dimensional echo images of the area under examination. Ultrasonography is a simple procedure that causes no discomfort to the patient and does not expose her to radiation.

The real-time gray-scale B-scanner provides not only image detail but shows fetal movement in utero. The B-scan can demonstrate a gestational sac as early as 5 weeks after the last menstrual period. By 9 weeks gestation the placenta can be identified, and by 14 weeks the fetal head is identifiable.

Indications:

- Pregnancy
  - Identifies intrauterine or ectopic pregnancy, determines fetal age, fetal position and size, locates placental position, and identifies anomalies, hydramnios, and multiple pregnancies
  - Used prior to amniocentesis, fetoscopy, and placental aspiration
  - Confirms or identifies nonviable pregnancies, such as hydatidiform mole or fetal death
  - Directly detects fetal abnormalities (*i.e.*, neural tube defects, urinary system abnormalities, skeletal dysplasia, abdominal wall defects, cardiac anomalies, conjoined twins)
  - Assesses gestational age
  - Aids in the correct interpretation of alpha-fetoprotein values
  - Evaluates oligo- or polyhydramnios
- Gynecology
  - Identifies ovarian cysts
  - Identifies ascites
  - Locates lost or misplaced IUD

At this time an understanding of tissue effects of ultrasound is incomplete. Prudent use of the Doppler for listening for fetal heart tones and limited use of ultrasonography whenever possible during the first trimester may be well advised.

Appendix A
Common Abbreviations in Maternity Nursing

GENERALLY USED ABBREVIATIONS

ABC	Alternative Birth Center
ACTH	Adrenocorticotropic hormone
ADH	Antidiuretic hormone (vasopressin)
AID	Artificial insemination, donor
AIH	Artificial insemination, husband
BBT	Basal body temperature
BP	Blood pressure
CBC	Complete blood count
CC	Chief complaint
CL	Corpus luteum
CNS	Central nervous system
CPD	Cephalopelvic disproportion
C/S	Cesarean section
CSF	Cerebrospinal fluid
CV	Cardiovascular
CVP	Central venous pressure
CX	Cervix
D&C	Dilatation and curettage
DNA	Deoxyribonucleic acid
DS	Dextrostix
EDC	Expected date of confinement
EFM	Electronic fetal monitoring
ESR	Erythrocyte sedimentation rate
FHR	Fetal heart rate
FHT	Fetal heart tone
FPD	Fetopelvic disproportion
FSH	Follicle stimulating hormone
FTA-ABS	Fluorescent treponemal antibody-absorption test for syphilis
GI	Gastrointestinal
GnRH	Gonadotropin releasing hormone
GTT	Glucose tolerance test
HCG	Human chorionic gonadotropin
HCS	Human chorionic somatomammotropin
HDL	High density lipoprotein

Hgb	Hemoglobin
HGH	Human growth hormone
HMD	Hyaline membrane disease
HPL	Human placental lactogen
ICN	Intensive care nursery
ICP	Intracranial pressure
IDM	Infant of diabetic mother
IM	Intramuscular
IRDS	Idiopathic respiratory distress syndrome (RDS)
IUD	Intrauterine device
IUFD	Intrauterine fetal demise
IUGR	Intrauterine growth retardation
IUP	Intrauterine pregnancy
IV	Intravenous
IVH	Intravascular hemorrhage
Kcal	Kilocalorie
kg	Kilogram
KOH	Potassium hydroxide
L&D	Labor and delivery
LBW	Low birth weight
LDL	Low density lipoprotein
LGA	Large for gestational age
LH	Luteinizing hormone
LMP	Last menstrual period
LUS	Lower uterine segment
MAS	Meconium aspiration syndrome
N&V	Nausea and vomiting
NEC	Necrotizing enterocolitis
NST	Nonstress test
OCT	Oxytocin challenge test
PAP	Papanicolaou smear
PG	Prostaglandin
PG	Phosphatidylglycerol
PID	Pelvic inflammatory disease
PIF	Prolactin-inhibiting factor
PIH	Pregnancy-induced hypertension
PKU	Phenylketonuria

PL	Prolactin
PMI	Point of maximal intensity
PMP	Previous menstrual period
PNMP	Previous normal menstrual period
PP	Postpartum
PROM	Premature rupture of membranes
RDS	Respiratory distress syndrome
RIA	Radioimmunoassay
RNA	Ribonucleic acid
ROM	Rupture of membranes
SAB	Spontaneous abortion
SGA	Small for gestational age
SROM	Spontaneous rupture of membranes
SS	Sickle cell disease
TPAL	Term pregnancy/premature/abortions/living children
TRIC	Trachoma inclusion conjunctivitis (chlamydia trachomatis)
TSH	Thyroid stimulating hormone
VS	Vital signs
WHO	World Health Organization

ABBREVIATIONS FOR FETAL POSITIONS

MA	Mentum (chin) anterior
LMA	Left mentum anterior
LMT	Left mentum transverse
LMP	Left mentum posterior
MP	Mentum posterior
RMA	Right mentum anterior
RMP	Right mentum posterior
RMT	Right mentum transverse
OA	Occiput anterior
LOA	Left occiput anterior
LOT	Left occiput transverse
LOP	Left occiput posterior
OP	Occiput posterior
ROP	Right occiput posterior

ROT	Right occiput transverse
ROA	Right occiput anterior
SA	Sacrum anterior
LSA	Left sacrum anterior
LST	Left sacrum transverse
LSP	Left sacrum posterior
SP	Sacrum posterior
RSP	Right sacrum posterior
RST	Right sacrum transverse
RSA	Right sacrum anterior

NOTES

Appendix B
Normal Values and Reference Tables

B-1 Normal Peripheral Blood Values at Different Ages

Age	Hemoglobin (g/dl)	Hematocrit (%)	MCV (fl)	WBC ($10^3/mm^3$)	Neutrophils (%)	Lymphocytes (%)	Platelets ($10^3/mm^3$)
Birth	13.5–21	42–65	100–140	9–30	60	30	100–300
1 wk	13.5–21	42–65	95–135	5–21	40	50	100–300
1 mo	10–16	30–48	85–125	5–21	35	55	100–300
Adult:							
Male	14–18	42–54	80–100	4–11	0	30	100–300
Female	12–16	36–48	80–100	4–11	60	30	100–300
Pregnancy	11.5–12.3	32–46	80–95	15–18	60 ± 10	34 ± 10	100–300

B-2 Blood Chemistries

Determination	Specimen	Age/Sex	Normal Value	
Acetone	Serum/plasma			
Qualitative			Negative	
Quantitative (acetone) and acetoacetic acid)			0.3–2.0 mg/dl	
Albumin (see Protein Electrophoresis)				
Aldolase	Serum	Newborn	4 × adult value	
		Adult	<11 IU/liter	
Alpha fetoprotein	Serum		<10 mg/dl	
Amylase	Serum	Newborn	5–65 U/liter	
		>1 yr	25–125	
Ascorbic acid	Serum		0.6–2.0 mg/dl	
Bicarbonate	Serum	Arterial	21–28 mmol/liter	
		Venous	22–29	
	Serum	Pregnancy	20.5–26	
Base excess	Whole blood	Newborn	(−10)–(−2) mmol/liter	
		Adult	(−3)–(+3)	
Bilirubin, total	Serum		*Premature (mg/dl)*	*Full-term (mg/dl)*
		Cord	<2	<2
		0–1 day	<8	<6

(continued)

B-2 Blood Chemistries (continued)

Determination	Specimen	Age/Sex	Normal Value	
		1–2 days	<12	<8
		2–5 days	<16	<12
		Adult	<2	0.2–1.0
		Pregnancy	Unchanged	
Bilirubin, direct (conjugated)	Serum		0.8–0.2 mg/dl	
Calcium, ionized	Serum, plasma, whole blood	Cord, newborn	5.5 ± 0.3 mg/dl	
		3–24 hr	4.3–5.1	
		24–48 hr	4.0–4.7	
		Adult	4.48–4.92	
Calcium, total	Serum	Cord, newborn	9–11.5 mg/dl	
		3–24 hr	9–10.6 mg/dl	
		24–48 hr	7–12	
		4–7 days	9–10.9	
		Adult	8.4–10.2	
		Pregnancy	7.8–9.3	
Carbon dioxide, partial pressure, pCO_2	Whole blood, arterial	Newborn	27–40 mm Hg	
		Infant	27–40	
		Pregnancy	27–32	
		Female adult	32–45	

Carbon dioxide (total CO_2)	Serum, venous	Cord	14–22 mmol/liter
		Premature (1 wk)	14–27
		Newborn	13–22
		Infant	20–28
		Adult	23–30
		Pregnancy	23–30 at term
Carbon monoxide	Whole blood		0.5%–1.5% saturation of Hgb (children and nonsmokers); symptoms > 20%
Carboxyhemoglobin (see carbon monoxide)			
β-Carotene	Serum	Infant	20–70 mcg/dl
		Adult	60–200
Chloride	Serum or plasma	Cord	96–104 mmol/liter
		Newborn	97–110
		Adult	98–106
		Pregnancy	slight elevation
	Sweat	Normal	0–35 mmol/liter
		Marginal	30–60
		Cystic fibrosis	60–200
Cholesterol, total	Serum	Cord	45–100 mg/dl
		Newborn	53–135
		Infant	70–175
		Adult	140–310
		Pregnancy	Elevated

(continued)

B-2 Blood Chemistries (continued)

Determination	Specimen	Age/Sex	Normal Value
Copper	Serum	Newborn–6 mo	20–70 mcg/dl
		Adult: M	70–140
		F	80–155
Cortisol	Plasma or serum	8 AM specimen	5–23 mcg/dl
		4 PM specimen	3–15
Creatine kinase, CK (creatine phosphokinase, CPK; 30°C)	Serum	Newborn	68–580 U/liter
		Adult: M	12–70
		F	10–55
			(higher after exercise)
Creatinine	Serum or plasma	Cord	0.6–1.2 mg/dl
		Infant	0.2–0.4
		Adult: M	0.6–1.2
		F	0.5–1.1
		Pregnancy	(0.47–0.7)
Creatinine clearance (endogenous)*	Serum or plasma and timed urine	Newborn	40–65 ml/min/1.73 m^2
		Under 40 yr	
		M	97–137
		F	88–128
			(decreases 6.5 ml/min/decade)
		Pregnancy	decreased
Disaccharide tolerance (dose: twice oral glucose tolerance test dose)	Serum		>20 mg/dl change in glucose concentration

Ethanol	Blood	0.0%	
		Toxic: 50–100 mg/dl CNS depression: >100 mg/dl	
Fatty acids, free	Serum or plasma	Adults	8–25 mg/dl
		Children and obese adults	<31
Fibrinogen	Whole blood	Newborn	125–300 mg/dl
		Adult	200–400
		Pregnancy	450
Folate	Serum	Newborn	7–32 ng/ml
		Adult	1.8–9 ng/ml
		Pregnancy	1.9–14
Follicle-stimulating hormone (FSH)	Serum/plasma	Birth–1 yr M	<1–12 mU/ml
		F	<1–20
		Adult F	5–30
		Premenopause	4–30
		Midcycle peak	10–90
Galactose	Serum	Newborn/Infant	0–20 mg/dl
		Adult	<5
Glucose	Serum	Cord	45–96 mg/dl
		Premature	20–60
		Neonate	30–60
		Newborn, 1 day	40–60
		Newborn, >1 day	50–90
		Adult	70–105
	Blood	Adult	65–95
	Urine		<0.5 g/d

(continued)

B-2 Blood Chemistries (continued)

Determination	Specimen	Age/Sex	Normal Value		
Glucose tolerance	Serum		*Time*	*Normal*	*Diabetic*
Dosages:			Fasting	70–105	>115
Child 1.75 g/kg of ideal weight,			60 min	120–170	≥200
maximum 75 g			90 min	100–140	≥200
Adult 75 g total dose			120 min	70–120	≥140
Growth hormone (HGH), fasting	Serum or plasma	Cord	10–50 ng/ml		
		Newborn	10–40		
		Adult: M	<5		
		F	<8		
Immunoglobulin levels	Serum		*IgA (mg/dl)*	*IgG (mg/dl)†*	*IgM (mg/dl)*
		Cord	0–5	760–1700	4–24
		Newborn	0–2.2	700–1480	5–30
		Adult	60–380	600–1600	40–345
IgD	Serum	Newborn		None detected	
		Adult		0–8 mg/dl	
IgE	Serum	M		0–230 IU/ml	
		F		0–170	
Insulin (12 hr, fasting) (RIA)	Serum, plasma	Newborn		3–20 mcIU/ml	
		Adult		7–24	

Insulin with oral glucose tolerance test	Serum		0 min: 7–24 mcIU/ml
			60 min: 18–276
			120 min: 16–166
			180 min: 4–38
Iron-binding capacity (TIBC)	Serum	Infant	100–400 mcg/dl
		Adult	250–400
		Pregnancy	300–450
Iron	Serum	Newborn	100–250 mcg/dl
		Infant	40–100
		Adult: M	50–160
		F	40–150
		Pregnancy	decreased
Lactate	Whole blood, venous		0.50–2.2 mmol/liter
	Whole blood, arterial		0.50–1.6
Lactate dehydrogenase (LDH)	Serum	Newborn	160–450 U/liter
		Infant	100–250
			60–170
		Adult	45–90
Lead	Whole blood	Child	<30 mcg/dl
		Adult	<40
		Acceptable for industrial exposure	<60
		Toxic	≥100
Lipase (Tietz method; 37°C)	Serum		0.1–1.0 U/ml
		Child	1–6 mIU/ml

(continued)

B-2 Blood Chemistries (continued)

Determination	Specimen	Age/Sex	Normal Value
		Adult:	4–14
		F, premenopause	4–25
		F, midcycle	25–250
		F, postmenopause	25–200
Magnesium	Serum	Newborn	1.2–1.8 mEq/liter
		Adult	1.3–2.1
Methemoglobin	Whole blood		0.06–0.24 g/dl
Osmolality	Serum		275–295 mOsm/kg H_2O
Oxygen capacity	Whole blood, arterial		1.34 ml/g hemoglobin
Oxygen partial pressure (pO_2)	Whole blood, arterial	Birth	8–24 mm Hg
		5–10 min	33–75
		30 min	31–85
		>1 hr	55–80
		1 day	54–95
		Adult	83–108 decreases with age
Oxygen, % saturation	Whole blood, arterial	Newborn	40%–90%
		Therafter	95%–99%
pH (37°C)	Whole blood, arterial	Premature (48 hr)	7.35–7.50
		Birth, Full term	7.11–7.36
		5–10 min	7.09–7.30
		30 min	7.21–7.38
		>1 hr	7.26–7.49

		1 day	7.29–7.45
		Mid Pregnancy	7.40–7.45
Phenylalanine	Serum	Premature/low birth weight	2.0–7.5 mg/dl
		Fullterm newborn	1.2–3.4
		Adult	0.8–1.8
Phosphatase, acid prostatic (RIA) Roy	Serum		<3.0 ng/ml
Brower & Hayden, 37°C			0.11–0.60 U/liter
Phosphatase, alkaline SKI method		Infant	50–155 U/liter
		Child	20–150
		Adult	20–70
		Pregnancy >50% rise	
Phospholipids (lipids P × 25)	Serum and plasma	Newborn	75–170 mg/dl
		Infant	100–275
		Adult	125–275
Phosphorus, inorganic	Serum	Cord	3.7–8.1 mg/dl
		Premature (1 wk)	5.4–10.9
		Newborn	4.3–9.3
		Adult	3.0–4.5
		Pregnancy	unchanged
Potassium	Serum	Newborn	3.9–5.9 mmol/liter
		Infant	4.1–5.3
		Adult	3.5–5.1
		Pregnancy	3.5–5.3
Protein, total	Serum	Premature	4.3–7.6 g/dl

(continued)

B-2 Blood Chemistries (continued)

Determination	Specimen	Age/Sex			Normal Value		
		Newborn			4.6–7.4		
		Adult, recumbent–0.5 g higher in ambulatory patients			6.0–7.8		
Protein, electrophoresis, (cellulose acetate)	Serum	*Total Protein (g/dl)*	*Albumin (g/dl)*	*α_1-glob (g/dl)*	*α_2-glob (g/dl)*	*β-glob (g/dl)*	*γ-glob† (g/dl)*
	Premature	4.3–7.6	3.0–4.2	0.1–0.5	0.3–0.7	0.3–1.2	0.3–1.4
	Newborn	4.6–7.4	3.6–5.4	0.1–0.3	0.3–0.5	0.2–0.6	0.2–1.0
	Infant	6.2–8.0	4.0–5.0	0.2–0.4	0.5–0.8	0.5–0.8	0.3–1.2
	Pregnancy	6.0–7.8	3.5–5.0 decreased 2nd and 3rd trimester	0.2–0.3 increased 2nd trimester	0.4–1.0 increased 2nd trimester	0.5–1.1 increased 2nd trimester	0.7–1.2 decreased 3rd trimester
Salicylates	Serum, plasma				Negative: <2.0 mg/dl Therapeutic: 15–30 Toxic: >30		
Sodium	Serum	Newborn			134–146 mmol/liter		
		Infant			139–146		
		Adult			136–146		
		Pregnancy			increased retention >500 over normal		

T_3 resin uptake (T_3RU)	Serum	Newborn	26%–36%	
		Adult	26%–35%	
		Pregnancy	decreased	
Testosterone	Serum	Adult: M	572 ± 135	
		F	37 ± 10	
Thiamine (vitamin B_1)	Serum		2.0 mcg/dl	
Thyroid-stimulating hormone (TSH)	Serum, plasma	Cord	3–12 mCU/liter	
		Newborn	3–18	
		Adult	2–10	
Transferrin	Serum	Newborn	130–275 mg/dl	
		Adult	200–400	
Triglycerides (TG)	Serum, after 12-hr fast		*M (mg/dl)*	*F (mg/dl)*
		Cord blood	10–98	10–98
		0–5 yr	30–86	32–99
		6–11	31–108	35–114
		12–15	36–138	41–138
		16–19	40–163	40–128
		20–29	44–185	40–128
		Recommended (desirable) levels for adults:	Male 40–160 Female 35–135	
Tyrosine	Serum	Premature	7.0–24.0 mg/dl	
		Newborn	1.6–3.7	
		Adult	0.8–1.3	

(continued)

B-2 Blood Chemistries (continued)

Determination	Specimen	Age/Sex	Normal Value
Urea nitrogen	Serum/plasma	Cord	21–40 mg/dl
		Premature (1 wk)	3–25
		Newborn	3–12
		Adult	7–18
Uric acid uricase	Serum	Child	2.0–5.5 mg/dl
		Adult: M	3.5–7.2
		F	2.6–6.0
Vitamin A	Serum	Newborn	35–75 mcg/dl
		Adult	30–65
Vitamin B_{12}	Serum	Newborn	175–800 pg/ml
		Adult	140–700
Vitamin C	Plasma		0.6–2.0 mg/ml
Vitamin E	Serum		5–20 mcg/ml
Volume	Whole blood	Premature	90–108 ml/kg
		Newborn	80–110
		Adult	72–100
	Plasma	Adult	49–59

* Endogenous creatinine clearance is expressed in ml per minute and is corrected to average adult surface area of 1.73 m^2.

$$\frac{UV}{P} \times \frac{1.73}{A} = \text{ml/min}$$

† Higher in blacks.

B-3 Urine Chemistries

Determination	Age/Sex	Normal Value
Catecholamines (24 hr)	Infant	
	Norepinephrine	0–10 mcg/day
	Epinephrine	0–2.5
	Adult	
	Norepinephrine	15–80
	Epinephrine	0.5–20
Chloride (24 hr)	Infant	2–10 mmol/day
	Adult	110–250
	(varies greatly with Cl intake)	
Creatinine (24 hr)	Infant	8–20 mg/kg/day
	Adult	14–26
	Pregnancy	elevated
Homovanillic acid (HVA) (24 hr)	Child	3–16 mcg/mg creatinine
	Adult	<15 mg/day
17-Hydroxycorticosteroids (24 hr)	0–1 yr)	0.5–1.0 mg/24 hr
	Adult: M	3.0–10.0
	F	2.0–8.0
17-Ketogenic steroids (17-KGS) (24 hr)	0–1 yr	<1 mg/day
	Adult: M	5–23
	F	3–15
17-Ketosteroids (17-KS) (24 hr)		
Zimmerman reaction	Infant	<1 mg/day
	Adult: M 18–30 yr	9–22
	>30 yr	8–20

(continued)

B-3 Urine Chemistries (continued)

Determination	Age/Sex	Normal Value
	F (decreases with age)	6–15
Lead		<80 µg/L
Osmolality (random)		50–1400 mOsmol/kg H_2O depending on fluid intake. After 12 hr fluid restriction >850 mOsmol/kg H_2O
Porphyrins		
Coproporphyrin (24 hr)		34–234 mcg/day
Porphobilinogen (24 hr)		0–2.0 mg/day
Protein, total 24 hr		1–14 mg/dl 50–80 mg/day (at rest) <250 mg/day after intense exercise
Reducing substances		<150 mg/dl (as glucose)
Specific gravity		1.002–1.030
Random void		
After 12-hr fluid restriction		>1.025
24 hr		1.015–1.025
Vanillylmandelic acid (VMA) 24 hr	Newborn	<1.0 mg/day
	Infant	<2.0
	Adult	2–7

B-4 Blood Coagulation Factors and Laboratory Tests for DIC

Laboratory Tests	Normal Test Results	Test Results in Conditions in Which Gross Bleeding Occurs	Change with DIC
Fibrinogen:			
Nonpregnant state	250 to 300 mg/dl	<100 mg/dl	
Pregnant state	400 to 500 mg/dl	<150 mg/dl	
Platelet count	200,000 to 300,000/mm^3	<50,000/mm^3	Lowered levels
Factor V	70 to 120%		
Factor VII	70 to 120%		
Factor VIII	70 to 120%		
Plasma Hgb			Increased level
Prothrombin time	<12 sec	>100 sec	
Partial thromboplastin time	35 to 50 sec	<100 sec	
Thrombin time	15 to 20 sec	<100 sec	Prolonged times*
Bleeding time	1 to 7 min	>15 min	
Coagulation time (Lee-White)	At 37°C—6 to 12 min At room temperature—10 to 18 min	>20 min	

(continued)

B-4 Blood Coagulation Factors and Laboratory Tests for DIC (continued)

Laboratory Tests	Normal Test Results	Test Results in Conditions in Which Gross Bleeding Occurs	Change with DIC
Euglobulin lysis time		<1 hr (primary) fibrinolysis) <2 hr (secondary fibrinolysis)	Shortened time
Fibrinogen and fibrin splint products			
Counter electrophoretic test (MISFI)	Negative	Positive	
Hemagglutination inhibition test	<16 μg/ml	>200 μg/ml	Positive tests
Staph clumping test	1:4 dilution	Positive at more dilutions	
Ethanol and protamine gel tests	Negative	Positive (secondary fibrinolysis) Negative (primary fibrinolysis	

*In early DIC these times are shortened because of the hypercoagulation state.
From Abouleish E: Pain Control in Obstetrics. Philadelphia, JB Lippincott, 1977.

B-5 Weight Conversion Table (Pounds and Ounces to Grams)

	Ounces															
lbs.	0	1	2	3	4	5	6	7	8	9	10	11	12	13	14	15
0	—	28	57	85	113	142	170	198	227	255	283	312	340	369	397	425
1	454	482	510	539	567	595	624	652	680	709	737	765	794	822	850	879
2	907	936	964	992	1021	1049	1077	1106	1134	1162	1191	1219	1247	1276	1304	1332
3	1361	1389	1417	1446	1474	1503	1531	1559	1588	1616	1644	1673	1701	1729	1758	1786
4	1814	1843	1871	1899	1928	1956	1984	2013	2041	2070	2098	2126	2155	2183	2211	2240
5	2268	2296	2325	2353	2381	2410	2438	2466	2495	2523	2551	2580	2608	2637	2665	2693
6	2722	2750	2778	2807	2835	2863	2892	2920	2948	2977	3005	3033	3062	3090	3118	3147
7	3175	3203	3232	3260	3289	3317	3345	3374	3402	3430	3459	3487	3515	3544	3572	3600
8	3629	3657	3685	3714	3742	3770	3799	3827	3856	3884	3912	3941	3969	3997	4026	4054
9	4082	4111	4139	4167	4196	4224	4252	4281	4309	4337	4363	4394	4423	4451	4479	4508
10	4536	4564	4593	4621	4649	4678	4706	4734	4763	4791	4819	4848	4876	4904	4933	4961
11	4990	5018	5046	5075	5103	5131	5160	5188	5216	5245	5273	5301	5330	5358	5386	5414
12	5443	5471	5500	5528	5557	5585	5613	5642	5670	5698	5727	5755	5783	5812	5840	5868
13	5897	5925	5953	5982	6010	6038	6067	6095	6123	6152	6180	6209	6237	6265	6294	6322
14	6350	6379	6407	6435	6464	6492	6520	6549	6577	6605	6634	6662	6690	6719	6747	6776
15	6804	6832	6860	6889	6917	6945	6973	7002	7030	7059	7087	7115	7144	7172	7201	7228
16	7257	7286	7313	7342	7371	7399	7427	7456	7484	7512	7541	7569	7597	7626	7654	7682
17	7711	7739	7768	7796	7824	7853	7881	7909	7938	7966	7994	8023	8051	8079	8108	8136
18	8165	8192	8221	8249	8278	8306	8335	8363	8391	8420	8448	8476	8504	8533	8561	8590
19	8618	8646	8675	8703	8731	8760	8788	8816	8845	8873	8902	8930	8958	8987	9015	9043
20	9072	9100	9128	9157	9185	9213	9242	9270	9298	9327	9355	9383	9412	9940	9469	9497
21	9525	9554	9582	9610	9639	9667	9695	9724	9752	9780	9809	9837	9865	9894	9922	9950
22	9979	10007	10036	10064	10092	10120	10149	10177	10206	10234	10262	10291	10319	10347	10376	10404

Appendix C
Medications and Drugs in Maternity Nursing

C-1 Drugs Used in Treatment of Preterm Labor

Drug	Dosage/ Route/Action	Maternal Side Effects	Fetal Side Effects	Nursing Implications
Ritodrine (Yutopar)	IV: 150 mg in 500 ml fluid yields concentration of 0.3 mg/ml. Dosage: 0.05 to 0.1 mg/min increasing every 10 minutes to maximum of 0.35 mg/min or until adequate response obtained. Oral: 10 mg every 2 hours for 24 hours (often started 30 min before IV administration discontinued), then decreased to 10 to 20 mg every 4 to 6 hours; not to exceed 120 mg/day. Stimulates sympathetic beta 2 receptors; inhibits uterine contractility.	ECG changes and cardiac arrhythmia; dose-related tachycardia; decreased blood pressure; increased pulse pressure; flushing; sweating; nausea and vomiting; tremors; headache Pulmonary edema (more frequent when used concurrently with corticosteroids and in cases of multiple gestation) Positional hypotension (may be exacerbated by anesthesia) Transient increases in serum isulin, glu-	Drug crosses placenta; increased FHR; hypoglycemia (infrequently); cardiac arrhythmia (occasionally)	Closely observe blood pressure and maternal and fetal heart rates; maternal heart rate should not exceed 135 bpm. Check apical heart rate for arrhythmia. Observe closely for signs of pulmonary edema; monitor input and output; maintain fluid restrictions. Ritodrine therapy may unmask occult heart disease and must be used with caution in hypertensive, diabetic, and preeclamptic patients.

	Metabolized by liver; 70% to 90% excreted in urine in 10 to 12 hr.	cose, and free fatty acids; decrease in serum potassium. Risk of overdose (signaled by exaggeration of cardiac and other side effects) Maternal deaths reported (from pulmonary edema)		Drug is contraindicated with active bleeding. Obtain maternal serum potassium, glucose, and ECG baselines before initiating IV therapy.
Betamethasone (Celestone) Dexamethasone Hydrocortisone Methylprednisolone	IM: 12 mg every 24 hr for two doses IM: 5 mg every 24 hr for two doses IV: 500 mg every 24 hr for two doses IM: 125 mg every 24 hr for two doses Increases lung maturity in fetus expected to be delivered preterm. Thought to bind with glucocorticoid receptors in alveolar cells to increase production of surfactant.	Increased white blood count; possibly decreased resistance to infection; increased risk of pulmonary edema if used concurrently with betamimetic therapy for preterm labor Possible production or exacerbation of maternal hypertension	Potential for fetal demise secondary to maternal HTN or placental insufficiency No documented long-term effects	All listed compounds *except* hydrocortisone are suspensions for IM use only; IV use is contraindicated. Monitor mother closely for signs of infection; ruptured membranes may be a relative contraindication, since medication may mask signs of developing infection.

(*continued*)

C-1 Drugs Used in Treatment of Preterm Labor (*continued*)

Drug	Dosage/ Route/Action	Maternal Side Effects	Fetal Side Effects	Nursing Implications
	Peak effect 48 hr after first dose; lasts 7 days.			
Terbutaline (Brethine, Bricanyl): experimental—not currently approved by FDA for use as tocolytic	IV: 5 mg/500 ml fluid. Initiate at rate of 1 mg/min to maximum of 8 mg/min; continue 8 to 12 hr. Then subcutaneously 2.5 mg every 4 hr for 24 hr. May be given orally for home management: 2.5 mg every 4 to 6 hr. Beta-adrenergic agent; suppresses uterine contractility. Partially metabolized by liver; excreted through gastrointestinal tract and kidneys.	Similar to those of ritodrine, but more severe.	Similar to those of ritodrine.	Similar to those for ritodrine.

C-2 Drugs Used for Analgesia in Labor

Drug	Dosage/Route	Maternal Side Effects	Fetal/Newborn Side Effects	Nursing Implications
Analgesics				
Morphine sulfate	8–15 mg IM or 1–2 mg IV; peak effect in 60 min after IM and 15–20 min after IV administration with duration 4–6 hours.	CNS depression, especially respiratory. Nausea/vomiting. Possible decrease in uterine activity early in labor	CNS depression; peak effect 2 hours after IM administration.	Not commonly used in labor. *Do not* administer if maternal respiratory rate is below 12/min or other signs of CNS depression are present. Avoid administration 1–3 hours before delivery; prepare to administer narcotic antagonist to neonate if depression is evident.
Meperidine hydrochloride (Demerol)	50–100 mg IM or 25–50 mg IV; peak effect in 40–60 min after IM and 5–10 min	CNS depression, especially respiratory. Nausea/vomiting.	Neonatal hypotonia; lethargy up to 72 hours after delivery.	Most commonly used narcotic drug for labor. Administered in active

(continued)

C-2 Drugs Used for Analgesia in Labor (*continued*)

Drug	Dosage/Route	Maternal Side Effects	Fetal/Newborn Side Effects	Nursing Implications
Analgesics				
	after IV administration with duration 3–4 hours	Mild oxytocic effect after initial decrease in contractility. Hypotension. Drowsiness, blurred vision		phase of labor, preferably at least 2 hours before delivery to minimize CNS depression in newborn. IV is most common administration route because onset is quicker. Parents may refuse the drug because of its side effects or because they wish to retain control.
Alphaprodine (Nisentil)	20–40 mg SC or 10–40 mg IV. Peak effect in 5–10	Slight amnesic effect; nausea; sedation; dizziness.	Slight CNS depression if administered too close to de-	Relative short-acting. Irritating to tissue when in-

	min after SC and 1–2 min after IV administration. May be repeated at 2–3 hours if needed.		livery. Pseudo-sinusoidal FHR pattern occasionally seen on electronic fetal monitor.	jected intra-muscularly.
Barbiturates				
Sodium secobarbital (Seconal) Sodium pentobarbital (Nembutal) Sodium phenobarbital (Luminal)	100 mg IM or orally	Reduced tension, release of inhibitions Lethargy, hypotension, decreased sensory perception. Restlessness in presence of pain or as idiosyncratic reaction in some patients.	CNS depression; neonatal hypotonia, delay in establishment of feeding.	Used to induce sedation during latent phase labor. *Note:* there is no available antagonist; avoid use in active labor when delivery can be anticipated.
Ataractics				
Promazine (Sparine)	25–50 mg IM or IV	Potentiates narcotic effects; antiemetic. Use with analgesic may produce pseudohypnotic effect.	Potentiates CNS depression	Monitor closely; institute standard safety measures for medicated patients (side rails, bed

(*continued*)

C-2 Drugs Used for Analgesia in Labor (*continued*)

Drug	Dosage/Route	Maternal Side Effects	Fetal/Newborn Side Effects	Nursing Implications
Ataractics				
				rest, frequent checking).
Promethazine (Phenergan)	25–50 mg IM or IV	As for promazine	As for promazine	As for promazine
Hydroxyzine (Vistaril, Atarax)	25–50 mg IM or IV	As for promazine	As for promazine	Spasmodic eye or neck movements suggest extra-pyramidal effect of phenothiazine; alert care provider.
Diazepam (Valium)	2–10 mg IM or IV	As for promazine	As for promazine	As for hydroxyzine; painful when administered IV.

C-3 Regional and General Anesthesia

Type	Method	Advantages	Disadvantages
Regional Anesthesia			
Pudendal Block	• Local anesthetic (lidocaine) is injected through the vaginal walls into the pudendal nerve.	• Anesthesia of lower third of vagina and perineum • Short duration for use during delivery and perineal repair • No fetal effects • No interference with uterine contractions or pushing	• May temporarily blunt the mother's bearing-down efforts • Contraction pain not relieved • May not produce adequate pain relief • Patient cooperation necessary
Paracervical Block	• Local anesthetic (procaine or tetracaine) is injected in lateral fornices.	• Simple procedure • Rare maternal side-effects • Good anesthesia for uterine contractions and cervical dilatation • Does not interfere with maternal pushing efforts	• Fetal bradycardia (25% to 85%) • Contraindicated in prematurity, compromised fetus, placental sufficiency, and with vaginal infection • Transient decrease in uterine activity for 20 to 30 minutes postinjection • Possible injection directly into the fetus when the cervix is dilated 8 cm or more

(continued)

C-3 Regional and General Anesthesia (*continued*)

Type	Method	Advantages	Disadvantages
Regional Anesthesia			
Subarachnoid Blocks			
• Spinal	• Anesthetic is introduced into cerebrospinal fluid in subarachnoid space (L4 and L5).	• Simple procedure • Effective 1 to 2 hours • Used at end of first stage and for delivery and fourth stage • Low failure rate • No direct effect on the fetus when maternal BP is maintained	• No pain relief in first stage • Maternal hypotension • Disruption of normal labor pattern and decreased bearing-down efforts • Increased use of forceps • "High" spinal block interferes with maternal respiration • Postspinal headache • Exacerbation of postpartum urinary retention
• Saddle	• Anesthetic is introduced into cerebrospinal fluid in subarachnoid space (S1 and S4).	• Loss of sensation in perineum, lower pelvis, inner thighs	• Uterine contractions remain painful • Delivery pain not completely eliminated

Epidural Blocks • Lumbar	• Anesthetic injected into the epidural space outside the dura (L-2 to L-4) • May be single or continuous injection. Repeated injection through a catheter inserted in the epidural space permits continuous pain relief.	• Produces blockade from T-10 to S-5 and provides complete pain relief from unbilicus to midthigh • No fetal effects • Fetal status may improve due to increased uterine blood flow and decreased pelvic resistance in second-stage labor. • Woman is awake and able to cooperate.	• Toxic response to the anesthetic agent • Requires considerable skill of operator • Maternal hypotension • Partial or total anesthetic failure • Woman will need assistance with pushing • Increased use of forceps
• Caudal	• Anesthetic is injected into the epidural space outside the dura through the sacral hiatus at S-4. It may be used continuously through a catheter as noted above.	• Rapid perineal anesthesia • Anesthesia for first and second stages as well as for delivery • No fetal effects • May be used in women with metabolic, lung, and heart disease	• Woman is awake • Loss of urge to push • Prolonged labor may occur in primigravida • Increased use of forceps • An anesthesiologist must inject and monitor the anesthesia.

(*continued*)

C-3 Regional and General Anesthesia (*continued*)

Type	Method	Advantages	Disadvantages
General Anesthesia	• Inhalation anesthesia (pain relief through administration of a gaseous agent mixed with oxygen and inhaled until loss of consciousness occurs)	• Produces overall relaxation useful in difficult forceps extraction and breech and cesarean deliveries • Reduces likelihood of convulsions in preeclamptic or eclamptic women • Can be rapidly administered in emergency situations when delivery must be immediate and pain relief is essential	• Delivery must occur within 5 to 7 minutes after administration because inhalation anesthetics rapidly cross the placenta and cause hypoxia and respiratory depression in the neonate • There is a risk of maternal aspiration of gastric contents, which may result in life-threatening pulmonary complications • Immediate postpartum recovery is more difficult, with nausea and vomiting and increased risk of uterine atony and postpartum hemorrhage • The mother is not alert for birth and the father may be excluded from the delivery room

Nitrous Oxide (40% nitrous oxide, 60% oxygen)	• Administered by face mask or inhaler • Produces analgesia but not true anesthesia	• Few side effects • Rapid, pleasant induction • Does not interfere with maternal physiology • Used for analgesia in second stage of labor and for induction of anesthesia in combination with other agents	
Halothane	• Infrequently used in obstetrics	• Rapid, predictable induction • Little or no nausea and vomiting • Moderate to good uterine relaxation	• May cause increased uterine contraction and risk of postpartum hemorrhage • Cardiac arrhythmia and respiratory depression may occur
Methoxyflurane (Penthrane)	• May be administered by inhaler for analgesia or in combination with other agents for anesthesia	• Provides a pleasant induction	• Induction and recovery is slower than with gas agents • Increased uterine relaxation • Restricted to low dose for short periods because of risk for uterine bleeding postpartum

(continued)

C-3 Regional and General Anesthesia (*continued*)

Type	Method	Advantages	Disadvantages
General Anesthesia			
Ketamine	• Intravenous induction Can be used as an induction agent for and in combination with inhalation anesthesia	• Produces analgesia, amnesia, and a sleeplike state (may be a disadvantage for some)	• Increase in maternal BP and pulse rate • May cause minimal respiratory depression • Confusion, delirium, and hallucinations may occur during emergence from anesthesia.
Pentothal Sodium	• An ultra short-acting barbiturate that produces CNS depression and loss of consciousness within 30 seconds of administration	• Rapid acting • Rapid induction of anesthesia for cesarean births	• Low potential for nausea and vomiting • Rapid recovery time • Does not produce anesthesia until doses are high enough to cause profound CNS depression. Rarely used alone The following are disadvantages of general anesthesia for use in the intrapartal period:

- Delivery must occur within 5 to 7 minutes after administration because inhalation anesthetics rapidly cross the placenta and will cause hypoxia and respiratory depression in the neonate.
- The risk of maternal aspiration of gastric contents with resulting life-threatening pulmonary complications is considerable.
- A skilled anesthetist or anesthesiologist is required for safe administration.
- Immediate postpartum recovery is more difficult, and there is nausea and vomiting and increased risk of uterine atony and postpartum hemorrhage.
- The mother is not alert for the birth, and the father is usually excluded from the delivery room.

C-4 Oxytocic Drugs Used to Control Postpartum Atony and Hemorrhage

Drug	Use	Dosage	Potential Side Effects and Contraindications
Oxytocin injection			
(Pitocin, Syntocinon, Uteracon)	To induce uterine contractions that reduce or prevent uterine atony and hemorrhage	SC, IM, IV: 0.3 ml as necessary IV drip: 10 to 40 U in 1000 ml diluent Nasal spray: 40 U/ml—1 spray in nostril 2 to 3 minutes before nursing or pumping breasts	Nausea, vomiting, uterine tetany, hypersensitivity, water intoxication, anaphylactic reaction Contraindications include cephalopelvic disproportion, placenta previa, prematurity, grand multiparity, primigravida over 35, previous cesarean delivery

Nursing Implications

When oxytocic drugs are used, a physician should be immediately available to manage possible complications. Fundal checks are done every 10 to 15 minutes to assess the quantity and quality of uterine contractions. When an IV infusion is used, a uterus that remains in a strong tetanic contraction is hypertonic, and the patient will complain of severe uterine pain. If this happens, the dose or the rate of the infusion is too high and should be slowed to a minimum. Notify the physician immediately.

When the uterus remains atonic (not contracted), the rate or dose of the infusion may be insufficient to effectively control uterine contractions. Notify the physician immediately.

Ergonovine maleate			
(Ergotrate maleate)	To produce uterine contractions to reduce or prevent postpartum hemorrhage due to atony	IV or IM: 0.2 mg every 2 to 4 hours up to a maximum of five doses Oral: 0.2 to 0.4 mg every 6 to 16 hours until atony passes (48 hr)	Nausea, vomiting, severe hypertensive episode, bradycardia, allergic reaction, shock Ergonovine is contraindicated in patients with hypersensitivity, infection, toxemia

Nursing Implications

Closely monitor and record the character of uterine contractions.
IM injections may cause vigorous contractions for 3 hours or more. The patient may be very uncomfortable and may need analgesia for pain relief.
Monitor the patient's blood pressure, pulse, and uterine response for 1 to 2 hours or until she is stabilized. Report any sudden blood pressure increase, pulse changes, and frequent episodes of uterine relaxation.
Patients receiving this therapy become more sensitive to cold. Exposure of the patient is to be avoided.
The use of IV therapy is limited to emergency situations because it causes a high incidence of nausea, vomiting, and hypertensive episodes.

(continued)

C-4 Oxytocic Drugs Used to Control Postpartum Atony and Hemorrhage (*continued*)

Drug	Use	Dosage	Potential Side Effects and Contraindications
Methylergonovine maleate			
(Methergine)	To induce uterine contractions that reduce or prevent uterine atony and hemorrhage (also used in management of subinvolution)	IM: 0.2 mg every 2 to 4 hours as necessary Oral: 0.2 mg three to four times daily for a maximum of 1 week IV (emergency use only): 0.2 mg given over 60-second period	Same as ergonovine

Nursing Implications

Monitor vital signs (particularly blood pressure) and uterine response during IV or IM use of this drug for 1 to 2 hours or until patient is stabilized.

If blood pressure suddenly increases or there are frequent periods of uterine atony, notify the physician.

C-5 Drugs Used in Neonatal Resuscitation

Drug	Action/Indication	Route/Dosage	Side Effects	Nursing Considerations
Sodium bicarbonate ($NaHCO_3$)	Used for correction of severe metabolic acidosis in asphyxiated infants *after* adequate ventilation is established	(2–5 mEq/kg body wt) 4 ml of 0.5-mEq/ml. concentration or 4.2% solution, *or* 2 ml of 1-mEq/ml concentration or 8.4% solution diluted 1:1 with 10% dextrose in water solution to decrease osmolarity.	Hypernatremia Intracranial hemorrhage secondary to too-rapid infusion and increased osmolarity. Fluid overload	Dilute 8.4% solution before use Assess adequacy of ventilation before use. Infuse at rate no faster than 1 mEq/kg/min. Monitor intake and output. Do not mix with calcium solutions: it causes precipitation.
Epinephrine	Used for treatment of asystole or severe bradycardia	0.5–1 ml of a 1:10,000 solution injected into the umbilical vein or directly into the heart. Dose may be repeated as necessary.		Do not inject directly into an artery. Evaluate adequacy of ventilation.

(*continued*)

C-5 Drugs Used in Neonatal Resuscitation (*continued*)

Drug	Action/Indication	Route/Dosage	Side Effects	Nursing Considerations
Isoproterenol	Used for treatment of bradycardia, hypotension, and low cardiac output	1–2 mg/100 ml of 5% dextrose in water solution. Adjust rate to maintain heart rate (usually 1 ml/kg/hr)		Monitor vital signs closely using cardiorespiratory monitor. Monitor intake and output. Use IV line *only* for isoproterenol administration. Do not use same line for rapid administration of other drugs.
Phenobarbital	Used for treatment of active seizures	With active seizures: 5–10 mg/kg body wt IV over several minutes. May give 2nd dose of up to 20 mg/kg if	Drowsiness Poor sucking and feeding Respiratory depression Circulatory	Monitor vital signs closely Observe for signs of respiratory or circulatory depression (decreased

		seizure activity continues.	depression Urinary suppression Interference with vitamin K effect on synthesis of clotting factors	respiratory rate, cyanosis, or pallor). Evaluate for adequacy of fluid and calorie intake.
	Used for maintenance therapy to prevent recurrence of seizures	Loading dose: 10–15 mg/kg in three divided doses IV or IM, then 5–8 mg/kg/day divided into two doses every 12 hrs to achieve therapeutic plasma level of 15–30 μg/ml		
Diazepam (Valium)	Used for acute control of seizures	With active seizures: 0.5–2.0 mg slow IV push.	Cardiac depression Respiratory depression Hypotension Drowsiness Interference with binding of bilirubin to albumin.	Monitor vital signs closely using cardiorespiratory monitor Observe for signs of respiratory and circulatory depression.

(continued)

C-5 Drugs Used in Neonatal Resuscitation (*continued*)

Drug	Action/Indication	Route/Dosage	Side Effects	Nursing Considerations
	Used for treatment of drug withdrawal	0.5–2.0 mg IM or orally PO until symptoms are controlled, then half dose administered every 12 hrs until discontinued (usually 2–7 days)	Drowsiness Rarely, circulatory or respiratory depression with oral doses in low dose range.	Observe for drowsiness. Monitor vital signs closely.
Digoxin	Used for treatment of congestive heart failure or supraventricular tachycardia	Digitalizing dose: Term infant: 0.04–0.07 mg/kg orally 0.03–0.05 mg/kg IM or IV Preterm infant: 0.03–0.04 mg/kg orally 0.02–0.03 mg/kg IM or IV	Decrease pulse Vomiting Diarrhea Signs of toxicity: Irritability P-R interval >0.16 seconds Sagging S-T segment Arrhythmia	Notify physician if pulse is below 90 Observe for vomiting & diarrhea. Observe for increased irritability. EKG should be done before digitalizing dose is given. Digoxin levels

		Maintenance dose: 1/3 to 1/4 of digitalizing dose divided into 2 equal doses every 12 hrs. (Usually 0.01–0.02 mg/kg/day)		should be checked regularly to determine if therapeutic level is maintained (1–2 ng/ml)
Furosemide (Lasix)	Used for treatment of pulmonary edema, cardiac overload and edema. Used for treatment of acute renal failure	Pulmonary edema or renal failure: 1–2 mg/kg IV or IM Maintenance: 1–4 mg/kg/day divided into 2–3 doses PO or IM	Electrolyte imbalances Lethargy Vomiting Anorexia Constipation Diarrhea Hyperglycemia Ototoxicity Blood dyscrasias Interference with bilirubin binding with albumin	Monitor vital signs closely Monitor intake and output Observe for lethargy, vomiting, diarrhea. Assess weight daily. Check urine for glucose Monitor serum electrolyte results.
Atropine	Used for treatment of bradycardia presumed to be of vagal origin	0.01 mg–0.03 mg/kg. IV, IM, or SC	Tachycardia Hyperpyrexia, especially in infants with CNS damage	Monitor vital signs closely using cardiorespiratory monitor.

(*continued*)

C-5 Drugs Used in Neonatal Resuscitation (*continued*)

Drug	Action/Indication	Route/Dosage	Side Effects	Nursing Considerations
			Erythema Dialted pupils Urinary retention	Monitor intake and output. Observe for lethargy.
Calcium gluconate	Used for treatment of severe bradycardia, cardiac arrhythmias, and low cardiac output	1–2 ml/kg of a 10% solution slow IV push. Give up to 5 ml in preterm infant and up to 10 ml in term infant.	With IV infusions, accidental infiltration into tissues causes necrosis and sloughing of tissues	Do not mix with sodium bicarbonate solutions: it causes precipitation. Do not give through umbilical vein line unless it is verified that tip is in inferior vena cava. Monitor vital signs closely using cardiorespiratory monitor. Observe IV infusion site closely for evidence of infiltration.

	Used for treatment of hypocalcemia	30–80 mg/kg/day of elemental calcium given over 24 hrs. IV or orally. Orally given in divided doses every 4 hr.	Hypercalcemia with IV infusions Bradycardia	Note that 1 ml of a 10% solution provides 9 mg of elemental calcium. Monitor electrolytes closely
	Used for treatment of seizures caused by hypocalcemia	0.1–0.2 gm/kg slow IV	Bradycardia	Stop infusion with bradycardia.
Dextrose	Used to reverse or prevent hypoglycemia	50% solution mixed in equal amounts with sodium bicarbonate. Inject solution through the umbilical vein (some neonatologists recommend infusion with 10% dexrose solution)	Inject slowly over 2–4 minutes	

(continued)

C-5 Drugs Used in Neonatal Resuscitation (*continued*)

Drug	Action/Indication	Route/Dosage	Side Effects	Nursing Considerations
Naloxone (Narcan)	Narcotic antagonist. Reverses neonatal CNS and respiratory depression caused by narcotic administration during labor.	0.01 mg/kg body wt. IM, IV into umbilical vein, or SC. May be repeated at 2-to-3-minute intervals until desired response is achieved. If no improvement after 3 doses, discontinue.	Irritability, tachycardia and prolonged prothrombin time noted with excessive use in some infants	Use with caution in infants of mothers with known or suspected narcotic addiction: it can cause severe withdrawal symptoms. Watch for reversal of therapeutic effects as medication is metabolized. Monitor respirations and heart rate closely.

C-6 Drugs Used in Neonatal Care

Drug	Action/Indication	Route/Dosage	Side Effects	Nursing Considerations
Silver nitrate 1% ophthalmic ointment	Bacteriocide used for prophylaxis against gonococcal conjunctivitis (ophthalmia neonatorum)	2 drops of a 1% solution (ophthalmic) to each eye one time for prophylaxis or gonococcal conjunctivitis	Chemical conjunctivitis Discoloration of skin coming into direct contact with solution.	Cleanse eyes of blood, mucus, and meconium before instillation. Separate upper and lower lids and place pool of solution between them. Allow solution to pool at least 30 seconds and make sure it comes in contact with all areas of conjunctiva. Remove excess from skin to prevent discoloration. Protect solution from light before use.

(*continued*)

C-6 Drugs Used in Neonatal Care (*continued*)

Drug	Action/Indication	Route/Dosage	Side Effects	Nursing Considerations
Phytonadione (vitamin K)	Prothrombogenic agent used for prophylaxis against hemorrhagic disease of the newborn	0.5 mg to 1 mg one time IM	Redness and swelling at injection site. Transient hyperbilirubinemia and jaundice have been observed in newborn after administration of vitamin K. Preterm infants who receive high doses are at greatest risk.	Protect solution from light before use. The preferred site for injection of Vitamin K in the neonate is the anterior thigh.
Erythromycin ophthalmic ointment	Antibacterial agent used as prophylaxis against gonococcal conjunctivitis (ophthalmia neonatorum)	1 strip 1 cm long of a 0.5% solution topically to conjunctival sac one time	Chemical conjunctivitis in approximately 20% of neonates	Cleanse eyes of mucus, blood, and meconium before instillation. Separate upper and lower lids to ensure instillation of ointment into conjunctival sac. Do not flush eye after instillation.

Appendix D
Drug Effects on the Fetus and Newborn

D-1 Reported Effects of Drug Exposure on the Fetus

Drugs	First-Trimester Effects	Second- and Third-Trimester Effects
Analgesics		
Acetaminophen	None known	None known
Narcotics	None known	Depression, withdrawal
Salicylates	Frequent reports, none proven	Prolonged pregnancy and labor; hemorrhage
Anesthetics		
General	Anomalies, abortion	Depression
Local	None known	Bradycardia, seizures
Anorexics		
Amphetamines	Anomalies	Irritable, poor feeding
Phenmetrazine	Skeletal anomalies	Unknown
Anti-Infection Agents		
Aminoglycosides	Skeletal anomalies	Nephrotoxic, ototoxic
Cephalosporins	None known	Decreased positive cultures
Chloramphenicol	None known	"Gray baby" syndrome (?)
Clindamycin	None known	Unknown
Erythromycin	None known	None known

Ethambutol	None known	None known
Ethionamide	Anomalies	None known
Isoniazid	None known	None known
Metronidazole	? Mutagenesis or carcinogenesis	None known
Penicillins	None known	None known; positive cultures
Rifampin	None known	None known
Sulfonamides	None known	Hemolytic anemia, thrombocytopenia, hyperbilirubinemia
Tetracyclines	Impaired bone growth	Impaired bone growth, stained teeth (enamel hypoplasia),
Anticoagulants		
Coumadin	Nasal hypoplasia, ophthalmic, abnormal epiphyseal stippling	Hemorrhage, stillbirth
Heparin	None known	Hemorrhage at placental site with possible stillbirth.
Anticonvulsants		
Barbiturates	Anomalies (?)	Bleeding, withdrawal
Carbamazepine	Anomalies	Bleeding withdrawal
Clonazepam	Facial cleft	Withdrawal, depression
Ethosuximide	None known	None known
Phenytoin	IUGR, craniofacial abnormalities, hypoplasia of phalanges	Hemorrhage
		Hemorrhage Depletion of vitamin K—dependent clotting factor
		Hemorrhage

(continued)

D-1 Reported Effects of Drug Exposure on the Fetus (*continued*)

Drugs	First-Trimester Effects	Second- and Third-Trimester Effects
Anticonvulsants		
Primidone	Same as barbiturates	
Trimethadione	IUGR, mental retardation, facial dysmorphogenesis	
Valproic acid	Unknown	Unknown
Cancer Chemotherapy		
Alkylating agents	Abortion, anomalies	Hypoplastic gonads, growth delay
Antimetabolites		
Folic acid analogs	Abortion, IUGR cranial anomalies	Hypoplastic gonads, growth delay
Pyrimidine analogs (Arabinoside)	Abortion	Hypoplastic gonads, growth delay
Purine analogs (Cytosine, 5-FU)	Abortion	Hypoplastic gonads, growth delay
Antibiotics (Actinomycin)	Abortion	Hypoplastic gonads, growth delay
Vinca alkaloids	Abortion	
Hormones	(See under Hormones)	
Cardiovascular Drugs		
Antihypertensives		
Alpha methyldopa	None known	Hemolytic anemia, ileus
Guanethidine	None known	None known

Hydralazine	None known	Tachycardia
Propranolol	None known	Bradycardia, hypoglycemia, IUGR with chronic use
Reserpine	None known	Lethargy
β-sympathomimetics	None known	Tachycardia
Digitalis preparations	None known	Bradycardia
Cold and Cough Preparations		
Antihistamines	None known	None known
Cough suppressants	None known	None known
Decongestants	None known	None known
Expectorants	Fetal goiter	None known
Diuretics		
Furosemide	None known	Death from sudden hypoperfusion
Thiazides	None known	Thrombocytopenia, hypokalemia, hyperbilirubinemia, hyponatremia
Fertility Drugs		
Clomiphene	Chromosomal anomalies (?)	Unknown

D-1 Reported Effects of Drug Exposure on the Fetus (*continued*)

Drugs	First-Trimester Effects	Second- and Third-Trimester Effects
Hormones		
Androgens	Masculinization (female fetus)	Adrenal suppression (?)
Corticosteriods	Cleft in animals, not in humans	Growth delay
Estrogens	Cardiovascular anomalies	None known
Progestins	Limb and cardiovascular anomalies	None known
Hypoglycemics		
Insulin	None known	Hypoglycemia (unlikely)
Sulfonylureas	Anomalies	Suppressed insulin secretion
Laxatives		
Bisacodyl	None known	None known
Dioctyl sodium sulfosuccinate	None known	None known
Mineral oil	Decreased vitamin absorption	None known
MOM	None known	None known

Psychoactive Drugs		
Antidepressants—tricyclics	CNS (?) limb defects	None known
Benzodiazepines	Facial clefts, cardiac	Depression
Hydroxyzine	None known	None known
Meprobamate	Facial clefts	None known
Phenothiazines	None known	None known
Sedatives	None known	Depression
Thalidomide	Phocomelia	None known
Thyroid Drugs		
Antithyroid		
^{131}I	Goiter, abortion, anomalies	Goiter, airway obstruction, hypothyroid, mental retardation
PTU	None known	None known
Tapazole	Aplasia cutis	Aplasia cutis
Thyroid USP	Does not cross	None known
Tocolytics		
Alcohol (ethanol)	Fetal alcohol syndrome	Intoxication, hypotonia, lethargy
Magnesium sulfate	None known	Hypermagnesemia, respiratory depression
β-sympathomimetics	None known	Tachycardia, hypothermia, hypocalcemia, hypo- and hyperglycemia

(continued)

D-1 Reported Effects of Drug Exposure on the Fetus (*continued*)

Drugs	First-Trimester Effects	Second- and Third-Trimester Effects
Vaginal Preparations		
Antifungal agents	None known	None known
Podophyllin	Mutagenesis (?)	Laryngeal polyps (?) CNS effects (?)
Vitamins (high doses)		
A	Renal anomalies	None known
B	None known	None known
C	None known	Scurvy after delivery
D	Mental retardation	None known
E	None known	None known
K	None known	Hemorrhage if deficiency

(Ians JD, Rayburn EF: Drug use during pregnancy. Perinatal Press 4: 134, 1980)

D-2 Medications in Breast Milk

Drug or Agent	Contra-Indicated	Prescribe With Caution	No Apparent Harm	Insufficient Information	Comment
Analgesics					
Acetaminophen			X		
Aspirin			X		
Propoxyphene (Darvon)			X		
Anticoagulants					
Ethyl biscoumacetate	X				Bleeding in infant
Phenindione	X				Bleeding in infant
Heparin			X		No passage into milk
Warfarin Na (coumadin)			X		
Bishydroxycoumarin (dicumarol)		X			

(continued)

D-2 Medications in Breast Milk (*continued*)

Drug or Agent	Contra-Indicated	Prescribe With Caution	No Apparent Harm	Insufficient Information	Comment
Anticonvulsants					
Phenobarbital			X		Low levels in infant
Primidone (Mysoline)			X		? Drowsiness
Carbamazepine				X	Significant infant levels; no reported effects
Diphenylhydantoin (phenytoin, Dilantin)			X		Low levels in infant, methemoglobinemia, 1 case
Antihistamines					
Diphenhydramine (Benadryl)			X		Small amounts excreted
Trimeprazine (Temaril)			X		Small amounts excreted
Tripelennamine (Pyribenzamine)			X		Small amounts excreted
Anti-Infective Agents					
Aminoglycosides (kanamycin, gentamicin)			X		Significant excretion in milk; not absorbed
Chloramphenicol	X				Bone marrow depression:

					gastrointestinal and behavioral effects
Penicillins			X		Possible sensitization
Sulfonamides		X			Hemolysis, G6PD deficiency, bilirubin displacement
Tetracyclines			X		Limited absorption by infant
Nalidixic acid		X			Hemolysis
Nitrofurantoin		X			Possible G6PD hemolysis
Metronidazole (Flagyl)		X			Low absorption but potentially toxic
Isoniazid		X			High levels in milk, possible toxicity
Pyrimethamine	X				Vomiting, marrow suppression, convulsions
Chloroquine			X		Not excreted
Quinine		X			Thrombocytopenia
Anti-Inflammatory					
Aspirin			X		
Indomethacin		X			Seizures, 1 case
Phenylbutazone		X			Low levels, ? blood dyscrasia
Gold	X				Found in baby; nephritis, hepatitis, hematologic changes
Steroids				X	Low levels with prednisone and prednisolone

(continued)

D-2 Medications in Breast Milk (*continued*)

Drug or Agent	Contra-Indicated	Prescribe With Caution	No Apparent Harm	Insufficient Information	Comment
Antineoplastic Agents					
Cyclophosphamide	X				Neutropenia
Methotrexate	X				Very small excretion
Antithyroid Agents					
Radioactive iodine	X				Thyroid suppression
Propylthiouracil	X				Thyroid suppression
Bronchodilators					
Aminophylline			X		Irritability, 1 case
Iodides	X				Thyroid suppression
Sympathomimetics				X	Inhalers probably safe
Cardiovascular Agents					
Digoxin			X		Insignificant levels
Propranolol			X		Insignificant levels
Reserpine	X				Nasal stuffiness, lethargy
Guanethidine (Ismelin)			X		Insignificant levels
Methyldopa (Aldomet)				X	

Cathartics					
Antnraquinones (Cascara, danthron)	X				Diarrhea, cramps
Aloe, senna		X			Safe in moderate dosage
Bulk agents, softeners			X		
Contraceptives, Oral*					
Diethylstilbestrol	X				Possible vaginal cancer
Depo-provera		X			May affect lactation
Norethisterone		X			May affect lactation
Ethyl estradiol		X			May affect lactation
Diuretics					
Chlorthalidone				X	Low levels, but may accumulate
Thiazides		X			May affect lactation; low levels in milk
Spironolactone			X		Insignificant levels
Ergot Alkaloids					
Bromocriptine	X				Lactation suppressed
Ergot	X				Vomiting, diarrhea, seizures
Ergotamine				X	
Ergonovine	X				Brief postpartum course may be safe

(continued)

D-2 Medications in Breast Milk (*continued*)

Drug or Agent	Contra-Indicated	Prescribe With Caution	No Apparent Harm	Insufficient Information	Comment
Ergot Alkaloids					
Methylergonovine	X				Brief postpartum course may be safe
Hormones					
Corticosteroids				X	Low levels with short-term prednisone or prednisolone
Sex hormones (see Contraceptives, Oral above)					
Thyroid (T_3 or T_4)			X		Excreted in milk; may mask hypothyroid infant
Insulin			X		Not absorbed
ACTH			X		Not absorbed
Epinephrine			X		Not absorbed
Narcotics					
Codeine			X		In usual doses
Meperidine (Demerol)				X	
Morphine			X		Low infant levels on usual dosage

Heroin	X				Addiction, withdrawal in infants
Methadone		X			Minimal levels
Psychotherapeutic Agents					
Lithium	X				High levels in milk
Phenothiazines		X			Drowsiness; chronic effects uncertain
Tricyclic antidepressants				X	Low levels; effects uncertain
Diazepam (Valium)	X				Lethargy, weight loss, EEG changes
Meprobamate (Equanil)	X				High levels in milk
Chlordiazepoxide (Librium)			X		Low levels in milk
Radiopharmaceuticals					
^{131}I	X				72 hr, no breast-feeding
Technetium (99M Tc)	X				48 hr, no breast-feeding
^{131}I albumin	X				10 days, no breast-feeding

(continued)

D-2 Medications in Breast Milk (*continued*)

Drug or Agent	Contra-Indicated	Prescribe With Caution	No Apparent Harm	Insufficient Information	Comment
Sedatives-Hypnotics					
Barbiturates		X			Short-acting, less depressant
Chloral hydrate		X			Drowsiness
Bromides	X				Depression, rash
Diazepam (Valium)	X				Depression, weight loss
Flurazepam				X	Chemically related to diazepam
Nitrazepam				X	
Social-Recreational Drugs					
Alcohol			X		Milk levels equal plasma, moderate consumption apparently safe, high levels inhibit lactation
Caffeine			X		Jitteriness with very high intakes

Nicotine		X	Low levels in milk
Marijuana		X	Minimal passage in milk
Miscellaneous			
Atropine	X		May cause constipation or inhibit lactation
Dihydrotachysterol	X		Renal calcification in animals

* Controversy in literature; long-term effects uncertain; one case of gynecomastia (Avery GB [ed]: Neonatology, 2nd ed, p 1216. Philadelphia, JB Lippincott, 1981)

Note: High doses of aspirin lead to metabolic acidosis in the infant.

Index

The letter f *following a page number indicates a figure; the letter* t *following a page number indicates a table.*